SOUTHWEST CONFERENCE on BOTANICAL MEDICINE

Lecture Notes

April 7 – 9, 2017

Southwest College of Naturopathic Medicine & Health Sciences

Tempe, Arizona

Produced by
Herbal Educational Services
555 Tyler Creek Rd
Ashland, OR 97520
Phone 541-482-3016
www.botanicalmedicine.org

Cover photo: Claret Cup Cactus by Mimi Kamp

*Note: Power points in this book have been edited—the downloadable version offers full power point presentations. Order from: **www.botanical-medicine.org***

Contents

Jill Stansbury, ND

David Winston, RH (AHG)

Eric Yarnell

SPEAKER CONTACT LIST

7Song
P.O. Box 6626
Ithaca, NY 14851
607-539-7172

Lise Alschuler
Tucson, AZ
LNAlschuler@comcast.net

Paul Bergner
PO Box 13758
Portland, OR 97213
720-841-3626

Mary Bove, ND
515 Fish Pond Rd
Colebrook NH 03576
802-380-7355

Phyllis Hogan
107 N San Francisco St. #1
Flagstaff, AZ 86001
928-774-2884

Mimi Kamp
PO Box 447
Naco, AZ 85620
520-432-9094

Jeffrey Langland, PhD
506 W. El Alba Way
Chandler, AZ 85225
480-518-4268

Rhonda PallasDowney
1131 S. 7th St.
Cottonwood, AZ 96326
928-639-3614

Kenneth Proefrock, ND
14991 W. Bell Rd.
Surprise, AZ 85374
623-977-0077

JoAnn Castigliego Sanchez
41921 North Central Ave.
New River, AZ 85086
623-465-7359

Katie Stage, ND
2164 E. Broadway Rd.
Tempe, AZ 85282
480-970-0000

Jill Stansbury, ND
408 E. Main St.
Battle Ground, WA 98604
360-687-2799

Jonathan Treasure, MNIMH
2305 Ashland Street Ste C258
Ashland, OR 97520
541-727-5103

David Winston, RH(AHG)
PO Box 553
Broadway, NJ 08808
908-835-0822

Eric Yarnell, ND, RH(AHG)
1207 N 200th St, Ste 210
Shoreline, WA 98133
206-542-4325

What was that Herb
again?
Cognitive support with
Botanicals

Lise Alschuler,
ND, FABNO

SW Botanical
Conference
2017

Disclosures

- Independent contractor providing educational services to healthcare and dietary supplement companies and nonprofit professional associations
- Executive Director of TAP Integrative, an educational non-profit with sponsorship from Integrative Therapeutics
- Medical Advisory Board member of Integrative Therapeutics, Gaia Herbs, Bioceuticals-Australia, Genova Labs
- Co-principle of Five to Thrive LLC. Five To Thrive which licenses a cancer survivorship web application to cancer centers.
- Co-principle of Thrivers LLC which hosts a weekly radio show for consumers and derives a small percentage of revenue from dietary supplement company sponsorships.

Overview

Cognitive decline: Setting the Stage

- Conventional management has limited success.
- Scientific and clinical research of natural treatments for cognitive issues is limited.
- There is a rich historical context of using herbs for memory loss and cognitive support.

Early Onset Dementia

- Can occur in any age adult
- Progressive cognitive impairment in one or more cognitive domains:
  - memory is usually affected
- Most common types are: Alzheimer disease (AD), vascular dementia and frontotemporal dementia
- Etiologies vary and include:
  - neurodegenerative - most common cause of slow, insidious disease (normal MRI)
  - vascular
  - infectious
  - autoimmune - multiple sclerosis
  - neurometabolic - important to distinguish cause –ie. Parkinsonism, Lewy body dementia
  - traumatic brain injury
  - genetic - Huntington disease

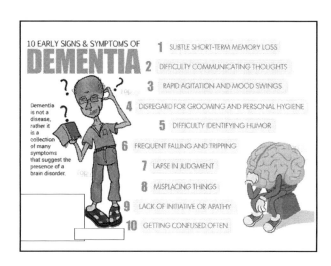

Prevalence

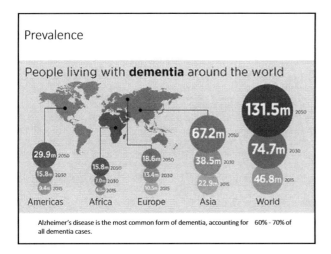

People living with **dementia** around the world

Alzheimer's disease is the most common form of dementia, accounting for 60% - 70% of all dementia cases.

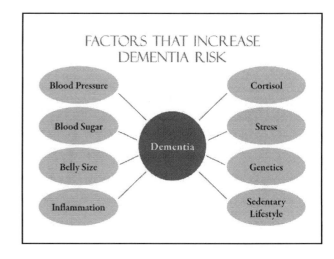

Alzheimer's Brain

Healthy microtubule
stabilizing protein tau

Alzheimer's microtubule
tangle of tau protein

pathophysiology

- Neurofibillary tangles (NFT) are intraneuronal cytoplasmic bundles of paired, helically wound filaments. They occur in large numbers in the Alzheimer brain, particularly in entorhinal cortex, hippocampus, amygdala, association cortices of the frontal, temporal, and parietal lobes, and certain subcortical nuclei that project to these regions.
- One subunit protein involved is the tau protein, a hyperphosphorylated protein that when bound to itself destabilizes microtubules and forms tangles. Other protein include MAP, a microtubule associated protein, ubiquitin, and amyloid β peptide (Aβ).
- Soluble Aβ is not toxic at physiologic concentrations, whereas oligomers (loose clumps of several Aβ molecules), small fibrils, or larger filaments may be toxic to neurons.
- Accumulating evidence implicates free radical oxidative stress in the pathogenesis of Alzheimer's disease.
  - Environmental toxins may contribute to this oxidation (heavy metals, pesticides, etc.)

Conventional management

Conventional approach to early onset dementia

- Treatment depends upon the cause
  - For example, autoimmune diseases are treated with steroids
  - Space occupying lesions are resected when possible
- Symptomatic treatment for dementia includes cholinesterase inhibitors and/or memantine, treatment of behavioral disturbances, counseling.

Cholinesterase inhibitors

- Cholinesterase inhibitors: used in Alzheimer disease (AD) patients who have reduced choline acetyl transferase leading to decreased acetylcholine synthesis and impaired cortical cholinergic function.
- Tacrine* (Cognex), donepezil (Aricept), rivastigmine (Exelon), and galantine (Razadyne) exert a small but clinically significant effect. In general, at best, these drugs slow progression by 1 to 1.5 years.
  - *First approved drug; no longer used due to hepatic toxicity and GI toxicity
- Only effective in about 25% and, while statistically significant, are of marginal clinical significance.
- Cholinergic side effects occur in 20%. Donepezil: mild (diarrhea, nausea, vomiting). Rivastigmine: moderate to severe (N/V, anorexia, headaches). Galantine: moderate (N/V/D, anorexia, weight loss)
- Effects typically decline after 2 years of treatment.

Arch Neurol. 2004;61(12):1852.
Ann Intern Med. 2008;148(5):379.
Birks JS. et al. Cochrane Database Syst Rev. 2015 Apr;4:CD001191.
Olin J. et al. Cochrane Database Syst Rev. 2001

Cholinesterase inhibition

Pharmacology of AChE INHIBITORS

Table 1. Pharmacological characteristics of cholinesterase inhibitors.				
Drug	Mechanism of action	Half-life	Protein-binding capacity	Metabolism
Donepezil (Aricept)	Selective reversible noncompetitive inhibitor of AChE*	58–90 hours	96%	CYP 2D6, CYP 3A4[‡]
Rivastigmine (Exelon)	Pseudo-irreversible inhibitor of AChE and BChE[†]	2 hours	40%	Non-hepatic, metabolized by AChE and BChE
Galantamine (Razadyne)	Reversible inhibitor of AChE, presynaptic modulator of nicotinic AChE	5–7 hours	18%	CYP 2D6, CYP 3A4

*AChE = acetylcholinesterase   [‡]CYP = cytochrome P-450
[†]BChE = butyrylcholinesterase   Adapted from Hsiung GYR, Loy-English I[²]

Memantine (a type of anesthetic)

- Memantine is a N-methyl-D-aspartate (NMDA) receptor antagonist, which exerts neuroprotective actions
  - Glutamate is the principal excitatory amino acid neurotransmitter in cortical and hippocampal neurons.
  - Glutamate activates NMDA receptor which is involved in learning and memory, but excessive stimulation induced by ischemia leads to excitotoxicity.
  - Blocking NMDA is though to protect against pathologic excitotoxicity and restore physiologic neuronal functioning
  - Most common side effect = dizziness
- Clinical trials have shown this drug to be well-tolerated and to reduce cognitive decline over study periods of 28 weeks to 1 year in moderate to severe AD.
  - Benefits and tolerability of long-term treatment is not known
- Patients with mild Alzheimer's disease do <u>not</u> appear to benefit from memantine.

N Engl J Med. 2003;348(14):1333.
Arch Neurol. 2006;63(1):49.

NMDA REceptors

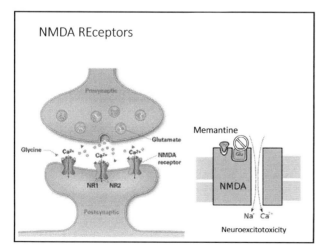

Lifestyle & Nutrient Approaches

Diet and Dementia

- Mediterranean diet high in vegetables and fruit is associated with lower risk of dementia
  - High flavonoid-containing berries are associated with slower rates of cognitive decline, with the highest quartile of intake associate with a delay of cognitive aging by up to 2.5 years.

Neurology. 2007;69(20):1921.
Alzheimers Dement. 2015;11(9):1007
Ann Neurol. 2012 Jul;72(1):135-43.

Exercise and dementia

- Moderate exercise increases cognitive performance including higher cortical function
  - 24 weeks of moderate exercise in healthy older adults (ages 65-95) resulted in improved function and reduced markers of oxidative stress and inflammation.
- Resistance training at least 2 times per week reduces white matter lesions in older women (ages 65-75) resulting in improved gait speed, but not improved executive functions.

Oxid Med Cell Longev. 2016;2016:2545168.
J Am Geriatr Soc. 2015;63(10):2052.

Melatonin: Circadian rhythm & Dementia

- Circadian rhythm is severely impaired in AD and results in sundowning (evening agitation) and disrupted sleep.
- Melatonin: Master regulator of circadian rhythm
- Melatonin attenuates beta-amyloid accumulation and also downregulates NFkB-induced inflammation in the hippocampus (center of memory)
- A Cochrane review found that studies (2) have failed to show benefit in sleep in patients with dementia
- However, a systemic review (4 RCTs and 5 case series) found that melatonin improves 'sundowning' behavior in patients with Alzheimer's

Sleep Sci. 2016;9(4):285
Neurosci Lett. 2016;621:39
Cochrane Database Syst. Rev. 2016;11:C009178
Int J Geriatr Psychiatry. 2010;25(12):1201

Antioxidants: Mild dementia

- AD brains contain elevated free radical exposure and upregulated endogenous antioxidant responses
- However, observational studies have failed to find a preventive benefit of supplementation of Vitamin E, C or beta-carotene or from diets high in these antioxidants.
- Vitamin E: 2000iu daily may delay functional progression in patients with mild to moderate AD.
  - No measurable effect on cognitive performance.

Cell Tissue Res. 1997;290(3):471.
JAMA. 2014 Jan;311(1):33-44.

Other nutrients for mild dementia

- Vitamins B6, B12, folate: supplementation lowers brain homocysteine levels, however over a mean of 5 years, there is no impact on cognitive domain scores.
- Vitamin D deficiency is associated with cognitive impairment; the effect of supplementation on preventing or improving cognition is unknown.
- Omega-3 fatty acids over many years of intake may decrease the risk of dementia and cognitive decline

Am J Clin Nutr. 2014 Jun;100(2):657-666.
Neurology. 2012;79(13):1397.
Arch Neurol. 2006;63(11):1545

botanicals

Ginkgo biloba

- Ginkgoaceae family; oldest tree species on earth (200-300 million years old)
- In medicinal use since 2,600 B.C.
- Leaves used
- Currently one of the most widely prescribed botanicals
- 375 published human clinical trials on ginkgo

Ginkgo biloba: active constituents

- ginkgo flavone glycosides
  - antioxidant, mild platelet aggregation inhibition
- proanthocyanidins
  - stabilize connective tissue, anti-inflammatory
- ginkgo specific terpene lactones
  - ginkgolide: enhances blood circulation, PAF antagonist activity
  - bilobalide: cognitive activation properties, neuroprotection

Glycosides : DeFeudis, FV *Ginkgo biloba extract (EGB 761): Pharmacological Activities and Clinical Applications*, Elsevier, Paris, 1991.
Ginkgolide: *Ginkgolides: Chemistry, Biology, Pharmacology and Clinical Perspectives*, vols 1 and 2 (Barcelona: JR Prous Science Publ), 1988.
Bilobalide: Itil, TM, Eralp E, Tsambis E, et al, *Am J Therm*, 1996; 3: 63-73.

Ginkgo biloba

- Improves uptake and utilization of oxygen and glucose by brain cells.
  - This is due, in part, to antioxidation.
- Enhances nervous system activity (nootropic actions) including stimulation of nerve transmissions by increasing both acetylcholine receptors and all neurotransmitters.
- Enhances cerebral blood flow via:
  - inhibition of platelet aggregation
  - regulation of artery tone and elasticity
  - stabilization of capillary permeability

Neurologic Psychiatrie, 1989; special issue 1:33-41.
Oberpichler, et al, Pharmacol Res Comm, 1988; 20:349-68.
Spinnewyn, et al, Recent Results in Pharmacology and Clinic,
Springer-Verlag Berlin; 1988:143-52

Ginkgo biloba and dementia prevention

- RDBPCT: In adults with normal cognition and with mild dementia, Gingko does not reduce the risk of dementia
  - 120mg twice daily of Ginkgo blob extract vs. placebo in 3069 adults at least 75 years of age
  - Median duration of study = 6 years
- Recent 6 month RDBPCT study of 29 postmenopausal women (ages 60-84) compared placebo to combination supplement containing 1g DHA, 160mg EPA, 240mg Ginkgo blob, 60mg phosphatidylserine, 20mg d-alpha-tocopherol, 1mg folic acid and 20 mpg B12.
  - Walking speed improved, shorter latencies in motor screening tasks and increased word recall in supplemented group (p<0.05)

JAMA. 2008;300(19):2253
J Geronotol A Biol Sci Med Sci. 2016;71(2):236-42.

Ginkgo biloba in dementia

- RCT from 1997 demonstrates Ginkgo's ability to stabilize dementia.
- One year, randomized, double-blind, placebo-controlled
  - 309 patients (202 patients provided data) with mild to severe Alzheimer's disease or multi-infarct dementia.
- After 1 year, in patients treated with 120mg EGb761 extract of Ginkgo, there was no change in memory, language, praxis, and orientation.
- Patients treated with placebo had significant deterioration of all of these parameters of cerebral functioning.
- Daily living and social behavior appeared to mildly improve in the Ginkgo group vs. the placebo group.
- There was no difference (or significant) side-effects in either the Ginkgo or placebo group.

JAMA, 1997, Oct. 22/29; 278:1327-32.

Ginkgo biloba

- A meta-analysis of five studies (1985-2000) on Ginkgo and dementia concluded that Ginkgo appeared to have a small, but significant effect on reducing symptoms of dementia.

Psychia Bulletin, 25(9), Sept. 2001

Ginkgo biloba

- The therapeutic results reported in the literature with Ginkgo biloba
  - utilize the standardized extract encapsulated form (24% gingko flavone glycosides and 6% terpene lactones) 120 - 240 mg daily
  - results are not usually seen until at least 6 weeks of continuous treatment and may take as long as 12 weeks to manifest
  - do not cause side-effects
- Ginkgo should not be combined with anti-coagulants (warfarin, coumadin) as it may cause retinal hemorrhage or other bleeding disorders.
- Other forms of ginkgo biloba may be used, but clinical data is limited.

Rosmarinus officinalis

- Labiatae family
- Herba used
- Historical use as a memory tonic

Rosmarinus officinalis

- Active constituents include:
  - Volatile oils (borneol, camphene, camphor, cineole, limonene, linalool and others)
  - Flavonoids (apigenin, diosmetin, diosmin and others)
  - Rosmarinic acid
  - Diterpenes
- The volatile oils in Rosemary are naturally occurring acetylcholinesterase inhibitors.
- Cineole stimulates the central nervous system
  - This effect has been demonstrated in rodents in their enhanced ability to negotiate a maze.
  - Also cineole has been shown to shorten reaction times as measured by brain wave activity.

Rosmarinus officinalis

- Rosemary also increases circulation, including circulation to the brain.
- Rosemary stabilizes the connective tissue of blood vessels leading to enhanced circulation and blood pressure.
- Rosemary is a lipid-soluable antioxidant and helps to regenerate vitamin E.

Rosmarinus: dose-dependent effect on cognition

- RPCDB cross-over study of 28 older adults, mean age 75
- The effects of dried rosemary leaf powder on cognitive performance was assessed at 1, 2.5, 4, and 6 hours following placebo and 4 different doses of rosemary
  - 7 day washout period
- Lowest dose (750mg) had a beneficial effect over placebo (p=0.01) whereas the highest dose (6000mg) had an significant impairing effect (p<0.01)
- Note: The lowest dose, 750mg = just shy of 1/2 teaspoon and can be achieved in the diet

J Med Food. 2012 Jan;15(1):10-7

Rosmarinus officinalis

- The essential oils of rosemary are readily absorbed into the bloodstream through application on the skin, through inhalation and through ingestion.
- Thus, it is conceivable to use Rosemary in shampoos, as an inhalant, or ingested in the form of food, tea, tincture or capsules for the treatment of dementia.

Rosemarinus officinalis

- Effective dosage for the treatment of dementia is unknown.
- Historical dosages:
  - 1/2 - 1 tsp. dried herb/ cup; 3 cups daily [1 tsp. = 2 g]
  - 1:5 tincture, 2 - 4 ml 3 times daily; maximum of 80 ml weekly
  - 2-3 times daily external application
  - 2-3 times daily inhalation.
- Essential oils are toxic therefore do not ingest isolated essential oil.
- Additionally, limit inhalation and topical application to no more than 3 daily applications.
- Long-term effects of chronic ingestion are unknown.

Eleutherococcus senticosus

- Araliaceae family
- Over 1000 papers have been published over the last 4 decades
- Has a long and continued history of use in Siberia and China to increase length and quality of life, prevent infection, improve memory and stimulate appetite.
- Bitter-warming and sweet-warming quality

Eleutherococcus senticosus

- **Active constituents**
  - Eleutherosides B and E
  - Phenylpropanes
  - Polysaccharide
  - Phenolic compounds

Eleutherococcus senticosus

- Classic adaptogen: Reduces the extent of HPA axis activation in response to stress and delays the exhaustive phase of the stress response.
  - decreases adrenal hypertrophy, corticosteroid production and hyperglycemia
- Antioxidant - eleutherosides inactive free radicals and accelerate lipid mobilization to exert a cellular protective effect

Phytomedicine.1994;1:63
Toxicologist.1983;2:51

Eleutherococcus in combination

- DBPCT - pilot study of a combination of Rhodiola rose, Schisandra chinensis and Eleutherococcus senticosus on mental performance.
- 40 females (ages 20-68) under self-assessed long term stress
- Intervention = single table of herbal combination or placebo
- Cognitive function was measured at baseline and 2 hours after the intervention
- Herbal combination resulted in a significant improvement in attention, cognitive processing speed and accuracy (p<0.05) compared to placebo
  - No adverse effects

Phytomedicine. 2010;17(7):494

Eleutherococcus and QoL in elderly

- Fatigue and asthenia in elderly are common symptoms and can be associated with cognitive decline
- DBRCT: 20 elderly (at least 65 years of age) adults were randomized to receive either 300mg/day of E. senticosus dry extract or placebo for 8 weeks.
- Several validated quality of life questionnaires were administered at 4 and 8 weeks
- At 4 weeks, there was higher social function in Eleutherococcus group (p = 0.02), but this difference disappeared at 8 weeks.
- These results suggest a short-term benefit of Eleutherococcus on mental health, with the benefits attenuating over time - this could be the result of dose habituation or HPA normalization.

Arch Gerontol Geriatr Suppl. 2004;9:69

Eleutherococcus senticosus

- Best dosed in morning and afternoon to match diurnal rhythm of HPA axis
- Standardized extract to greater than 1% eleutheroside E: 200 - 400mg daily
- 1:5 tincture - 5mL twice daily
- 24:1 liquid extract - 10-20 drops twice daily
- solid extract - 1/4 teaspoon twice daily

Centella asiatica

- Common name: Gotu kola
- Mackinlayaceae family
- Historically used throughout the India, Asia and Africa
- Above ground parts used
- Active constituents:
  - triterpenoid saponins (asiaticoside, centelloside, madecassoside, asiatic acid)
  - volatile oils
  - flavonoids
  - tannins
  - phytosterols

Centella asiatica

- Centella is primarily used for vascular insufficiency and to accelerate wound healing due to its effects on increasing collagen cross-linking in vessels.
- Centella also can regenerate neuronal axons

Int J Clin Pharmacy Res. 1990;10:229
J Pharm Pharmacol. 2005;57:1221

Centella asiatica: cognition and mood

- RDBPCT of 28 healthy elderly participants.
- Once daily dosing of either 250mg, 500mg, 750mg or placebo for 2 months
- The 750mg dose enhanced working memory and increased self-rated mood.

J Ethnopharmacol. 2008;116(2):325.

Centella asiatica: Anxiety

- Anxiety is a common attribute of cognitive decline.
- Pilot observational study of 33 adults with generalized anxiety disorder.
- All were given 70% hydro-ethanolic extract of Centella asiatica was evaluated on 1000mg twice daily for 2 months
- Changes over baseline: reduced anxiety (p<0.01), reduced self-perceived stress (p<0.01)

Nepal Med Coll J, 2010;12(1):8

Centella asiatica: Health-related QoL in healthy elderly

- RDBPCT of 80 healthy elderly (ages 55-80) in Thailand received either placebo or standardized extract of Centella asiatica at 250mg, 500mg or 750mg once daily for 90 days.
- Physical health was evaluated with 30s chair stand test, hand grip test and 6 min walk test. Quality of life was assessed with SF-36.
- Beginning at 2 months, C. asiatica at doses of 500mg and 750mg improved physical strength (p<0.0001) . These improvements were lost after 1 month of discontinuance of the intervention.
- There was a trend towards improved QoL beginning at 2 months, but this did not reach statistical significance.

Evid Based Complement Alternat Med. 2011;2011:579467

Centella asiatica

- Standardized extracts (standardized to asiaticoside, asiatic acid and madecassic acid): 60-120mg

- 1:5 tincture, 10-20mL daily

- Crude herb: 0.5 - 6g daily

- Pharmacokinetic studies indicate maximum plasma levels (asiatic acid) in 4 - 4.5 hours with daily dosing resulting in increased plasma concentrations, longer half-life and greater area-under-the-curve values.

- Can cause GI upset, nausea and isolated reports (Argentina) of jaundice and elevated liver enzymes following Centella ingestion

J Ethnopharmacol. 1990;28:235

Hericium erinaceus (Lion's mane mushroom)

- Edible mushroom
- Native to China
- Family: Hericiaceae
- Fruiting body contains:
  - Meroterpenoids such as hericenones A-H
  - Cyathane diterpenoids such as erinacines
  - cyclic dipeptides
  - indole alkaloids
  - pyrimidines
  - flavones
  - anthraquinone
  - phenolics
  - amino acids

Hericium

- Hericenones and erinacines from fruiting body stimulate nerve growth factor (NGF).
- NGF, in turn, stimulates cholinergic nerve activity, protects against neuronal cell death, reduces oxidative stress and facilitates neuronal protection from degeneration

Furukawa S. et al. Tetrahedron Lett. 1994;35:1569
Mizuno T et al. Phytother Res. 2009;23:367

Hericium and cognition

- DBRPCT of 30 Japanese adults ages 50-80 - all diagnosed with mild cognitive impairment
- Randomized to receive tablet of dried powder or placebo x 16 weeks
- At weeks 8, 12 and 16, the Hericium group had significantly increased scores on cognitive function scale compared to placebo and the improvement correlated with duration of intake.
  - After 4 weeks without intervention, scores declined to baseline.
  - No adverse effects noted.

Phytother Res 2009;23:367

Hericium and mood

- RDBPCT of 30 menopausal women
- 2g daily of powdered extract for 4 weeks
- Reduced depression and anxiety - presumed to be the result of increased NGF
- Liquid extracts: 20-50mL per week of a 1:2 liquid

Biomed Res.2010;31(4):231

Hericium: Other actions (In-vivo)

- Cardioprotective: reduces oxidation of LDL, inhibits platelet aggregation
- Antidiabetic: reduces serum glucose and may reduce neuropathic pain
- Anti-fatigue: activates metabolism, specifically supporting glycogen storage in muscle and liver tissue
- Hepatoprotective: antioxidant, specifically in liver
- Anticancer: in-vitro activity against many cancer cell lines, exerts antiproliferative effect, synergistic with doxorubicin chemotherapy
- Immunomodulatory: activates dendritic cells and augments Th1 immunity

BioMed Res Intern, 2014;828149.
Phytomedicine. 2010;17(14):1082
BMC Complement Altern Med. 2013;13:253
Exp Ther Med. 2015;9(2):483
J Agri Food Chem. 2015;63(32):7108
Process Biochem. 2013;48(9):1402

Crocus Sativus (Saffron)

- Family: Iridaceae
- Origin: Iran, India, Greece
- Part Used: Flower pistils
- Active constituents: more than 150 volatile and aroma-yielding compounds mainly terpenes, terpene alcohol, and their esters.
- Medicinal Actions: antihypertensive, anticonvulsant, antitussive, antigenototoxic, anxiolytic, aphrodisiac, antioxidant, antidepressant, antinociceptive (analgesic), anti-inflammatory, and relaxant.

Pharmacogn Rev. 2010;4(8):200

Saffron

- Saffron may inhibit the aggregation and deposition of amyloid B in the human brain
- DBRCT of 46 adults with mild-moderate AD randomized to saffron 30mg/day (15mg twice daily) or placebo for 16 weeks.
- Saffron produced improvement in cognitive function over placebo (P=0.04).

J Clin Pharm Ther. 2010;35(5):581

Bacopa monnieri (Brahmi)

- Family: Plantaginaceae
- Origin: India, Australia, Indochina, Sri Lanka
- Part(s) Used: Leaves
- Active Constituents: triterpenoid saponins (bacosides), alkaloids (brahmine, nicotine, herpestine), flavonoids (apigenin, luteolin)
- Medicinal Actions: antioxidant, acetylcholinesterase inhibition, increases cerebral blood flow, neuroprotective

HerbalGram. 2011;91:1

Bacopa monnieri (Brahmi)

- Bacopa has anxiolytic, nootropic and adaptogenic effects.
- Meta-analysis of the cognitive effects of Bacopa
- 9 high quality studies met inclusion criteria, total of 437 subjects
- Results: Bacopa results in improved cognition (p<0.001) and decreased choice reaction time (p<0.001) compared to placebo

J Ethnopharmacol. 2014;151(1):528

Meta-analysis of 6 studies conducted over 12 weeks.
Results: Bacopa improves memory free recall at dosages of 300-450mg daily (standardized to 10-20% bacopa glycosides)

J Altern Complement Med. 2012; 18(7):647

Bacopa: memory

- RDBPCT of 98 healthy participants over the age of 55y
  - Randomized to 300mg Bacopa monnieri extract (BacopaMind; 20:1 alcohol extract standardized to contain 40-50% bacosides) or placebo x 12 weeks
  - Bacopa improved verbal learning, memory acquisition, and delayed recall, total learning (p= 0.001)
  - Bacopa did cause increased stool frequency, abdominal cramps and nausea in some participants.
- RDBPCT of 54 adults over age 65y (mean age 73y) without clinical signs of dementia.
  - Randomized to 300mg Bacopa monnieri extract (methanol-extracted extract with minimum of 50% bacosides A and B) or placebo x 12 weeks
  - Bacopa participants had enhanced delayed word recall scores as well as decreased depression and anxiety.
  - Small percentage of participants experienced mild nausea

J Altern Complement Med. 2010; 16(7):753
J Altern Complement Med. 2008; 14(6):707

Melissa officinalis: memory

- DBRPCT of 42 adults (ages 65-80) with Alzheimer's disease randomized to 60 drops of 1:1 Melissa officinalis liquid extract or placebo for 4 months.
- At 4 months, Melissa officinalis produced improved cognition on cognition measures than placebo (p<0.0001) and Melissa participants demonstrated less agitation than placebo participants.

J Neurol Neurosurg Psychiatry. 2003;74(7):863

Other Important consideration: Antioxidation

- Silybum marianum (milk thistle)
  - antihepatotoxic
- Camellia sinensis (green tea)
  - enhances cP450 Phase II enzymes, anticarcinogenic
- Crataegus oxycantha (hawthorne)
  - bioflavonoids protect vasculature against peroxidation
- Rosa canina (rose hips)
  - vit. C and bioflavonoids are water soluable antioxidants

Other Important Consideration: Anti-inflammation

- Bupleurum falcatum (Chinese thoroughwax)
  - enhance activity of corticosterone, stimulates adrenocortical function, suppress granulation tissue, inhibits PGE2 production
- Glycyrrhiza glabra (licorice)
  - increases half-life of cortisol, enhances cortisol receptor sensitivity
- Dioscorea villosa (wild yam)
  - diosgenin is a precursor to adrenocortical hormones, anti-spasmodic
- Curcuma longa (turmeric)
  - curcuminoids cross BBB and reduce NFkB activation
- Boswellia serrulata (Indian frankincense)
  - inhibits 5-lipoxygenase inflammation

Conclusions

- There are viable botanicals for the improvement of cognitive function in adults with early dementia or cognitive decline.
- The scientific data on most of these herbs is limited.
- Conventional medications, however, offer limited benefits
- Treat the person with dementia rather than the dementia in the person.
- Begin treatment as early as possible!

Happiness

Applying the Science and Holism of Happiness to Transform clinical practice

Lise Alschuler, N.D., F.A.B.N.O.

CNDA 2014

Topics

- Why Happiness?
- The tenets of happiness
  - A primer on Positive Psychology
- The Power of Positive
  - Implications of happiness to patient care and wellness
- A New Model for the Clinical Encounter
  - To include my favorite herbs to elevate mood

We are practitioners, why bother with happiness?

- While relieving symptoms in our patients is a significant step towards wellness, assisting them even further along the wellness pathway towards joy and contentment is ultimate healing.
- Happy patients are:
  - Healthier
  - Able to sustain healthy lifestyles
  - Willing to adhere to treatment plans
  - Able to generate greater insight to help explain their health issues
  - Creative in solving health challenges
  - More fun and gratifying to work with

Today's Practice of Medicine – the opportunity

- Oriented around complaint, unwellness and disease
- Is good at alleviating the symptom – either by masking it (allopathic) or by addressing the cause (naturopathic)
- However, this approach reinforces weakness and neglects rejuvenation
- There is an opportunity to transform the practice of medicine to one that includes the alleviation of suffering and extends beyond this to establishing deeply exuberant living.

Positive Psychology: the study of Happiness

- Developed by Martin Seligmann, PsyD. in 1998
- The purpose was to use research to understand the positive, adaptive, creative and emotionally fulfilling aspects of human behavior.
- Positive psychology
  - = the scientific study of ordinary human strengths and virtues
  - = the scientific study of what enables individuals and communities to thrive
- Positive Psychology assesses the factors that most contribute to a well-lived and fulfilling life, "the good life"
- Focuses on what is right, rather than what is wrong

Compton W. and E. Hoffman. Positive Psychology, 2nd ed. 2013 (Belmont CA: Wadsworth, Cengage Learning): 1-3.

Happiness is a set of practices

- Positive Subjective States: positive emotions such as joy, happiness, satisfaction, love, contentment
  - Positive emotions are independent of negative emotions (i.e. they don't substitute each other out)
  - Thus, freedom from anxiety or depression doesn't automatically result in happiness.
  - In fact, negative emotions are vital for self-understanding and personal growth, and challenges can be deeply enriching experiences.
- Self-acceptance
- Personal Growth and Autonomy
- Positive relationships and helping others
- Hope: A sense of agency, or having sufficient drive to reach important goals, and believing that there are pathways available to reach those goals.

Lambert M and D Erekson. J Psychother Integration. 2008;18(2):222.
Woolfolk R. J Theoretical Philosoph Psychol. 2002;22(1):19.

Ultimate happiness

- "Breathing a sense of wonder, sacredness, and true understanding into one's perception of the world, into one's relationships, and into one's actions."

Biswas-Diener R. Practicing Positive Psychology Coaching, 2010 (John Wiley & Sons: New Jersey):78.

Determinants of Happiness

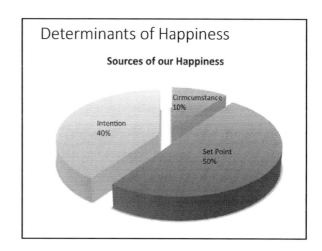

Happiness Set Point

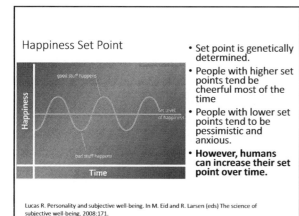

- Set point is genetically determined.
- People with higher set points tend be cheerful most of the time
- People with lower set points tend to be pessimistic and anxious.
- **However, humans can increase their set point over time.**

Lucas R. Personality and subjective well-being. In M. Eid and R. Larsen (eds) The science of subjective well-being. 2008:171.
Headley B. Social Indicators Res. 2008;86(2):312.

Moving targets of Happiness

- Positive emotions broaden our awareness thereby facilitating our ability to learn from these experiences and to build our personal resources in order to have continued positive emotions.
- You know you are happy when...
  - **Mindfulness**: paying attention, awareness, openness, flexibility
  - **Flow**: unified flowing from one moment to the next without worry and with effortless concentration
  - **Playfulness**: emotional, humorous, social and creative engagement
  - **Savoring**: an awareness of pleasure and delighting in it
  - **Peak performance**: moments of performance beyond our normal level of functioning
  - **Compassion**: observing and practicing kindness, altruism and care of others
  - **Loving relationships** with at least 2 of 3: Passion, Intimacy, Commitment

Compton W. and E. Hoffman. Positive Psychology, 2nd ed. 2013 (Belmont CA: Wadsworth, Cengage Learning): 1-3.

A new model for the clinical encounter

- Create a Culture based on Strengths
- Acknowledge weaknesses, or chief complaints
- Engage your patients' brains
- Grease the Skids
- Take in the Good
- Create goals
- Set the agenda
- Walk our Talk

Why establish strengths?

- Associated with higher happiness and less depression and anxiety
- Establishing strengths is associated with faster and more complete recovery from illness
- And, quite simply, most people just don't get authentic and relevant positive feedback in their lives.

Seligman M, et al. American Psychologist. 2005;60(5):410-12
Peterson C, et al. J Positive Psychology. 2006;1(I):17-26

1. Identify strengths

- All of us have pre-existing capacities (thoughts, feelings, behaviors) which are energizing and lead to authentic happiness.
- Many of us neglect our strengths
- Patient Exercise:
  - Ask your patient to focus on a time when they worked on improving their health (specific to chief complaint, if possible)
  - Have the patient describe this effort
  - Listen and identify the underlying capacities – identify those to the patient
- Take note of these strengths in your patient record and reference them going forward.
- Example…

Reframing a Chief Complaint into an Awesome Attribute

- Another way to reinforce patients innate strengths is to accentuate the positive aspects of their current health issue.
- Ex. A patient with long-standing IBS might say, "My intestines are my weakest organ – all my stress goes there."
- Reframe: "Perhaps your intestines are your strongest system as they are both a barometer of stress and contain its effects. Your intestines appear to be, not your weakest organ, but your warrior organ."

2. Immediately follow weaknesses / chief complaints with strengths

- Reinforces the importance of addressing the complaints and models their co-existence with the patient's strengths

Weakness

- Patient with cancer: "My immune system is weak."
- Doctor response: "We do need to recalibrate your immunity, and I am excited that you have no markers of inflammation and no signs of insulin resistance. These pathways are healthy and are helping you to control cancer growth.

Strength

- **Focusing on both strengths and weaknesses is essential to create and maintain health.**

Extracting Strengths

- What are some things about your health of which you are the most proud?
  - I had a terrible sledding accident when I was a teenager. My brother broke his leg, but, miraculously, none of my bones broke.
- What parts of your health energize you now?
  - I sleep soundly and with ease.
- What are you looking forward to experiencing with regards to your health in the (near) future?
  - Regular bowel movements without gas and bloating

Extracted Strengths

Adventurous
Powerful
Strong

Trusting
Serene

Assimiliator
Sifter
Willing to be nourished

When strengths are established

- Result: patient should visibly demonstrate a boost in energy, alertness, engagement and, ultimately, motivation.
- Signs to look for:
  - Quicker and higher pitched speech
  - Straighter posture
  - Increased use of metaphors in their descriptions
  - Smiling
  - Greater eye contact
  - Increased use of hand gestures
- Create a safe environment to acknowledge strengths
  - ≠ to bragging
  - Not creating a sense of invulnerability or superiority
  - Goal is to balance challenges and issues with strengths and capacities

Lima C. Behav Res Methods. 2013 Dec;45(4):1234-45.

3. Engage our Brains - Capturing Positivity

What just happened?

- Story created happiness
- And with that, feelings of interest, optimism, enthusiasm, warmth, generosity...
- That is all happening in your brain right now!

- Don't be afraid to tell stories and to give inspirational examples during clinic visits

What flows through the mind sculpts the brain; immaterial experiences leave material traces

- The brain:
  - 80-100 billion neurons
  - A trillion glial cells
  - Half a quadrillion synapses
- With all of this, the brain demonstrates experience-dependent neuroplasticity
- The mind:
  - The brain processes sensory information in neuronal networks that are shaped by experience, particularly during early life, but not exclusively, to optimally represent the internal and external milieu.
  - With conscious awareness and repetition of mental states, neural networks are established that facilitate these mental states into becoming neural traits
  - Neurons that fire together wire together   Castren E. JAMA Psychiatry. 2013 Sep;70(9):983-9.

Brain's Negativity Bias

- **Amygdala** = Alarm bell: reacts to a perceived threat and activates the sympathetic nervous system and the hypothalamus
  - 65% of the amygdala reacts to threats, or negative stimuli
- **Hypothalamus** activates the stress response via HPA axis
  - Cortisol stimulates and sensitizes the amygdala
- The **hippocampus** makes visual-spatial short term memories and imbeds a neural trace of the experience into cortical memory networks so we can learn from the experience later
  - Hippocampus ultimately facilitates homeostasis by reducing amygdalar hyperreactivity and reducing hypothalamic (and, ultimately, cortisol) activation
- Our brains have a built-in negativity bias as a survival mechanism
  - Ready for full response to perceived threats
- Therefore, as happiness and resilience come from positive experiences (such as the story you just heard), to override this negative bias, we need to pay sustained attention to these positive experiences in order to transform momentary happiness into a more permanent neuronal pathways.

Graeff F. Braz J Med Biol Res. 1994 Apr;27(4):811-29.

Processing Emotions

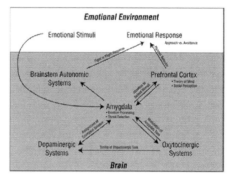

Neurochemistry of Happiness

- Fresh positive experiences stimulate the release of dopamine
- **Dopamine** signals the hypothalamus to produce oxytocin which is stored and released by the posterior pituitary gland.
  - **Oxytocin** creates feelings of comfort, safety, attraction and attenuates the fear response of the amygdala
  - This is supported by sufficient serotonin
- Sustained release of dopamine helps the amygdala to more consistently respond without eliciting fear or aggression and also signals the hippocampus and prefrontal cortex
- The hippocampus essentially hard wires this response, resetting the proclivity towards happiness of the individual.
  - Serotonin supports hippocampal activity
- The left prefrontal cortex overlays reasoning and recall to the emotional experience while suppressing negative emotions
- This focus on promoting "the good" increases stimulation of the nucleus accumbens (a collection of neurons in the midbrain)
  - Rich in dopamine receptors
  - This initiates a sense of agency (ownership and control), motivation and spurs action towards a person's goals

Kienast T. Pharmacopsychiatry. 2013 Jun;46(4):130-6.
Asan E. Histochem Cell Biol. 2013 Jun;139(6):785-813.

Oxytocin – the love hormone

- Oxytocin is synthesized in hypothalamus, stored and released into the peripheral venous bloodstream by the posterior pituitary and **to the amygdala where it attenuates amygdalar hyperactivity.**
- OXT decreases anxiety, decreases stress and facilitates social encounters
- Caveat: when social cues in the environment are interpreted as "safe" oxytocin may promote prosociality but when the social cues are interpreted as "unsafe" oxytocin may promote more defensive and, in effect, "anti-social" emotions and behaviors.
- OXT influences:
  - Social emotions such as trust, generosity, altruism and empathy
  - Strength of social bonds, especially mother-child and romantic relationships

Labuschagne I, et al. Neuropsychopharmacology. 2010;35:2403-13.
Olff M, et al. Psychoneuroendocrinology. 2013 Sep;38(9):1883-94

Molecules of happiness

- Serotonin
  - Receptors exist throughout the brain and especially in the hippocampus where serotonin influences positive mood and reduces depression
  - High levels are associated with serenity, optimism and spiritual experiences
- Norepinephrine
  - Excitatory and induces physical and mental arousal and heightens mood; involved in flight or fight response
- Dopamine
  - Controls arousal and is vital for motivation, pleasure and reward
- Opiates/Endorphins
  - Modulate pain, reduce stress and promote a sensation of bliss
- Oxytocin
  - is released by the posterior pituitary and is implicated in social bonding, trust and love

Ashby F. et al. Psychol. Rev. 1999;106:529.
Farrell P. et al. Medicine Sci Sports Exercise. 1987;19(4):347.
Urry H. et al. Psychological Sci. 2004;15(6):367.

4. Greasing the skids

- As people implement positive lifestyle and attitudinal changes, integrative therapies can alter brain chemistry and facilitate positive emotions.
- Mood enhancing nutrients include:
  - Vitamins and Minerals
  - L-theanine
  - Phosphatidylserine
  - SAMe
- Botanicals:
  - Holy basil
  - Lavender
  - St John's Wort
  - Chamomile
  - Schisandra
  - Lemon balm

Neurotransmitter support with vitamins and minerals

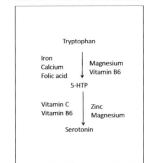
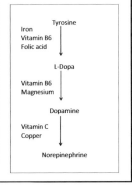

L-theanine

- L-theanine (γ-glutamyl-ethylamide) is a unique amino acid present almost exclusively in the tea plant (*Camellia sinensis*) (1-2% of dry weight of tea leaves) [i]
- L-theanine **increases dopamine and serotonin production and GABA activity** and generates alpha waves in the central nervous system resulting in reduced blood pressure and anxiety (**causing a relaxed yet alert state**). [ii]
- 100mg TID

(i) L-theanine Monograph. Altern Med Rev. 2005 Jun;10(2):136-8.
(ii) Ito K, et al. Effects of Ltheanine on the release of alpha-brain waves in human volunteers. *Nippon Nogeikagaku Kaishi* 1998;72:153-157.

Phosphatidylserine

- Derived from soy or sunflower lecithin
- Supplemental phosphatidylserine reduces ACTH, CRH and cortisol levels
  - Also reduces epinephrine and norepinephrine
  - Donates choline and supports dopamine production
- RPCT: 4 groups of 20 subjects x 3 weeks and then exposed to a mental and emotional stressor (standardized stress test):
  - 400mg, 600mg, 800mg soy-derived PS or placebo
  - Primary Outcome measure: Spielberger State Anxiety Inventory stress subscale
- 400mg blunted serum ACTH and cortisol and exerted a positive effect on emotional responses to the stress test.
  - Larger doses did not result in the same effects.

Hellhammer J. et al. Stress. 2004;7(2):119-26.

S-adenosyl-L-methionine (SAMe)

- Donates methyl groups to:
  - Dopamine (from Tyrosine)
  - Serotonin (from Tryptophan)
- Relieves depression
- Take with B-vitamin complex to reduce build-up of homocysteine
- SAMe dosing: 800mg – 1600mg daily

Papakostas GI, Can J Psychiatry. 2012 Jul;57(7):406-13.
Bottiglieri T. Psychiatr Clin North Am. 2013 Mar;36(1):1-13

Holy basil

- Ocimum sanctum (syn. O. tenuiflorum)
- Also known as Tulsi
  - Considered a sacred plant by Hindus
- Lamiaceae (mint) family
- Native to Asia
- Actives: eugenol, caryophyllene, triterpenoic acids (ursolic and oleanolic acids)
- Medicinal uses: common cold, bronchitis, malaria, skin diseases, insect bites, reduces anxiety and stress, improves mental clarity

Holy Basil: Medicinal Actions

- Hepatoprotective (Adhvaryu M. World J Gastroenterol. 2007;13(23):3199)
- Antiproliferative (Manikandan P. Singapore Med J. 48(7):645)
- Antioxidant -prevents GSH depletion (Bhartiya U. Indian J Exp Biol.2006;44(8):647-52)
- Reduces cholesterol (Gupta S. Indian J Exp Biol. 2006;44(4):300)
- Improves memory (Joshi H, M Parle. Indian J Exp Biol. 2006;44(2):133)
- Anti-ulcer (Goel R. Indian J Exp Biol. 2005;43(8):715)
- Normalizes corticosteroid levels with stress exposure (Archana R, A Namasivayam. Phytother Res. 2002;16(6):579)
- Reduces stress-induced behavioral despair, cognitive dysfunction and immune suppression (Muruganandam A. Indian J Exp Biol. 2002;40(10):1151)
- Hypoglycemic (Vats V. J Ethnopharmacol. 2002;79(1):95)

Holy basil: anxiolytic

- 35 adults, average age 38.4 years (21 male, 14 female) took 500mg Holy Basil twice daily after meals
- Holy Basil resulted in a significant decrease in generalized anxiety and reduced feelings of stress and depression (p<0.001)
- Holy Basil also increased motivation to make lifestyle changes and facilitated the ability to change perception of current circumstances.

Bhattacharyya D. Nepal Med Coll J. 2008;10(3):176-9

Holy basil: Immunosupportive

- DBRC cross-over trial of 24 healthy volunteers
- 300mg of ethanolic extract of Holy basil or placebo x 4 weeks
- Holy basil increased IFN-gamma (p=0.039), IL-4 (p=0.001), % T-helper cells (p=0.001) and % NK cells (p=0.017)

Mondal S. J Ethnopharmacol. 2011;136(3):452-6

Holy Basil: Hypoglycemic

- RPC cross-over single blind trial of patients with DB2
- Following a fixed dose of Ocimum sanctum:
  - Fasting blood glucose decreased by 21.0 mg/dL (p<0.001); a reduction of 17.6%
  - Post-prandial glucose decreased by 15.8 mg/dL (p<0.02); a reduction of 7.3%

Agrawal P. et al. Int J Clin Pharmacol Ther. 1996;34(9):406-9

Holy Basil as a Happiness herb

- Mentally clarifying
- Increases mental clarity and focus
- Facilitates a shift in perspective
- Reduces mental inertia and even depression
- Restores hope and optimism

Holy Basil: Dosing

- Tincture 1:5. 3ml-5ml TID
- Tea 1 tsp./8 oz hot water; steep x 10m covered TID
- Capsules: Extracts standardized to total eugenols and rosmarinic acid.
  - 150mg capsule (equivalent to 1.5g crude herb)
  - 1 capsule BID
- CI: Use with caution during pregnancy (conflicting information on toxicity to fetus)

Lavender angustifolia

- Contains volatile oil, primary active constituents of which are linalool and linalyl acetate – considered responsible for the anxiolytic effects
- Potentiates $GABA_A$ receptors, inhibits glutamate binding in brain
- Over 440 RCTs on lavender and anxiety
- Recent review included 15 RCTs, involving 1565 participants
  - 8 trials investigated the effects of lavender inhalation, with 4 reporting a significant positive effect for at least one anxiety measure
  - 3 trials assessed oral lavender
- Conclusion: oral lavender supplements may have therapeutic effects
  - methodological issues limit the strength of the conclusions drawn.
- Effective studied dose = 20-80mg per day

Perry R. et al. Phytomedicine;2012 Jun;19(8-9):825-35.

Lavender

- Silexan was studied in DBRCT (Jadad = 4)
- N = 221 (212 were evaluated) adults with subclinical anxiety
- 80mg lavender oil (WS 1265) daily or placebo x 10 weeks
- Primary outcome measure: Hamilton Anxiety Rating Scale and Pittsburgh Sleep Quality Index
- Anxiety decreased significantly more in the Silexan group over placebo (p<0.01)and was found to be superior to placebo regarding the percentage of responders (76.9 vs. 49.1%, P<0.001) and remitters (60.6 vs. 42.6%, P=0.009).
  - Silexan had a significant beneficial influence on quality and duration of sleep and improved general mental and physical health without causing any unwanted sedative or other drug specific effects.

Kasper S. Int Clin Psychopharmacol. 2010 Sep;25(5):277-87.

Lavender as a Happiness Herb

- Establishes serenity
- Creates calmness and increased resistance to stress
- Facilitates peacefulness

St. John's Wort

- Hypericum perforatum
- Native to Europe and naturalized to N. America
- Part used: flowering tops
- Active constituents include: hypericin, hyperforin, xanthones, flavonoids, essential oils
- Medicinal actions: anti-inflammatory, astringent, vulnerary, nervine, anti-depressant, antimicrobial
- Traditional uses: SJW has been used throughout Europe and historically was thought to 'ward off evil spirits'. SJW has been used to treat wounds and burns.

SJW: Clinical indications

- Reduces depression and anxiety
  - *Hypericum* extract has demonstrated synaptosomal serotonin, dopamine and norepinephrine uptake inhibition and weak monoamine oxidase A and B inhibition.
- Insomnia due to restlessness
- Irritability
- Neuralgia (i.e. herpetic neuralgia)
- Migraine headaches
- Sciatica, pain, inflammation (topical and internal)
- Incontinence
- Anti-viral

Bombardelli E, Morazzoni P, Fitoterapia, 1995;66:43

SJW: depression meta-analysis

- Hypericum has been tested in over 3,000 patients against placebo and various controls.
- A meta-analysis of 23 randomized trials of Hypericum with a total of 1,757 outpatients with mild to moderate depression revealed that Hypericum is significantly superior to placebo and comparably effective to standard antidepressants while producing fewer side effects.
  - Of these studies comparing Hypericum with placebo, approximately 55% of patients receiving Hypericum improved, vs. 22% receiving placebo
  - In those studies comparing Hypericum with standard antidepressants, 64% of patients receiving Hypericum improved while 58% of patients receiving standard anti-depressants improved.

Linde, K, et al, British Medical Journal, 1996;313(7052):253

SJW: depression

- RDBPCT of adults aged 18-65 (n=72) diagnosed with mild-moderate major depressive disorder according to DSM-IV criteria
- Oral doses of Hypericum standardized extract WS 5572 (contains 0.3% hypericin) 300 mg three times per day or identical placebo for 42 days
- "Group differences in favor of WS 5572 were descriptively apparent as early as day 7 of randomized treatment and were statistically significant at days 28 (p=0.011) and day 42 (p<0.001)...The results indicate that Hypericum extract WS 5572 is an effective and well-tolerated drug for the treatment of mild to moderate major depressive disorder."

Kalb R, et al. Pharmacopsychiatry 2001; 34:96-103.

SJW vs. Celexa

- RDBPCT of adults aged 18-70 years (n=388) with moderate depression diagnosed according to DSM-IV criteria
- Oral dose of Hypericum extract 900 mg, citalopram (Celexa) 20 mg or placebo daily for six weeks
- "The statistical significant therapeutic equivalence of Hypericum extract to citalopram (p<0.0001) and the superiority of this Hypericum extract over placebo (p<0.0001) was demonstrated."

Gastpar M, et al. Pharmacopsychiatry 2006; 39(2):66-75.

SJW vs. Prozac

- RDBCT of 240 adult outpatients with a current diagnosis of mild to moderate depression
- Oral dose of Hypericum 250 mg (standardized to 0.5 mg hypericin per 250 mg tablet) twice daily or fluoxetine (Prozac) 20 mg daily for six weeks
- "Hypericum and fluoxetine are equipotent with respect to all main parameters used to investigate antidepressants in this population. Although Hypericum may be superior in improving the responder rate, the main difference between the two treatments is safety. Hypericum was superior to fluoxetine in overall incidence of side effects, number of patients with side effects and the type of side effect reported."

Schrader E, et al.. International Clinical Psychopharmacology 2000; 15:61-68

SJW vs. Paxil

- RDBCT of 251 men and women aged 18-70 years diagnosed with severe acute major depression according to DSM-IV criteria
- Oral doses of hypericum extract WS 5570 (contains 0.3% hypericin) 300 mg three times daily or paroxetine (20 mg once daily) for six weeks. In non-responders, the initial dose was doubled after two weeks.
- This study "...showed non-inferiority of Hypericum and statistical superiority over paroxetine. In the treatment of moderate to severe major depression, Hypericum extract WS 5570 is at least as effective as paroxetine and is better tolerated."

Zegedi A,et al.. BMJ 2005; 330(7490) :503.

St. John's wort as a happiness herb

- The doctrine of signatures for this plant aptly describes its effect.
- The leaves are perforated – holding this leaf to the sunlight, one can see that the leaf 'lets the light in'. This is appropriate for people with mild depression who have lost a sense of hope.
- SJW is most indicated in people who need inspiration and motivation to be happier
- SJW can also be considered to facilitate enlightenment – developing a more profound and deeply appreciative sense of life.

SJW: Clinical dosing

- Standardized extract: 180mg standardized to 0.8-1mg hypericins, 3 capsules daily
- 1:5 tincture, 1-4 mL TID
- Infusion 2-4g/cup, QD – TID (1 tsp = 1.8g)
- The clinical effect of SJW may take 2 to 8 weeks to manifest
- Toxicity: Photosensitivity occurs in susceptible individuals at the highest therapeutic doses. Approximately 2.4% of patients report side effects which include: gastrointestinal irritations, allergic reactions, tiredness and restlessness.
- CI: People with a diagnosis of bipolar disorder or hypomania should avoid St. John's wort as it may trigger a manic episode
- Interactions: SJW is a strong inducer of cytochrome p3A4, which is a common metabolic enzymes for drug activation and/or elimination. Some known contraindications, based on this activity:
  - Iirinotecan chemotherapy
  - Oral contraceptives
  - Digoxin
  - Anesthesia (discontinue 2 weeks prior to planned surgery)
- SJW should also be avoided with SSRIs

Chamomile (Matricaria recutita)

- Asteraceae
- Cultivated in Europe and N. America
- Part used: Flowers
- **Constituents**: volatile oil (0.3-1.5%) containing: alpha bisabolol oxides, sesquiterpenes (anti-inflammatory, anti-spasmodic) such as chamazulene; flavonoids (anti-spasmodic, anti-inflammatory) inc.: methoxylated flavones and flavonols, apigenin, luteolin, quercetin
- **Medicinal actions**: Gentle sedative (relaxant, restorative), anti-spasmodic, anodyne, anti-inflammatory, antipyretic, antiseptic, anti-diarrheal, anti-emetic, carminative, anti-microbial, anti-anaphylactic, vulnerary

Chamomile Medicinal Uses

- The volatile oils, such as chamazulene, appear to be due in part to activation of the pituitary-adrenal axis.
- Azulene also is a gentle sedative, restoring the nervous system to a calmer state.
- The volatile oils, such as alpha-bisabolol is anti-inflammatory and anti-spasmodic specifically enhancing prostaglandin production thereby strengthening the mucosal protective barrier (therefore protective against ulcers).
- Chamazulene inhibits lipid peroxidation
- Matricaria is therefore useful in the treatment of IBS and colitis (for its anti-spasmodic, anti-ulcer, and nervine effects).

Carl W and L Emrich. J Prosthet Dent. 1991;66(3):361-9
McKay D and J Blumberg, Phytother Res. 20(7):519-30
Rekka E, et al. Res Commun Mol Pathol Pharmacol. 1996;92(3):361-4.

Chamomile: Hot Flushes

- DBRCT of 55 postmenopausal women with hot flushes and not taking hormonal therapy.
- Women were randomized to chewable Chamomile tablets (5 chewed daily) or placebo x 12 weeks.
  - The women completed a (Kupperman) questionnaire assessing the frequency and intensity of menopausal symptoms, prior to and throughout the study. All women underwent hormone profile measurements and transvaginal ultrasonography evaluation before and after treatment.
- "There was a significant difference between the study group and the control group in the decrease in number and intensity of hot flushes from baseline to completion of treatment (90-96% vs 15-25%, p < 0.001). In the study group, a response was already noted during the first month of treatment (68% +/- 2% reduction of hot flushes during the day and 74% +/- 4% during the night). There was also a marked alleviation of sleep disturbances and fatigue."

Kupfersztain C. et al. Clin Exp Obstet Gynecol. 2003;30(4):203-6.

Chamomile as a Happiness Herb

- Chamomile is a gentle, restorative herb
- It is indicated in people who feel irritable and desire contentedness and peacefulness.
- Chamomile is also indicated for people who have somatized psychological distress as gastrointestinal and hormonal complaints.

Chamomile: Dosing

- Infusion: 1-2 tsp./cup water; steep 3-5 min. covered; sig 1 cup TID [1 tsp. - 1 g; 1 TB - 2.5 g]
  - Light tea- sweet (good for ulcers)
  - Strong tea (steeped longer) and cool tea- bitter (good for G.I. conditions)
  - Hot tea will be dispersed throughout the body.
- Tincture 1:5 45% EtOH sig 1-4 ml TID; max. weekly dose 100 ml
- Liquid extract 1:1 45% EtOH sig 1-3 ml TID
- Capsules: 350-700 mg (1-2 OO caps) TID
- Baths, Steams, Enemas
- Note: Matricaria is best dosed on the low end of its dosage range over a long period of time.
- Matricaria is a smooth muscle relaxant and therefore may cause miscarriage in pregnant women, especially before 12 weeks.

Schisandra chinensis
wu-wei-zi

- **Botanical description**: Schisandra is a Chinese climbing shrub.
- **Historical uses**: This berry has been used in China as a tonic herb, known as "five-taste fruit" which acts on all organ systems by being sweet, sour, salty, bitter and pungent.
- **Parts used**: dried berry
- **Constituents**: Schizandrins (biphenyl octenoid lignans) including wuweizisu C, wuweizichun B, schisantherin A, B, C and D.
  - There are over 200 identified constituents in Schisandra berry
- **Medicinal actions**: Astringent, sedative, aphrodisiac, kidney and skin tonic, anxiolytic, hepatoprotective

Schisandra: medicinal uses

- Schisandra strengthens the lungs, kidneys and adrenals.
- In TCM, Schisandra "calms the shen" making it useful for anxiety, insomnia, night sweats, palpitations and forgetfulness and worry due to excessive stress.
- The lignans improve concentration, fine coordination and sensitivity.
  - Improves vision, hearing and skin sensory discrimination
- Hepatoprotective; in the presence of toxins Schisandra reduces liver damage, improves protein synthesis and accelerates liver repair.
  - Schisandra elevates liver microsomes which increase the ability of the liver to detoxify foreign substances in the body.
  - Schisandrin lignans lower SGPT levels and Schizandra is a useful remedy in chronic hepatitis

Evans, W.C., Trease and Evans' Pharmacognosy, (WB Saunders Co. Ltd: London), 14th ed., 1996:438

Schisandra: adaptogen

- Traditionally used to prolong life, retard the aging process, increase endurance and energy and improve libido.
- Schisandra reduces the effects of stress, namely fatigue and weakness, by lowering elevated cortisol and by accumulating phenolic secondary metabolites that activate maximum work capacity.
- Chronic administration of schisandra lignans have been demonstrated to inhibit p-SAPK/p-JNK formation during stress. Note: a single dose activates this pathway, indicating support to the organism to initially respond to, and then chronically adapt to, stressors.

Panossian A. et al. Drug Target Insights. 2007;2:39-54

Schisandra: stress-induced HTN

- 30 day DBRCT of 40 military personnnel with cardiovascular maladaptation to stress (HTN).
- All subjects received lifestyle counseling and were, in addition, randomized to receive a proprietary extract blend of Rhodiola rosea, Schisandra chinensis and Eleutherococcus senticosus or placebo
  - 2 capsules provide 1,750mg
- The adaptogens produced significant improvement over placebo in cardiovascular function, notably reduced blood pressure.

Ciumasu-Rimbu M. et al. Rev Med Chir Soc Med Nat Iasi. 2012;116(3):790-3.

Schisandra: Illness Recovery

- DBRPCT of 60 adults ages 18-65 years with acute nonspecific pneumonia.
- All patients received SOC (cephazoline, bromhexine and theophylline). 30 patients also received standardized combination of a proprietary extract blend of Rhodiola rosea, Schisandra chinensis and Eleutherococcus senticosus or placebo.
  - 2 capsules provide 1,750mg
- Results:
  - mean duration of treatment with antibiotics was 2 days shorter in the intervention group over placebo
  - QOL was significantly higher at all time points in the intervention group
- "Clearly, adjuvant therapy with ADAPT-232 has a positive effect on the recovery of patients by decreasing the duration of the acute phase of the illness, by increasing mental performance of patients in the rehabilitation period, and by improving their QOL. "

Narimanian M. et al. Phytomedicine. 2005;12(10):723-9

Schisandra: Hepatoprotection

- 5 month DBRPCT of 40 adults with boderline high ALT (40-60 U/L) or AST (40-60 U/L)
- Intervention was a mixture of Schisandra extract and sesamin given as 4 tablets daily or placebo.
- "Intervention of SCH clearly reduced the levels of ALT and AST, but it made no change in the total bilirubin and direct bilirubin.
- "Intake of SCH also greatly increased the antioxidant capacity and decreased the values of thiobarbituric acid reactive substances, total free radicals, and superoxide anion radicals in the plasma. The activities of glutathione peroxidase and reductase in the erythrocytes were significantly increased.
- "In addition, the lag time for low-density lipoprotein oxidation, an inflammatory marker, was evidently increased. Fatty liver was found to have been significantly improved in this study. SCH proved to have the effects of antioxidation and improving liver function."

Chiu H. et al. Phytother Res. 2013;27(3):368-73

Schisandra: Liver Transplant

- Liver transplant recipients are often placed on Tacrolimus to prevent allograft rejection.
- 2 phase RCT clinical trial of 46 liver transplant recipients.
  - Phase 1: all patients received equal doses of Tac
  - Phase 2: 21 patients received Schisandra extract and either the same dose of Tac or a lower dose of Tac.
- Co-administration of Schisandra with Tac increased the blood concentration of Tac from 183% -227%, improved liver function as evidenced by lower LFTs (p<0.01) and decreased Tac side effects of diarrhea and agitation.

Jiang W, et al. Int J Clin Pharmacol Ther. 2010;48(3):224-9.

Schisandra as a Happiness herb

- Schisandra transforms a worrier into a warrior
- Schisandra helps people increase their perception and awareness, clarity of perspective and to develop mindfulness

Schisandra: dosing

- Standardized extract to 20mg lignan (equivalent to 1.5g crude schisandra); 500mg – 2g daily
- 3 -5 dried berries daily
- Schisandra induces cytochrome P450 2C9 and may increase the metabolism of drugs that primarily utilize this enzyme.
  - Of note: celecoxib, Ibuprofen, tamoxifen, warfarin

Melissa officinalis

- Lemon balm
- Labiatae
- Native to Europe
- **Part used**: Herba
- **Constituents:** Volatile oil (0.02%-0.3%): monoterpenes (>60%) sesquiterpenes (>35%) with over 70 components identified Flavonoids; Polyphenolic compounds; Triterpenic acids; Rosmarinic acid; Chlorogenic and caffeic acids

Melissa: medicinal actions

- Melissa has been in use throughout European history.
- It was used as a herb for longevity, memory, fertility, rheumatism, as a sedative and spasmolytic, and to create happiness.
- Hyperthyroidism: Melissa interferes with the binding of TSH to thyroid cell membrane receptors. Melissa also inhibits iodothyronine deiodinase and thus prevents the incorporation of iodine into thyroxine synthesis.
  - Additionally, Melissa blocks the auto-antibodies produced in Grave's disease from binding to the thyroid. Melissa is often the leading herb in formulas for Grave's disease.
  - The sedative effects of Melissa may be due in part to the anti-thyroid effects
- Reduces oxidative stress in the face of radiation exposure

Zeraatpishe A, Toxicol Ind Health. 2011;27(3):205-12

Melissa: medicinal actions

- Potent antioxidant properties
- Affinity for binding to cholinergic (nicotinic and muscarinic) receptors in human brain cortex tissue is present in some extracts thereby improving cognition
- Sedative
- Melissa may be contraindicated in hypothyroidism as it interferes with TSH binding and inhibits iodothyronine deiodinase thus preventing the incorporation of iodine into thyroxine synthesis

Mantle D. et al. J Ethnopharmacol. 2000;72(1-2):47-51
Wake G, et al. J Ethnopharmacol. 2000;69(2):105-14
Zeraatpishe A, Toxicol Ind Health. 2011;27(3):205-12

Melissa: medicinal actions

- As a sedative, Melissa is most indicated in a someone with symptoms typical of hyperthyroidism: anxiety, restlessness, palpitations, headache, and excitability.
- In addition, Melissa is a mild anti-depressant. The volatile oils act on the limbic system in such a way as to cause a lifting of depression and anxiety.
- Melissa is well indicated in stress-induced migraine headaches, palpitations, and insomnia.
- The carminative effects of Melissa combined with its sedative and anti-depressant actions make Melissa particularly useful in intestinal colic secondary to or associated with anxiety, stress or depression.
- Over all, Melissa is trophorestorative to the nervous system.

Lemon Balm: Pediatric Insomnia

- Open, multicenter 4 week study of 918 children under the age of 12 (average age = 8.3y) with restlessness and impaired sleep (sleep latency, night terrors, etc.)
- Investigators and parents rated core symptoms on scale from moderate/severe to mild or absent.
- Intervention was 4 tablets daily of an 4-5:1 extract from the dried roots of Valerian (160mg) and 4-6:1 extract of dried Melissa leaves (80mg)
- 80.9% of patients experienced an improvement in sleep
- 70.4% of patients experienced improvement of restlessness
- Overall toleration was very good without any adverse events reports.

  Muller S and S Klement. Phytomedicine. 2006;13(6):383-7

Melissa: adaptogen

- DBPCR cross-over trial of 18 healthy adults.
- Doses: standardized M. officinalis extract 300mg, 600mg and placebo separated by 7 day washout.
  - Extract of dried leaves extracted up to exhaustion in a 30:70 methanol:water mixture, evaporated and homogenized to a soft extract
- Modulation of mood was assessed pre-dose and 1 hour post-dose with completion of the 20 minute Defined Intensity Simulation (DISS) battery of concurrent cognitive and psychomotor tasks.
- The 600mg dose of Melissa ameliorated the negative mood effects of the DISS, with increased self-reports of calmness (p=0.02) and alertness (p=0.006). In additional, cognitive processing speed increased as measured by task performance.

  Kennedy D, et al. Psychosomatic Med. 2004;66(4):607-613

Melissa: agitation in dementia

- 4 week DBPCRT of 72 people with severe dementia and significant agitation.
- Randomized to aromatherapy with Melissa essential oil or placebo (sunflower oil) as an applied oil in a base lotion applied to face and arms twice daily by caregiving staff
- Changes in clinically significant agitation (Cohen-Mansfield Agitation Inventory [CMAI])
  - 60% of tx group vs. 14% of placebo group achieved 30% reduction of CMAI score with an overall improvement in agitation of 35% in Tx group vs. 11% in placebo group.
- Quality of life indices (percentage of time spent socially withdrawn and percentage of time engaged in constructive activities, measured with Dementia Care Mapping) improved significantly in the melissa group (p<0.0001)

  Ballard C, et al. J Clin Psychiatry. 2002;63(7):553-8

Melissa as a happiness herb

- Melissa brings joy to the heart
- Creates a sense of relaxed, calm alertness

Melissa: dosing

- 2-4 gm herba daily (powdered capsules)
- 2-3 tsp. dried herba or 4-6 fresh leaves covered with just boiled water; drink 1 cup of this tea BID – prn
- 2-6 ml TID of 1:5 tincture
- Topically: poultice, compress

Happiness herbs

- Holy Basil: mentally CLARIFYING
- Lavender: establishes safe SERENITY
- St John's Wort: Lets in light and HOPE
- Chamomile: gently restores PEACEFULNESS
- Schisandra: Creates the DRIVE to be happy and mindful
- Lemon balm: brings JOY to the heart

Reinforce Happy Brain Chemistry

- Actively respect your patient (lays the framework)
- Express gratitude to and for your patient – specific and authentic
- Ask patient to express gratitude for 1-3 things that they have experienced today.
- With any improvement in health status, reinforce with the patient the things that they did to achieve the greater health. Praise the patient!
- Smile!!
- Introduce levity in your appointments
  - Self-depreciating humor
  - Gentle and kindly teasing
- Touch your patients (professionally, of course!)
- Bring random acts of kindness into your daily practice

5. Taking in the Good

- Create a positive mood by pairing a feeling with an experience, examples:
  - **Gratitude** when gazing at the mountain view
  - **Contendedness** with a cat purring in your lap
  - **Safety** in the quiet splendor of your backyard garden
  - **Pleasure** at the taste of home-prepared dinner
  - **Love** while holding a partner's hand, or when gazing in the mirror
  - **Enjoyment** with discovering new solutions to challenges at work
- Savor the positive experience for 10-30 seconds to better develop the neural networking
- We can encourage this during each patient encounter – solicit the virtue in association with an attribute of physical wellness from the patient and then take 10 seconds to savor it.
  - "I haven't had a headache in 2 weeks." "How does that feel?" "Great, so freeing." "Let's appreciate your pain-free head for a few moments and really savor how free you feel.

6. Create goals

- "We are not pushed by the past so much as we are pulled by the future."
  - – Martin Seligman, founder of Positive Psychology
- Goals are future-oriented benchmarks that help us to organize our behavior.
- Goals are:
  - short-term achievable landmarks and
  - visions (tapestry of longer term goals)
  - measurable and achievable
  - reinforcements of optimism, engagement and agency (empowerment)

Realistic goals

- Goals should be based upon your and the patient's realistic expectations
  - Temper overly-optimistic goals, i.e. false hopes
    - Ex. 50 year old man with metastatic lung cancer
      - "I want cure my metastatic cancer with natural means."
        - Maybe, but what if the therapies don't work? How long will this take? When can we say, I've done everything I can.
      - "I want to have enough energy to walk my son to school every day."
        - Focuses efforts on a meaningful life experience – for the sake of what!
        - Requires active and effective anti-cancer therapies
        - Positions the patient for success in the daily achievement of this goal – every day builds upon his success.
  - Make sure that you and the patient have the resources needed enjoy success

7. Setting the agenda

- Pitfall of 'Physicians who Listen' is letting the patient dictate the agenda of each encounter
  - Limits the emphasis and scope of the visit to the patient's agenda which is influenced by:
    - Recent and long-standing problems
    - Limited self-knowledge
    - Reinforced incapacity
    - Complaints and lacks
  - And, yes, listen to your patient: good doctoring rests upon your ability to know how your patient is faring.
- While the patient informs the visit, the doctor directs the experience on behalf, and for the good, of the patient.

Agenda setting strategies

- "I am so tired of feeling sick and tired."
  - Remind the patient of progress made
    - "When you first came to see me, you couldn't go to work without 4 cups of coffee. Now you only drink one cup."
  - Point out what is working right
    - "I know you are still feeling tired, but I am so impressed with your improved sleep quality."
  - Reframe complaints
    - "Some of your fatigue is now the result of the energy that you are expending on healing."
  - Set appropriate expectations
    - "With today's recommendations, one month from now, I expect you to have 50% more energy that is sustained throughout the day."
  - Go back to established goals
    - "You have walked your son to school every day since we started working together and that was your top priority."

8. Walk our Talk

- Positive doctoring is good for the patients and good for the doctor. Just as we encourage our patients to:
  - Evaluate their strengths
  - Set goals and maintain perspective
  - Promote hope and positivity
  - Increase joy
- So should we for ourselves.
- And, establish a pre-visit ritual that helps you to gain presence, joy and compassion

Happy Patients, Happy Practice

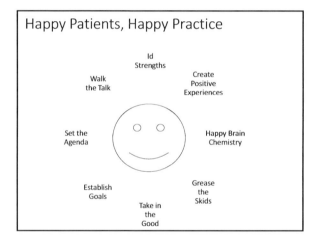

The brain is wider than the sky.
- Emily Dickinson

82

Herbs & Resetting the 24 Hour Circadian Cycle

Dr. Mary Bove
SW Herbal Conference 2017

Human Circadian Cycle

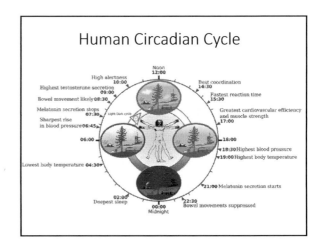

Human Biological Rhythms

Some biological rhythms in humans

Wake-sleep cycle
The rhythm of wakefulness and sleep is tied to the daily 24-hour period of the Earth's rotation.

Body heat
The heat of the body varies throughout the day. However, body temperature falls to its lowest point during the very early morning hours.

Oxygen intake
Regulated by a control center in the brain, oxygen intake increases during the body's normal peak hours of activity, even in the absence of activity.

Heartbeat rate
The heartbeat rate, about 70 beats per minute, dips somewhat between the evening and early morning hours.

Adrenal-gland output
The secretion of cortisone and other adrenal hormones involved in metabolism is low during sleeping hours but increases before waking to ready the body for normal activity.

Kidney excretion
Sodium, potassium, and other metabolic wastes are usually removed from the blood by the kidneys during the afternoon hours.

Blood-cell count
White blood cells called eosinophils are most numerous during the early morning hours when most other rhythms are at their lowest levels. Thus the eosinophil rhythm is out of phase with the body's typical activity rhythms.

Reproduction
The reproductive cycle is not a daily rhythm. Eggs are released from the ovaries of the female about once every 28 days, in phase with the lunar cycle.

© 2010 Encyclopædia Britannica, Inc.

CIRCADIAN RHYTHMS Effect all Organs and Systems

https://www.non-24pro.com/physiology-of-non-24.php

Circadian Sleep/Wake Brain

Circadian nocturnal sleep-daytime wakefulness:
• changes in peripheral cytokines
• immune function
• endocrine influences

The interaction between the circadian sleeping/waking brain and the cytokine-immune-endocrine system are integral to preserving homeostasis.

Circadian Sleep Rhythm

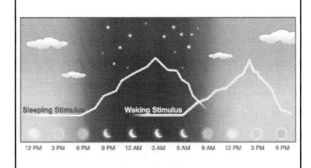

Restoration Happens at Night

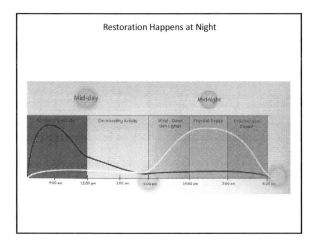

Pineal Secretes Melatonin

The pineal gland is activated in the dark, and actively produces melatonin (N-acetyl-5-methoxytryptamine) and its precursor, serotonin (5-hydroxytryptamine)

Tryptophan is required for the body to manufacture melatonin.
Found in Fenugreek, Spearmint, Fennel Seeds

Meditation can also increase melatonin.

Med Sci Monit. 2004 Mar;10(3):CR96-101. Epub 2004 Mar 1. The effects of long meditation on plasma melatonin and blood serotonin. Solberg EE(1)
http://www.ncbi.nlm.nih.gov/pubmed/14976457
http://www.sandhillsneurologists.com/2015/04/melatonin-and-sleep/

Glucose Dysregulation

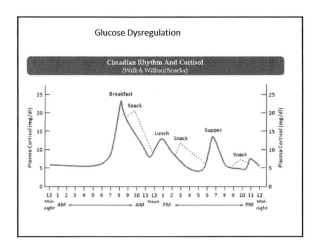

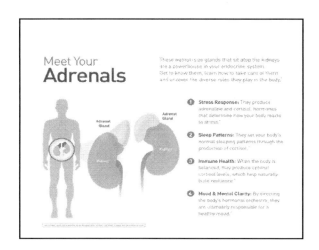

Adrenal Dysregulation

Common Terms:
- Adrenal Fatigue
- Adrenal Exhaustion
- Adrenal Maladaptation
- Adrenal Dysregulation

ICD-10: Hypoadrenia

Role of Cortisol

- Cortisol has two modes of operation:
  - Proactive mode - It promotes coordination of circadian events, such as the sleep/wake cycle and food intake and is involved in processes underlying selective attention, integration of sensory information, and response selection.
  - Reactive mode - It facilitates our ability to cope with, adapt to, and recover from stress; cortisol promotes learning and memory processes.

Lopen-Duran NL, et al. Hypothalamic pituitary adrenal axis functioning in reactive and proactive aggression in children. *J Abnorm Child Psychol.* 2009; 37: 169-182.
Koolhaas JM, et al. Coping styles in animals: current status in behavior and stress physiology. *Neurosci Biobehav Rev.* 1999; 23: 925-35.

Role of Cortisol: Stress Adaptation

- When cortisol levels are chronically too low or too high, hippocampal transmission is impaired and therefore hippocampal outflow is reduced.
- This results in a myriad of symptoms related to energy, mood, memory and food cravings.
- It is at this point that cortisol ceases to be beneficial and begins instead to enhance vulnerability to damage.

Oei NY, Everaerd WT, Elzinga BM, van Well S, Bermond B. Physhosocial stress impairs working memory at high loads: an association with cortisol levels and memory retrieval. Stress. 2006 Sep;9(3):133-41.
Rimmele U, Meier F, Lange T, Born J. Suppressing the morning rise in cortisol impairs free recall. Lern. Mem. 2010. 17:186-190.

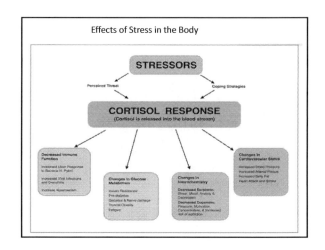

Effects of Stress in the Body

Adrenal Immune Connection

- HPA axis has direct effect on immune system health and function

- Disruption of the adrenal axis (HPA) and cytokine relationships lead to a predisposition and aggravation of allergies and autoimmune disorders.*

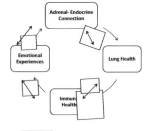

* These statements have not been evaluated by the Food and Drug Administration. This product is not intended to diagnose, treat, cure or prevent any disease.

Adrenal Compromise
Immune Signs

- Increase in allergies
- Increase in respiratory infection eg chronic sinusitis
- Link to immune dysregulation diseases
- Gum inflammation
- Changes in microbiome health*

Common Symptoms

- Stress
- Anxiety
- Irritability
- Mental fog
- Fatigue
- Hyperactivity
- Suppressed immune system
- Depression
- Insomnia

- Difficulty getting up in the morning
- Decreased stamina
- Sugar or salt cravings
- Headaches
- Low energy around 3-4pm, but after dinner energy increases. Winding down for bedtime is difficult

Phases of Adrenal Gland Fatigue

Healthy Adrenal Response (Cortisol levels within range with desired rhythm)	Phase 0
Acute Fight or Flight (Increased HPA tone)	Phase 1
HPA Axis Dysfunction (Zig Zag patterns)	
Early Adrenal Fatigue (Elevated/high range AM with HPA blunting thereafter)	
Evolving Adrenal Fatigue (Suboptimal or low AM cortisol with HPA blunting thereafter)	Phase 2
Established Adrenal Fatigue/Hypoadrenia (Hypofunctioning HPA axis)	Phase 3

Adrenal Exhaustion

- HPA activity falters
- Cortisol level falls
- DHEA level falls
- Worsening organism response and ultimately death

HPA Axis

DIURNAL CURVE

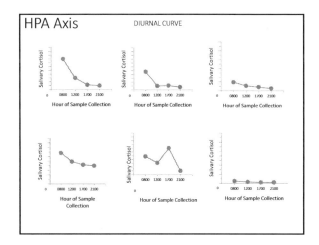

Cortisol Circadian Cycle

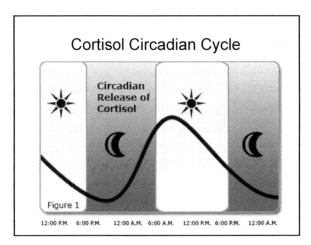

Figure 1

12:00 P.M.   6:00 P.M.   12:00 A.M.   6:00 A.M.   12:00 P.M.   6:00 P.M.   12:00 A.M.

Normal 24 hour Circadian Cortisol Cycle

Cortisol is released in a circadian rhythm pattern. This means that the levels of cortisol change based on the time of day

Cortisol levels are highest in the morning, decline sharply by noon, flatten out in the afternoon, and slightly decline before bed

This type of pattern suggests a properly functioning Hypothalamic-Pituitary-Adrenal (HPA) Axis

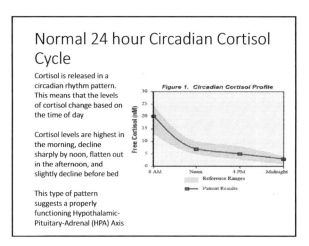

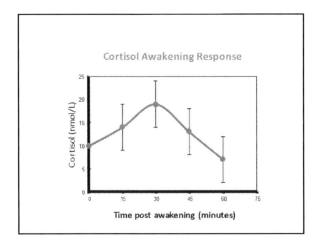

Cortisol Awakening Response

Restoring the Adrenal 24 Hour Cycle

- Regulating Adrenal and HPA axis communication
- Homeostasis of cortisol patterns & influences
- Glycemic Regulation and Stability
- Healthy Sleep Wake Cycle
- Application of Specific Adaptogen agents in the 24 hour cycle
  - Morning
  - Night
  - Daytime

Adaptogens
What are they?

Coined in 1947 by the Soviet Union's Ministry of Health, to define a narrow class of botanical medicines and must fulfill 3 categories:

1. It must be non-toxic to the body's physiological functions;
2. It must increase the body's resistance to adverse influences, not by a specific action but by a wide range of physical, chemical, and biochemical factors;
3. It must have an overall normalizing effect, improving all kinds of conditions and aggravating none.

A pharmacotherapeutic group defined as:

"Herbal preparations that increased attention and endurance in fatigue, and reduced stress-induced impairments and disorders related to the neuro-endocrine and immune systems."

Sources: 1. Nikolai Vasilyevich Lazarev;
2. Panossian, A.; Wikman, G. Evidence-based efficacy of adaptogens in fatigue, and molecular mechanisms related to their stress-protective activity. Current Clin.Pharmacol. 2009, 4, 198–219

Not All Adaptogens are Created Equal

While all adaptogens share some basic characteristics, adaptogens work on the body in different ways. Gaia is using different adaptogenic actions in each HPA Axis formula to reach specific results.

Physically & emotionally supporting: Such as Rhodiola, Holy Basil & Schisandra. Support your body's ability to naturally protect against daily stressors, supporting your daily circadian rhythm.*

Regulating, calming & restoring: Such as Magnolia Bark, Ashwganda, Mimosa Bark & Cordyceps. Work on the body to balance adrenal function, restoring the body's nighttime circadian rhythm.

Physically & emotionally motivating: Such as Eleuthero, Korean Ginseng, Rhaponticum & Licorice Root. While not stimulating like caffeine, they awaken the body and set in motion internal activity that can help people power through their day.*

Phases of Adrenal Gland Fatigue	
Healthy Adrenal Response (Cortisol levels within range with desired rhythm)	Phase 0
Acute Fight or Flight (Increased HPA tone)	Phase 1
HPA Axis Dysfunction (Zig Zag patterns)	
Early Adrenal Fatigue (Elevated/high range AM with HPA blunting thereafter)	
Evolving Adrenal Fatigue (Suboptimal or low AM cortisol with HPA blunting thereafter)	Phase 2
Established Adrenal Fatigue/Hypoadrenia (Hypofunctioning HPA axis)	Phase 3

HPA Axis Daytime Maintenance

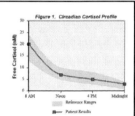

Chronic Acute Stress Mode

- 42 yr old man, with a family and a busy work schedule with lots of stress and responsibility. He often feels uptight and experiences a racing heart much like he drank too much coffee.

- He has trouble falling to sleep, sometimes it takes hours, he sleeps 4-5 hours/night, wakes with a start and a sense of dread sometimes. He has headaches more than ever and tends to be anxious and worrisome as of late. He finds himself more irritable at home and with the kids. No sexual energy.

Phase 1
Adaptogens &Supportive Botanicals

nse
- Ashwagandha
- Rhodiola
- Maca
- Schisandra Berry
- Holy Basil

Nervines
Lemon Balm
Blue Vervain
Skullcap
Chamomile Flowers
Avena

Rhodiola rosea: Actions in the Brain

Brain Stem:
Reticular Activating System

Cognitive Stimulation:

Improves: Norepinephrine & 5-HT (Serotonin)

Cerebral Cortex
Improves: Cognitive Functions

Prefrontal & Frontal Cortex
Improves: Attention Memory Learning

Emotional Calming:

Improves: Norepinephrine 5-HT (Serotonin) Dopamine Acetylcholine

Limbic System Pathways
(Regulates Emotional Tone & Mood)

Hippocampus
Emotion Memory Vigilance

Amygdala
Emotion Memory

Hypothalamus
decreases: CRF

Pituitary
decreases: corticotrophin

Forebrain Reward System
Pleasure, Satiety Energy & Drive

Adrenal Gland
decreases: Release of Cortisol, Norepinephrine, and Epinephrine

Brain & Heart

HPA Imbalance

Super Mom

- 36 year old with 2 young children under the age of 6, just weaned youngest child.
- Works full time as manager in large company, describes her job as high stress and her life very busy.
- Sleep is disrupted due to kids, often feels tired upon waking and gets anxious easily which can lead to heart palpations.
- Not able to put on a little needed weight, vegetarian, and finds herself to startle easy and worry more.

Chronic Acute Stress Mode

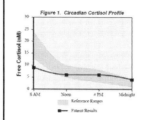

Figure 1. Circadian Cortisol Profile

- Allostatic Load is Heavy
- More than the NeuroEndocrine Stress Response can handle in a healthy way.
- System is over taxed
- Stress maladaptation response
- Breakdown of Healthy & Wellness

Night Owl

- Never seems to get enough sleep, wakes up tired but able to get up and going.
- Always has a low time midafternoon looking for a sweet or caffeine to boost their energy.
- Notes that they feel tired soon after they evening meal or may even fall asleep for a short time while putting the kids to bed.
- After that she gets a second wind and may stay up to 1-2am doing things as the house is quiet and this is "her time."
- Struggles with weight issues even though she exercises regularly.

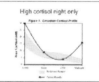

Phase 2
Adaptogens & Supportive Botanicals

Adaptogens
- Ashwagandha
- Rhodiola
- Holy Basil
- Schisandra Berry
- Cordyceps
- Elethrococcus

Nervines
- Passionflower
- Valerian
- St John'swort
- Magnolia
- Mimosa Flowers

Night Cycle Adaptogen Formula

Cordyceps

Scientific names: *Cordyceps sinensis & militaris*

Aka Caterpillar mushroom

In nature, this parasitic fungus grows on the caterpillar larvae of a moth.

Grows in the highlands (10,000 feet) of China, Tibet and Nepal

Recently, cultivated varieties (*Cordyceps militaris*) have been developed. These Cordyceps fruiting bodies are cultivated on nutritious barley substrate, and they are therefore vegan. Research has shown that *C. militaris* and *C. sinensis* provide similar support, and they are used interchangeably in TCM and other branches of herbalism.* Our Cordyceps (*C. militaris*) are processed by hot water extraction into a fine powder.

Cordyceps

Bioactive compounds:

Cordycepic acid (aka D-mannitol)

Many polysaccharides demonstrating lipid-lowering ability, blood sugar-lowering effect, immunostimulating and radioprotective activity

18 amino acids, many micronutrients

Saponin compounds researched for their tumor-inhibiting effects

---

Cordyceps

Action:

Anti-inflammatory, antioxidant, anti-tumor, adaptogen, immunomodulatory, endocrine modulator, hypolipidemic, tonic

Promotes restoration and regeneration

Sourcing:
We use only fruiting bodies not substrate.

Cordyceps in nature

Cordyceps

- Decreases fatigue and increases physical endurance, vigor, and energy
- Enhances athletic performance and training
- Builds vitality when recovering from stress
- Oxygen free-radical scavenger
- Regulates testosterone and cortisol

  - Supports liver function and acts to protect the liver from stressors, aids regeneration
  - Immune regulating, building, and supporting to normal cell growth and development

Safety: Research on this mushroom shows complete safety when consumed in recommended doses

---

Magnolia

Magnolia officinalis
Bark

Anxiety and Adrenals

- Magnolia (Magnolia officinalis),
- Overweight premenopausal women
- A decrease in transitory anxiety, although salivary cortisol levels were not significantly reduced.
- Magnolia has been demonstrated to improve mood, increase relaxation, induce a restful sleep and enhance stress reduction.

Nutrition Journal 2008;7:11:1-6.
J Pharm Pharmacol 1998;50:819-826.

Magnolia Binds to Several Important Targets Associated With Drowsiness:

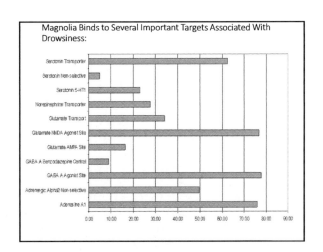

Magnolia References

- Cortisol and Mood
  http://www.ncbi.nlm.nih.gov/pubmed/23924268
- Anti-inflammatory Suppresses NF-kB
  http://www.ncbi.nlm.nih.gov/pubmed/24893579

- Honokiol, a Multifunctional Antiangiogenic and Antitumor Agent
  http://www.ncbi.nlm.nih.gov/pmc/articles/PMC2842137/

- Enhanced GABAergic Neurotransmission in Hippocampal Neurons
  http://www.ncbi.nlm.nih.gov/pmc/articles/PMC3652012/

Magnolia

Dose: 160 mg to 500 mg depending on weight/condition of patient

- Refers to total neolignans (usually magnolol plus honokiol), which are usually at 1-10% of a basic bark extract
- Centuries of Traditional Use

Caution : Safety data is not substantial. Avoid in pregnancy due to possible oxitocic effects

Mimosa
Albizia julibrissin

Scientific name: Tree of Happiness

"Calms the spirit"

"Relieves constrained emotions"

Parts used: Bark and flower

Has an acrid taste

Actions: Anxiolytic,
anti-microbial, anti-oxidant, anti-inflammatory, anti-asthma, nervine, hepatoprotective and lipid-lowering

Mimosa Tree

Bioactive Compounds:

- High in saponins in many forms: triterpenes, monoterpenes, flavone saponins, alkaloids and flavonoids
- Flowers high in Quercetin and Isoquercetin

Mimosa Bark

Nervine with immune-regulating and cancer-inhibiting effects.

5-HT receptor binding – depression, anxiety, irritability

Neurotransmitter mechanisms via GABA, dopamine and serotonin

Supports:
- Person with low blood pressure, low mood, low thyroid, anxiety and poor energy
- Parasympathetic-dominant person
- Low thyroid function with female hormonal aggravation and low mood
- Linking endocrine system to the nervous system via the pituitary gland
- Decreases sleep latency
- Poor memory, mind chatter

Who Might That Be

- Adrenal Exhaustion, Fatigue, Maladaptation
- At this point the adrenal system is failing, they may have dizziness with bending over or getting up to fast, may have anxiety or panic attacks for no specific reason, sleep disruption often waking a number of times in the night with the best sleep coming in the morning hours, difficult waking in the morning, Deals with anxiety, fatigue, brain fog, depression and forgetfulness. Chronic pain and discomfort get in the way of activities and exercise.

Wired and Tired

- This person wakes in a fog, takes a long time to wake up "has to have their caffeine fix", feels draggy most of the day, finding hard to focus and concentrate until later in the day.
- They get more energized as the day goes and finds the evening a high energy time.
- They have difficulty winding down from the day and though they may feel tired at 11pm they don't fall asleep until 1am most nights.
- Has a very active mind that goes into overdrive once in bed

---

Who Might That Be

Adrenal Burnout

This person has had life challenging situations for several years. Examples of this could be graduate student, very stressful job, several pregnancies with breastfeeding periods close together, PTSD, chronic fatigue issues, super athlete for several years coupled with acute injury to body over that time and a very busy life

---

Phase 3
Adaptogens & Supportive Botanicals

- Licorice
- Rhaponticum
- Cordyseps
- Ashwagandha
- Rhodiola
- Holy Basil
- Korean Ginseng

Nervines
- Lavender flowers
- Mimosa
- Blue Vervain
- Magnolia Bark
- Tonic Nervines
    Scutelleria, Avena, etc

Day Cycle Reinforcing Adaptogen Formula

Support the cortisol cycle

- Licorice Root – helps decrease the breakdown of cortisol thereby effectively increasing cortisol levels. If your cortisol levels are very low then you may benefit from licorice root supplementation at the appropriate times of the day
- Adaptogens to support anabolic metabolism

Rhaponticum

Rhaponticum carthamoides

Common name: Leuzea or Maral Root, derived from the fact that the Maral deer fed on this plant.

Root

Herbaceous plant native to the sub-alpine and alpine meadows of Siberia.

Traditionally used as an energizing or tonic remedy after long Siberian winters

This plant was often combined with *Rhodiola rosea* in traditional Siberian folk medicine and is still used by modern Russian athletes.

Rhaponticum

Active Constituents:

Levseins (over 10 different ecdysterones), which increase activity of the cellular compartments where protein synthesis takes place, thus enhancing muscle protein synthesis

25 years of research and clinical study has gained this plant entry to the *Official Russian Pharmacopoeia.*

Recommended for: increasing work efficiency, athletic performance and recovery after muscular workloads. Stimulates muscle growth by increasing protein synthesis in the muscle.

The Real Deal: A synthetic version was manufactured in Russia and the US, but the Rhaponticum extract proved superior to both synthetic versions.

Rhaponticum

How does Rhaponticum affect the physiology?

- Promotes anabolic metabolism, preserves mitochondria
- Increases working capacity of skeletal muscle and their content of glycogen for fuel and increases ATP
- Increases glycogen to the brain, liver and muscles; has mental and physical anti-fatigue effects
  - Increases oxidative enzyme systems, decreases lipid peroxidation acting as a free-radical scavenger
  - Enhances protein synthesis in muscle tissue, builds lean muscle mass
  - Increases muscle recovery, supports structural integrity of muscle
  - Decreases fat deposition
  - Restoration of lowered IgG, IgA and C3 concentrations, improving humoral immunity

---

Reishi

Active constituents:
- Polysaccharides
- Immunomodulating proteins
- Steroidal saponin glycosides

Influences:
- Adrenal-hypothalamic-pituitary axis
- Regulates inflammation
- Circadian rhythm
- Sleep cycles
- Reduces stress

Botanical Nervines

- CNS relaxant (mild)
  - Anti-epileptic
  - Analgesic
  - Anxiolytic
- Hypnotic (mild)
- Sleep architecture improver
- Anti-spasmodic
- Balance autonomic nervous system
- Influence neurotransmitter production
- Not sedating
- Anti-addiction (maybe)

Botanical Nervine Summary

- Lemon Balm
  - Attention, focus, cognitive function, memory
  - Insomnia, restlessness, hyperactivity
  - Mood elevation, anxiety
- Passion Flower
  - Insomnia
  - Generalized anxiety
  - Hyperactivity, nervousness
- American Skullcap
  - Nervous irritation, fear, anxiety
  - Depression
  - Substance withdrawal
- Chamomile Flowers
  - Agitation, worry, nervousness, anxiety
  - Insomnia, restlessness
  - Mood elevation

Herbal Protocol for 24 Hour Support

	Recover & Rebalance	Daily Support	Sleep Support
Possible Botanicals of Relevance	Asian Ginseng, Cordyceps, Eleuthero, Licorice, Prickly Ash, Rhaponticum, Rhodiola, Schisandra	Ashwagandha, Holy Basil, Oats, Rhodiola, Schisandra	Ashwagandha, Cordyceps, Lemon Balm, Magnolia, Mimosa, Reishi, Vervain
Mechanism Intention	Deep support of the HPA Axis, for those in state of adrenal fatigue/exhaustion.	Adatogens to help the HPA Axis deal with and adapt to everyday stressors; Foundational and supports adrenal function;	Restores HPA Axis function at night promoting a healthy sleep cycle, repair, growth and restoration
Dosage/ Usage	Short term use, 8-12 weeks until HPA Axis achieves a state of homeostasis. Then move to a daily support formula.	Daily dose, in the morning or before noon intended for long-term use	Daily dose, in the evening after dinner. Take in conjunction with a daytime formula.

Herbs to Balance Sleep & Circadian Rhythms

Ashwagandha
Reishi
Cordyceps
Mimosa
Magnolia
Vervain
Lemon Balm
Cinnamon

Passionflower
Kava Kava
American Skullcap
Valerian
California Poppy
Hops
Gotu Kola
Jujube date

By Rolf Engstrand – Own work, CC BY-SA 3.0,
https://commons.wikimedia.org

Adrenal Nutritional Treatment Guidelines

Phase 0	• Multivitamin/Multi-mineral • Omega 3 EFAs • Consider vitamin D, iodine and probiotics
Phase 1	• Phosphorylated serine • Melatonin if cortisol levels elevated at night. • Vitamins B5, C, B6, E • Lifestyle modification: deep breathing, stress management, exercise, optimal diet, etc.
Phase 2	• Vitamins B5, C, B6, E • Adrenal glandular and/or herbal adaptogens in morning and at noon. • Lifestyle modification: deep breathing, stress management, exercise, optimal diet, etc.
Phase 3	• Vitamins B5, C, B6, E • Adrenal glandular and/or herbal adaptogens in morning and at noon. • Cortef or hydrocortisone supplementation at physiological dosages. • Lifestyle modification: deep breathing, stress management, exercise, optimal diet, etc.

Childhood Constipation: How Herbs Can Help

Dr. Mary Bove
IWH January 2017

Disclosure

- Director of Medical Education
- Member, Scientific Advisory Board
- Sponsored today by Gaia Herbs

Childhood Constipation

- Fewer than 2 bowel movements a week
- Or hard, dry, and small bowel movements that are painful or difficult to pass

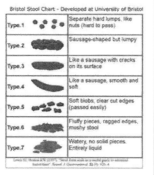

Constipation in Kids

Normal bowel habits
- Up to 1 year old: 2.2/day
- 1–4 years old: 1.4/day

Constipation
- More common in boys girls over age 3
- Up to 25% of school-age children
- 95% of cases functional
- 5% are gluten enteropathy, cystic fibrosis, lead toxicity

Parents Worry

Child's stools are:
- too large
- too hard
- not frequent enough
- painful to pass

Constipation in Kids

- Dietary factors: food sensitivity
  - Fibers
  - Fluids
- Gut ecosystem health and development
- Gut-brain connection: enteric nervous system
- Emotional connections
  - Control, shame, fear, anger triggers
- Pain/discomfort connection

Contributing Factors

- Ignoring urge
- Painful bowel movement
- Toilet training issues
- Changes in diet
- Changes in routine
- Cow dairy intolerance
- Family history
- Medication
- Medical conditions

Functional Constipation (FC)

- History
  - Differentials Hirschsprung Dx: constipation issues since birth, chronic within the first 4-5 months of life, 50% don't pass meconium at birth
  - Onset, duration, pain, bleeding
  - Fecal incontinence
  - Withholding of stool

Withholding Behaviors

Often associated with avoidance of pain with stool:

- Squatting
- Crossing ankles
- Stiffening the body
- Holding on to furniture or person
- Flushing, sweating, and crying
- Hiding during defecation

Common Onset Timing

- **Infants**: at time of dietary transition

- **Toddlers**: at time of toilet training or after illness with severe diaper dermatitis or dehydration

- **Older children**: when entering school, due to avoidance using bathroom at school

Complications for Constipation

- Anal fissures (extremely painful)
- Rectal prolapse
- Stool withholding
- Stool avoidance, impaction

Early Life Experiences & the Gut

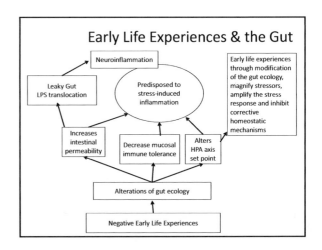

Brain-Gut Interactions

- Disturbances at every level of neural control of the GI tract can affect modulation of GI motility, secretion, and immune functions.
- Also perception and emotional response to visceral events.
- Stress and emotions may trigger neuroimmune and neuroendocrine reactions via the brain-gut axis.

"Intestinal reactivity to words with emotional content ..."

- Study compared healthy controls with nonpsychiatric irritable bowel syndrome patients and IBS patients with comorbid phobic anxiety disorders with respect to rectal wall reactivity during exposure to everyday words with emotional content.
- Outcomes showed that 70.3% of the subjects responded either with increased or decreased rectal tone during exposure to anger words, 75.0% when exposed to sadness words, and 76.6% when exposed to anxiety words.
- We observed significant group differences in the frontal brain to sadness (P < 0.001) and anxiety (P = 0.013) distracter words, and threshold significant group difference to anger (P = 0.053) distracter words.
- Rectal wall reactivity during the word series significantly predicted frontal amplitude to the same word series, indicating a close interaction among mind, brain, and gut.

Blomhoff S, Spetalen S, Jacobsen MB, et al, Dig Dis Sci (2000 Jun) 45(6):1160-5, ISSN: 0163-2116

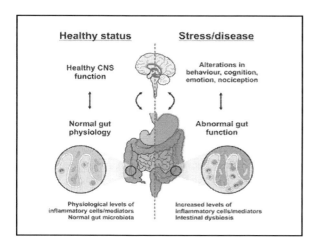

Medications for FC

- Osmotic laxatives produce an osmotic effect in the colon that results in distention and promotes peristalsis:
  - Polyethylene glycol (MiraLAX, Dulcolax Balance)
  - Magnesium hydroxide (Phillips' Milk of Magnesia)
  - Lactulose (Constulose, Generlac)
  - Sorbitol (alcohol of of glucose) colonic flora fermentation
  - Magnesium citrate (Citroma)
  - Sodium acid phosphate (OsmoPrep, Visicol)

Medications for FC

- Lubricants: mineral oil
- Stool Softeners
  - Docusate sodium (Colace)
- Stimulating laxatives
  - Senna AC sennosides (Ex-Lax, Senokot, Little Tummys)
  - Bisacodyl (Dulcolax, Bisco-Lax)

Herbs Can Help

- Microbiota health
- Mucosal health and function
- Nerve function
- Visceral relaxants
- Reduce symptoms of pain, spasm, irritation
- Bowel-stimulating action

Constipation in Kids
General Considerations

The Story of Liam

Constipation in Kids
General Considerations

- Carminative agents
- Botanical nervines
- Bulking agents: seeds, pectin, gums
- Botanical autonomic visceral relaxants
- Anthraquinone herbal laxatives
- Magnesium considerations

Functional Constipation
3-year-old girl

- Constipation episodes for 9 months
- Increase in incidents over last 3 months
- Treated w/ glycerin suppository prn
- 1–2 stools/week, formed, not hard/dry
- Dairy-free diet, breast-fed 1.5yrs
- Fluid intake adequate
- New sister, 6 months old

Constipation in Kids

- 3-year-old Sadie
  - Probiotics: mix strain 20 billion/day
  - Elderberry juice w/ 125 mg magnesium citrate powder
  - Pumpkin, fig, hemp oil puree 2–3 tbsp/day
  - Herbal GI Relaxant Tea
    - Chamomile flowers, Fennel seeds, Lavender flowers, Lemon Balm, Catnip, Cramp Bark, Spearmint, and *Rumex crispus* tincture prn*
    - Steep 1 tsp in 1 cup boiling water for several minutes; dilute with water or dark fruit juice.
      *Anthraquinone compounds

Digestive Analgesics & Antispasmodics

- *Lavandula spp:* Lavender flowers
- *Eschscholzia californica*: California Poppy
- *Piscidia piscipula:* Jamaica Dogwood
- *Valeriana officinalis*: Valerian root
- *Nepeta cataria*: Catnip

Autonomic Visceral Relaxants

- Relaxes tension in the bowel and digestive viscera
- Not stimulating to the bowel
- Restores normal bowel tension
- Can be used more long-term than anthraquinones containing herbs

Catnip
Nepeta cateria

- Nepetalactone
- Catnip essential oil contains mostly nepetalactone, but also citral, geraniol, citronellol, nerol, thymol and limonene
- Traditionally used as carminative, anti-spasmodic, muscle relaxant and mild sedative

Highbush Cranberry (Guelder Rose)
Viburnum opulus

Active compounds:
- Hydroquinones: aurbutin
- Coumarins: scopoletin, scopoline
- Tannins: mainly catechins

Highbush Cranberry

- Scopoletin: coumarin compound, the major constituent responsible for antispasmodic action
- Viopudial: Contributes to antispasmodic action

Scopoletin
(antispasmodic)

Highbush Cranberry

- Proanthocyanidins extracted from *Viburnum opulus* protected gastric mucosa on exposure to ingested ulcerating substances.
- The study suggested that *Viburnum opulus* proanthocyanidins decreased lipid peroxidation, while increasing nitric oxide and antioxidant activity. This resulted in an overall protective effect

Zayachkivska O, Gzhegotsky M, Terletska O, Lutsyk D, Yaschenko A, Dzhura O. Influence of *Viburnum opulus* proanthocyanidins on stress-induced gastrointestinal mucosal damage. *Journal of Physiology and Pharmacology: an Official Journal of the Polish Physiological Society* 2006;57 Suppl 5:155-167.

Jamaican Dogwood
Piscidia piscipula

- Phytochemistry: isoflavones, glycosides, tannins, resins, organic acids, volatile oils and β-sitosterol
- Actions: analgesic, anti-inflammatory, antispasmodic, nervine, sedative
- *Piscidia piscipula* produced a pharmacological effect between the sedative action of *Valeriana* and the anti-anxiety activity of *Passiflora*.

Riv-Neurol 1981 ; 51 : 297-310

Jamaican Dogwood
Dosing

- Use 1-3 times daily
  - Decoction of the dry roots 1-2 grams
  - Tincture: 1:5, use 3-5 ml/dose
  - Fluid extract: 1:1 use 1-2ml/dose
  - Solid extract: 500 mg/dose

Digestive Nervines

- *Avena sativa*: Milky Oats
- *Lavandula spp*: Lavender flowers
- *Melissa officinalis*: Lemon Balm
- *Matricaria chamomila*: Chamomile flowers

Chamomile
Matricaria chamomila

- Asteraceae family
- Part used: Flowers and essential oil

- Active constituents
  - Flavonoids: apigenin, rutin, quercetin
  - Coumarins: umbelliferone
  - Polysaccharides: heteroglycans
  - Sesquiterpene lactones: matricin, matricarin

Chamomile

Clinical studies indicate:

- Chamomile essential oil inhalation: sedative and mood enhancing effect
- Chamomile Infusion: induction of deep sleep
- Chamomile Extract: increased T-lymphocyte rosette formation
- Polysaccharides/heteroglycans: demonstrate immunostimulating activity

Braun, L ."Herbs and Natural Supplements: An evidence-based guide." Elsevier Australia 2007, 215-221

Chamomile

Therapeutic application:

- Insomnia
- Relaxing, calming to restlessness
- Mood-elevating
- Anxiety, worry, agitation, nervousness
- Stress-related dermatitis
- Ulceration of gastrointestinal tract, mucous membranes
- With pectin, diarrhea in children

Chamomile

- Chamomile may have modest anxiolytic activity in patients with mild to moderate GAD

  J Clin Psychopharmacol. 2009 Aug;29(4):378-82. doi: 10.1097/JCP.0b013e3181ac935c. **A randomized, double-blind, placebo-controlled trial of oral *Matricaria recutita* (chamomile) extract therapy for generalized anxiety disorder.** Amsterdam JD[1], et al.

- Chamomile may provide clinically meaningful antidepressant activity that occurs in addition to its previously observed anxiolytic activity.

  Altern Ther Health Med, 2012 Sep-Oct;18(5):44-9. **Chamomile (*Matricaria recutita*) may provide antidepressant activity in anxious, depressed humans: an exploratory study.** Amsterdam JD et al.

Chamomile

- Actions
  - Anti-inflammatory, antioxidant
  - Sedative, anti-spasmodic, relaxant
  - Anti-ulcer, vulnerary

- Dose
  - Dry flower infused 2-8 grams TID
  - Tincture 1:5 3-10 mls TID
  - Essential oil inhalation 5-7 drops/16 oz

- Contraindications and Safety
  - General considered safe
  - Avoid if hypersensitivity to Asteraceae family

Chamomile

- A mouthwash with chamomile showed the good performance in reducing the plaque index

LINS, R. et al. **Clinical evaluation of mouthwash with extracts from aroeira (*Schinus terebinthifolius*) and chamomile (*Matricaria recutita* L.) on plaque and gingivitis.** *Rev. bras. plantas med.* [online]. 2013, vol.15, n.1, pp. 112-120. ISSN 1516-0572. http://dx.doi.org/10.1590/S1516-05722013000100016

Oats
Avena sativa

- Alkaloid: gramine
- Organic acids, flavonoids, triterpenes, saponin
- Inhibits the secretion of proinflammatory cytokines IL-6, chemokines IL-8
- Traditional uses nervous irritation, depression, sleeplessness, nervous exhaustion, nervous weakness

Actions of Aromatic Compounds

- Carminative action
  - Reduces flatulence
  - Relieves colic
  - Supports digestion
- Encourages saliva and digestive enzyme secretion
- Supports peristalsis
- Anti-spasmodic/analgesic

Aromatic Compounds

- Lemon Balm: *Melissa officinalis*
- Lavender flowers: *Lavandula spp.*
- Spearmint: *Mentha spicata*
- Fennel: *Foeniculum vulgare*

Lemon Balm
Melissa officinalis

- Labiatae family
- Medicinal Uses and Indications:
  - Insomnia, restlessness, hyperactivity
  - Anxiety, nervousness, agitation
  - Improves cognitive function
  - Antiviral: herpes, bacteria and fungi
  - Antispasmodic, analgesic

Lemon Balm

Active Constituents

- Phenolic acids: rosmarinic (up to 6%), coumaric, caffeic and chlorogenic acids
- Essential oil (0.02–0.37%) composed of monoterpenes and sesquiterpenes
- Terpenoid components: citral, citronellal, eugenol, geraniol, nerol, linalool, farnesyl acetate, humulene
- Flavonoids, tannins

Braun, L ."Herbs and Natural Supplements: An evidence-based guide." Elsevier Australia 2007, 452-455

Lemon Balm

Dosing
- Capsules: Take 300, 600, 900 mg dried lemon balm TID
- Tea: 1.5–4.5 grams/150 ml water infused TID
- Tincture: 1:5, 3-5 ml TID
- Fluid Extract: 1:1, 2-3 ml TID
- Topical: Apply topical cream to affected area, 3 times daily or as directed

Contraindications and Safety
- Generally well-tolerated
- No known toxicity or drug interaction
- No clinical studies on thyroid-inhibiting effects

Botanical Nervine Summary

- **Lemon Balm**
  - Attention, focus, cognitive function, memory
  - Insomnia, restlessness, hyperactivity
  - Mood elevation, anxiety
- **Lavender**
  - Pain, discomfort
  - Generalized anxiety
  - Hyperactivity, nervousness
- *Avena sativa*
  - Nervous irritation, fear
  - Depression
  - Sleeplessness
- **Chamomile**
  - Agitation, worry, nervousness, anxiety
  - Insomnia, restlessness
  - Mood elevation

Anthraquinone Compounds

- Bitter in taste
- Short-term use; 8-14 hours activation time
- Glycoside: aglycone and sugar
- 1-2 year curing of plant material
- Presence of bile and microbiota for activation and absorption
- Enters bloodstream → targets bowel wall cells → impacts protein and enzyme synthesis → release of PGL → bowel wall irritation → increase bowel muscle contraction and peristaltic movement.

Anthraquinone Herbs

- *Rumex crispus*: Yellow Dock root
  - .25 ml for ages 3-5, .5 ml for ages 5-8, 1 ml ages 10-12
  - 1–2 doses/day; 8–12 hours prior to sitting time
- *Rheum p.*: Rhubarb root
- Aloe vera: as a juice ½–2 tsp/day
- *Rhamnus spp*: Cascara Sagrada, Buckthorn
- *Cassia spp*: Senna
- Caution: short-term use, combine with a carminative such as Fennel

Herbal FC Formula for 8 yr boy
stool holding due to pain avoidance/school bathroom

- Piscidia
- Viburnum
- Spearmint
Equal parts, 2.5 mls BID
- Aloe vera juice 1 oz with fennel tincture 10 drop/d for 2-4 weeks
- Tincture of Rumex c., viburnum opulus & poppy, equal parts 2.5 ml dose, prn evenings
- Exercise, diet, and breath work

Summary Points for FC in Kids

- Time to shift
- Naturopathic Detective Skills
- Consider Botanicals Agents
  - GI Nervines
  - Autonomic Visceral Relaxants
  - Anthroquinones combined with carminatives
  - Avoids over doing bulking agents

Aromatic Compounds

Dr Mary Bove

SW Herbal Conference 2017

Aromatic Agents

- Aromatic plants are rich in volatile oils high in terpene phenols, and esters compounds. Many of these acting as anti- viral/bacterial agents, anti-oxidants, warming mucolytic
- Consider using Aromatic Agents in Cold and Flu Prevention Formula

- Propolis Extract
- Thymus vulgaris
- Garlic – Allium sativa

Traditional Herbal Medicine

- *Synergy*- important concept in herbal medicine.
- Plant compounds which are not active themselves can act to improve the stability, solubility, bioavailability, or half-life of the active constituents.
- A single compound in pure form may have only a fraction of the pharmacological activity of that of the whole plant matrix.
- Whole Plant is more than the sum of the parts
- Whole Plant action
  - Synergy interaction between all chemical compounds

Terpene Compounds

Hydrocarbons & Oxygenated Compounds
- Monoterpenes
  - Highly volatile, irritating in nature, aromatic, colorless
  - Alcohols, hydrocarbons, aldehydes, ketones
  - Camphor, borneol, limonene, menthol, thymol
  - Iridoids – bitter tasting, catnip=nepetalactone
- Sesquiterpenes
  - Largest grp in plants
  - Greater molecular wgt
  - Less volatile
  - Azulenes, bisabolol, farnesene
  - Subgroup – Sesquiterpene lactones - highly active compounds; tumor inhibition, immunostimulating

---

Terpene Compounds

- Diterpenes
  - Resins- crystalline solids
  - Higher plant species and fungi
  - Ginkgolide A, carnosol, forskolin, marrubiin
- Triterpenes
  - Roots, foliage and seeds
  - saponins, sterols
- Tetraterpenoids
  - Carotenoids – carotene, capsanthin, lycopene

Actions of Terpene Compounds

- Carminative action
  - Reduces flatulence
  - Relieves colic
  - Supports Digestion and peristalsis
- Encourages saliva and digestive enzyme secretion
- Expectorant
- Circulatory Stimulant
- Anti-spasmodic/Analgesic
- Antiseptic Properties
  - Anti-bacterial
  - Anti-fungal
  - Anti-viral

Polyphenol Compounds

- Tannins – hydrolysable / condensed
- Flavonoids
- Salicylates- Phenolic acid
- Cinnamic acids – caffeic, curcumin
- Coumarins
- Naphthaquinones and Anthraquinones
  - Overall laxative action
  - Age raw herb 1-2 years
- Hydroquinone – simple phenolic, arbutin glycoside
- Lignans and Lignins

Common Aromatic Benzene Ring "A basic polyphenol structure"

Benzoic Acid   Benzoin

Polyphenol Compounds

- Common aromatic benzene ring
- Water-soluble(majority) or lipophilic
- Occur as glycosides
- Bring color, scent, flavor to plant
- Antioxidant, free-radial scavenger activity
- Anti-inflammatory
- Anti-microbial

Simple Phenolic Compound

- Salicylates – methyl salicylate, salicylic alcohol, salicylic acid →
  - Anti-inflammatory
  - Anti-pyretic
  - Analgesic

Plants high in salicylates;
- Willow/ Salix spp
- Wintergreen/ Gaultheria procumbens
- Meadowsweet/ Filipendula ulmaria

Acetylsalicylsalicylic Acid

Essential Oils

- Specific phytocompounds found in plants
- Aromatic terpene and phenolic compounds
- Concentrated form of a plant constituent which contains many aromatic plant compounds
- Distillation Extraction
- Safety and Caution
  – Internal verses External
  – Purity and EO quality

Aromatic Plants of Interest

- Holy Basil
- Lavender Flowers
- Lemon Balm
- Oil of Oregano
- Rosemary
- Sage
- Spearmint

Sage Tea for Bone Health

- Salvia officinalis
- Dried leaves of sage strongly inhibit bone resorption
- Contains borneol, thymol, and camphor which are directly inhibitory in osteoclast resorption

Bone, 2003 Apr;32(4):372-80

Thyme
Thymus vulgaris L.

- Antibacterial, antioxidant, expectorant, spasmolytic, and topical anti-microbial
- Essential oil – thymol and carvacrol
  - Synergistic effects with thymol & carvacrol
- Rosmarinic acid
- Flavonoids and phenolic glycosides
- Broad spectrum anti-bacterial effect on URI
- Dose 3-5 times daily .5-3 mls dose to age

Rosemary
Rosmarinus officinalis

- Active constituents include:
  - Volatile oils (borneol, camphene, camphor, cineole, limonene, linalool and others)
  - Flavonoids (apigenin, diosmetin, diosmin and others)
  - Rosmarinic acid
- DiterpenesThe volatile oils in rosemary are naturally occurring acetylcholinesterase inhibitors.
- Cineole stimulates the central nervous system
  - This effect has been demonstrated in rodents in their enhanced ability to negotiate a maze.
  - Also cineole has been shown to shorten reaction times as measured by brain wave activity.

Rosmarinus officinalis

- Rosemary for Remembrance

- Essential oils are easily absorbed into the bloodstream through application on the skin, scalp, inhalation and ingestion

- Rosemary also increases circulation, including circulation to the brain.

- Rosemary stabilizes the connective tissue of blood vessels leading to enhanced circulation and blood pressure.

- Rosemary is a lipid-soluable antioxidant and helps to regenerate vitamin E.

Rosmarinic Acid

Romanic Acid Also Shows a Binding Affinity for Graves Auto-antibodies

Grave's antibodies mimic TSH and bind to TSH receptors leading to excessive stimulation of the thyroid.

Melissa has been shown to inhibit the ability of a TSH receptor antibody to promote intracellular cyclic AMP responses

Rosmarinic Acid for Hyperthyroidism

Rosmarinic acid is a phenolic compound derived from caffeic acid

Most common in Lamiaceae and Boraginacea family plants including:

Melissa officianalis (Lemon Balm)

Lycopus virginia (Bugleweed)

All have been traditionally used for hyperthyroid symptoms

Rosmarinic acid

RA in Autoimmune Inflammatory States

Rosmarinic acid appears to reduce:

Autoimmune responses,

Auto antibody production

Autoimmune processes contributing to Graves Dz

Rosmarinic acid appears useful in other immune and autoimmune diseases including:

- Asthma
- Allergies

Spearmint Mentha spicata/verdis

Tolerance, bioavailability, and potential cognitive health implications of a distinct aqueous spearmint extract

- Subjects consumed 900 mg/day spearmint extract for 30 days.
- Tolerability parameters were assessed at baseline and end of treatment visits.
- Computerized cognitive function tests were completed and blood was drawn at pre- and post-dose (0.5 to 4 h) timepoints during baseline and end of treatment visits. Subjective cognition was also assessed at end of treatment.

- *Functional Foods in Health and Disease 2015; 5(5):165-187 Page 165 of 187*

Spearmint and Cognitive Health

- **Conclusions**: The results from this pilot trial suggest that the spearmint extract, which contains higher rosmarinic acid content relative to extracts from typical commercial lines, was well-tolerated at 900 mg/day. In addition, the extract was bioavailable and further investigation is warranted regarding its potential for supporting cognitive health

- Plasma vanillic, caffeic, and ferulic acid sulfates, rosmarinic acid, and methyl rosmarinic acid glucuronide were detected in plasma following acute administration of the spearmint extract.

Spearmint Tea & PCOS
2 cups/day

	Active (* $p < 0.05$)	**Placebo**
TT (pg/ml)	- 0.19*	- 0.07
FT (ng/ml)	- 4.8*	- 0.49
DHEAS (mcg/ml)	-1.2 (NS)	+ 3.8
LH (mIU/ml)	+ 1.98*	- 0.24
FSH (mIU/ml)	+ 0.98*	- 0.08
DQLI	- 6*	- 3

Grant P. *Phyto Res* 2010;24:186-188

Lemon Balm Tea Melissa officinalis

- Carminative and Anti-colic Effects
- Calming Effects for Insomnia & Hyperactivity
- Anti-anxiety and Mood Elevating
- Cognitive Function
- Alzheimer's disease

Lemon Balm

Active Constituents

- Phenolic acids-rosmarinic [up to 6%], coumaric, caffeic and chlorogenic acids
- Essential oil (0.02–0.37%) composed of monoterpenes and sesquiterpenes
- Terpenoid components-citral, citronellal, eugenol, geraniol, nerol, linalool,farnesyl acetate, humulene
- Flavonoids, tannins

Braun, L ."Herbs and Natural Supplements: An evidence-based guide". Elsevier Australia 2007, 452-455

Lemon Balm

Dosing
- Capsules: Take 300, 600, 900 mg dried lemon balm TID
- Tea: 1.5 - 4.5 grams/150mls water infused TID
- Tincture1:5, 3-5 mls TID
- Fluid Extract 1:1, 2-3 mls TID
- Topical: Apply topical cream to affected area, 3 times daily or as directed

Contraindications and Safety-generally well tolerated, no known toxicity
or drug interaction.
No clinical studies on thyroid inhibiting effects

Holy Basil
Ocimum sanctum

- Lamiaceae family
- Mental cloudiness from use of drugs and marijuana
- As a sacred plant and goddess
- Uplifting/Anti-despair
- Enhancing mental clarity and meditation

Holy Basil as a Happiness Herb

- Increases mental clarity and focus
- Facilitates a shift in perspective
- Reduces mental inertia and even depression
- Restores hope and optimism

Holy Basil

Actions:
- Adaptogen, analgesic, anodyne, antiviral, antibacterial, antifungal, anti-allergic, galactogogue, radioprotective, hypoglycemic, hypocholesterolaemic, anti-inflammatory, COX-II anti-inflammatory agent, cortisol regulator, tonic, immunomodulating,

Active Constituents:
- Alkaloids, oleanolic acid, ursolic acid, tannins rosmarinic acid , eugenol , carvacrol , linalol, β-caryophyllene, saponins, flavonoids,

Holy Basil

Preparations:
- Dried powder-250-1000mg/d
- Fresh leaf
- Herbal tea
- Tincture-4-10mls/day1:5 LE
- Mixed powdered herb with ghee

Oregano (*Origanum vulgare*)

- Oregano leaves are used dry or fresh as a culinary herb. In foods and beverages, oregano is used as a culinary spice & a food preservative
- Uses - **Orally**:
  - Respiratory tract infections (influenza, the common cold, & croup)
  - Respiratory conditions (cough, asthma, allergies, sinusitis, & bronchitis)
  - Gastrointestinal disorders (dyspepsia, bloating, & intestinal parasites)
  - Dysmenorrhea, rheumatoid arthritis, urinary tract disorders (UTIs), headaches, diabetes, bleeding following tooth extraction, heart conditions, & hyperlipidemia
- Uses - **Topically**:
  - Acne, athlete's foot, dandruff, insect & spider bites, canker sores, gum disease, toothache, psoriasis, seborrhea, ringworm, rosacea, muscle & joint pain, varicose veins, wounds, warts, & insect repellent

Oil of Oregano - Parasites

Oregano oil for six weeks resulted in eradication of several intestinal parasites (*Blastocystis hominis*, *Entamoeba hartmanni*, and *Endolimax nana*)

- 14 adult patients with enteric parasites were administered four tablets providing 200mg of emulsified oil of *Origanum vulgare* (with meals) three times daily (for a total of 600mg daily) for six weeks

Results:
- Complete disappearance of *Entamoeba hartmanni* (four cases), *Endolimax nana* (one case), and *Blastocystis hominis* (eight cases)
- *Blastocystis hominis* scores declined in three additional cases
- In the 11 patients who had tested positive for *Blastocystis hominis*, gastrointestinal symptoms improved

Ref: Force M, et al. 2000 May; 14(3):213-4

Oil of Oregano - Wound Healing

- RDBPCT - 3% Oregano (*Origanum vulgare*) extract ointment on wound healing

  - N=40; Individuals who were undergoing dermatologic excisions on the trunk and upper and lower extremities were included
  - Randomized to apply either a 3% oregano extract ointment or petrolatum ointment to the excision site twice daily for 12 ± 2 days

- Results: Oregano extract ointment reduced the incidence of bacterial contamination and infection and improved scar appearance

Ragi J, et al. J Drugs Dermatol. 2011 Oct;10(10):1168-72

Oil of Oregano - Dosages

Adult
- *Oral*:
  - **Intestinal infections and infestations**: A specific emulsified oregano leaf oil product 200 mg orally three times daily with meals
- *Topical*:
  - **Wound healing**: An ointment containing 3% of an aqueous extract of oregano has been applied to wounds from minor dermatological surgery twice daily for 10 days to 12 days

Children
- Insufficient available evidence

Standardization & Formulation
- There is insufficient reliable information available about the standardization of Oregano

Adverse Effects: GRAS

Bee Propolis

- Over 300 constituents
- Biological active compounds include flavonoids, terpenes, caffeic, ferulic and cumaric acids and esters.
- Antimicrobial activity against a wide range of microorganisms (bacteria, fungi and viruses)
- Anti-inflammatory, analgesic, vulenary, vasoprotective, antioxidant, anti-ulcer and hepatoprotective activities

Propolis

- Clinical application

  Acute Otitis Media- acute/prevent

  Acute Bronchitis

  Acute Asthma Reaction

  Strep Throat, Tonsillitis

  Acute Rhinopharyngitis
  Rom J Virol, 1995 Jul-Dec;46(3-4):115-33

  Upper Respiratory Infection- acute and prevention

  Mix with Honey to avoid sticking to everything and teeth staining; .5-2 mls/dose 1:5 extract

Botanical Essential Oils

- Unique olfactory brain relationship
- Inhalation of the fragrances bypasses organs and tissues
- Enters directly into cerebral circulation
- Regulates mood, emotion, and mental states
- Regulates sleep cycles
- Supports alertness and cognation

How to use Botanical Essential Oils

- Direct skin application- neat or diluted, test patch
- Nasal ointment – lipid based, decrease colonization in nasal passages
- Air Diffused – atomize or diffuse
- Bathing – emulsify or add to salt
- Steam Inhaled – direct application to nasal passages
- Internal – Oil of Oregano, as an emulsion
- Personal Hygiene Products

Carrier Oils

- The use of a carrier oil with EO aids in the application of the EO, helps to protect the skin from the strong effects of the EO on the skin and allows it to time release into the skin over a longer period of time with out evaporating
- Common carrier oils include;
  - Almond
  - Coconut
  - Jojoba
  - Sesame
  - Rosehip or Sea Buckthorn

Botanical Essential Oils

- As strong and effective anti-microbials
- Essential oils can provide secondary benefits for healing from infections:
  - immune support
  - tissue regeneration
  - reduction of swelling
  - lymphatic cleaning and support.

Essential oils that are active against Staph and MRSA include:

- Tea Tree
- Oregano
- Thyme
- Cinnamon
- Clove

- Eucalyptus
- Rosemary
- Lemongrass
- Geranium
- Lavender

Blends of Essential Oils

- Staph or MRSA may not respond to a single oil, blending several essential oils can bring added benefits from treatment
- Blends combine the benefits of several different essential oils into a single formula
  - Complementary constituents can be specific to target area of infection
  - Broadest spectrum of action of all the antibacterial oils[1]
  - Allows for synergistic action
  - Provides secondary benefits, such as
    - tissue healing
    - enhanced immune response properties.

Tea Tree Oil
Melaleuca alternifolia

- A high quality oil will contain over 100 phytochemical constituents
- In one study superior to standard medical chlorhexidine treatments or a silver preparation for eliminating MRSA colonization Tea tree is considered at safe alternative to drug therapies for treating MRSA skin infections (Journal of Hospital Infection (2004;56:283–6)
- This oil is most commonly used for direct application onto skin infections. It's also popular in natural antibacterial hand soaps, sanitizing sprays and other household products. so mild, it's a great choice for babies, infants, the elderly and sensitive skin areas.

Topical Tea Tree Oil

- 4% tea tree oil (TTO) nasal ointment and 5% TTO body wash (intervention) with a standard 2% mupirocin nasal ointment and triclosan body wash (routine) for eradication of methicillin-resistant *Staphylococcus aureus* (MRSA)
- More patients in the intervention than in the control group cleared infection

Antimicrob. Chemother. (2003) 51 (2): 241-246.

Ravensara Aromatica

Ravensara essential oil; from a large rainforest tree native to Madagascar, traditionally thought of as a "Cure All"

•Essential oils contains many terpene compounds; alpha pinene, delta carene, caryophyllene, germacreme, limonene, linalool, methyl chavicol, methyl eugenol, sabinene and terpineol.

•Ravensara Essential Oil actions include analgesic, anti-allergenic, antibacterial, antimicrobial, antidepressant, antifungal, antiseptic, antispasmodic, antiviral, diuretic, expectorant, relaxant, and tonic

Anti-MRSA Essential Oil Blend

- Tea Tree 15 drops
- Lavender 15 drops
- Ravensara 15 drops
- Rosemary 10 drops
- Clove 5 drops

Mix with 20 drops of castor oil, shake well before using

Apply 1-3 times daily directly to lesion

Add 10-20 drops to bath, steam inhalants, and nasal ointments

Turmeric Clay Paste with Essential Oils

1 teaspoon turmeric powder

1 teaspoon bentonite clay powder

1-2 teaspoons soft coconut oil

5-10 drops essential oil blend

Blend turmeric, clay, and coconut oil until smooth and well mixed, stir in essential oil blend. Store in air tight jar.

Apply directly to lesion 2-4 times daily

Chamomile Flower EO

Chamomile essential oil inhalation: sedative and mood enhancing effect

- Generalized anxiety disorder – 6-8wks
- Depression with long term use 12 wks or greater
- Irritable bowel syndrome– bisabolol and chamazulene
- Gingivitis, canker sores, dental plaque- oral mouthwash
- Dermatitis in creams, lotions, washes, and bath

Chamomile Herb Profile, Engels and Brinckmann; Herbalgram, Issue 108, Nov. 2015, p 8-17

Chamomile Medicinal Uses

- The volatile oils, such as chamazulene, appear to be due in part to activation of the pituitary-adrenal axis.
- Azulene also is a gentle sedative, restoring the nervous system to a calmer state.
- The volatile oils, such as alpha-bisabolol is anti-inflammatory and anti-spasmodic specifically enhancing prostaglandin production thereby strengthening the mucosal protective barrier (therefore protective against ulcers).
- Chamazulene inhibits lipid peroxidation
- Matricaria is therefore useful in the treatment of IBS and colitis (for its anti-spasmodic, anti-ulcer, and nervine effects). Carl W and L Emrich. J Prosthet Dent. 1991;66(3):361-9
  McKay D and J Blumberg, Phytother Res. 20(7):519-30
  Rekka E, et al. Res Commun Mol Pathol Pharmacol. 1996;92(3):361-4.

Chamomile Cream

- Azulene compounds
- Partially dbl-blind randomized trial
- Half-side comparison w/0.5% hydrocortisone
- 2 week treatment duration

  Outcome showed the Chamomile cream mildly superior to the 0.5% hydrocortisone or placebo

Patzelt-Wenczler R, Pounce-Poschl E, Eur J Med Res 2000;·5(4):171-5

Colic Rub

- 5 drops lavender EO
- 5 drops Chamomile EO
- 5drops Lemon Balm EO
- 1 oz of carrier oil such as almond, jojoba, sesame, coconut

Massage over baby's abdomen in a clockwise direction, back, and buttock

Cord Wipe

- 1 oz rosewater
- 1 oz distilled witch hazel
- 5 drops lavender EO
- 5 drops ravensara EO

Mix well in a 2 oz bottle, use to wipe the umbilical cord stub and area, several times daily.

Aromatic Bath for Sleepless Babes

2 drops each
- Lemon balm EO
- Chamomile EO
- Clary Sage EO

Mix all the essential oils into 2 teaspoons of epson salts. Use 1 tsp per bath soaking child for 10-15 minutes.

Aromatic Air Spray

- 5 drops Eucalyptus EO
- 5drops Neroli EO
- 5 drops Peppermint EO
- 5 drops Clary Sage EO
- 2 oz OrangeFlower Water (rose or lavender ok)
- 2 Tbsp rubbing alcohol

Mix all into a spray pump bottle and shake well before use.

Aromatic Spray & Wipe

- 2 Tbsp white vinegar
- 2 Tbsp liquid castile soap
- 5 drops lemon EO
- 5 drops rosemary EO
- 5drops Siberian fir EO
- Lemon juice from one freshly squeezed lemon.

Mix all in a 8 oz spray bottle and fill up with hot water, mix well.

Anti-Head Lice Oil

Combine equal amounts of

- Rosemary EO
- Lavender EO
- Tea Tree EO
- Eucalyptus EO
- Rose Geranium EO

Use mixture in hair shampoos and rinses, apply to hairbrush, combine with coconut oil and apply to hair for several hours, rinse out and thoroughly dry hair with a hairdryer.

A Peek Inside My Medicine Bag

Phyllis Hogan
Founding Director
Arizona Ethnobotanical Research Association

It was in the early 1970's when I began learning how Native elders used medicinal plants. Taking herbs from the desert and gaining knowledge of their healing properties was incredible, and my passion for the practice bloomed. The Sonoran desert, seemingly desolate and dry, became full of life and magic; it became my home. In the early spring and summer the landscape came alive with all sorts of strange life forms that, to my amazement, were the tried and true pharmacy of the people who lived close to the earth. My keen interest and my respect for the land was noticed, and the grandparents shared with me the age-old tradition of folk medicine. I was taken to secret places in remote areas: we waded through hidden springs and trekked forgotten mountaintops. These were the gardens the healers had tended to for generations, where they would collect herbs for their *medicine bags,* their stores of plants and knowledge.

From the top of the mountain to the desert's green edge, this presentation is a glimpse inside *my* medicine bag, the one that I've relied upon for over 40 years. This class will be a glimpse into some of the traditional plant medicines that have been used with success by native people in Arizona for centuries. I have selected a few of the medicinal plants that are readily available in the Southwestern United States.

From the roads running south to North in our Arizona, the spirit of the abalone mountain winds through the rivers, becoming a confluence of traditional wisdom and today's medical needs. I would like to share these plants with you as a means of cultural preservation, and to honor the people and plants native to this region.

We will take a multisensory journey with these plants by viewing specimens, sampling tinctures and teas, and breathing in their aromas. This hands-on approach will provide a tactile relationship between the plants and people. We will also look at ways to give offerings and use sustainable wildcrafting techniques as a method to show reverence in our interactions with the plants.

From tribal lands to the thriving desert oasis, I present my ethnobotanical knowledge gained from my home in the Winter Sun. I invite you to join me in the experience of traditional medicines of our land.

The Plants of my Medicine Bag:

Cliff Rose
Purshia stansbariana
Family: Rosaceae
Due to the bitter taste of the leaves, Cliff Rose is sometimes called "quinine bush", and is best known as a tea for coughs. There are six species of this many-branched evergreen in Arizona, and are common in Pinion-Juniper forests. It grows up to eight feet tall with an intoxicatingly sweet-smell, and has cream-colored flowers that produce long, showy plumes. It has shreddy bark that has been used historically by the Navajo and Hopi for ropes, clothing, cradleboard padding, menstrual padding, fire starters, and sleeping mats. The Navajo make a strong infusion of Cliff Rose and Juniper leaves to induce vomiting in order to cleanse out a sour stomach. Topically, the leaf tea is used to wash wounds

and treat skin problems such as impetigo, chicken pox sores, gunshot wounds, and arrow wounds. The Navajo use the leaves and twigs as a natural dye that gives textiles a lovely golden shade.

Ephedra, Mormon Tea, Popotillo, Osvi, Tl'oh asihi libahiggii
Ephedra viridis
Family: Ephedraceae

This is a small to medium sized shrub with young trigs that are bright green and broom-like. The leaves are reduced to bracts and have yellow, flower-like cones. They are dioecious, meaning that there is a male plant and a female plant. The cones form clusters at the joints, and is topped by a spore producing strobilus. Ephedra can be found growing on dry mesas, often forming shrubby clumps. It is often used by hikers, who chew a twig of it in their mouths to give a slight energy boost. Ephedra is one of the oldest known medicinal plants in the Southwest. Its fibrous twigs preserve well in archeological sites, and have been found in medicine bundles with other objects used in healing ceremonies, dating back a thousand years or more.

One unique application of ephedra tea is to help women during childbirth. The Navajo shepherds who lived in the remote areas of the Painted Desert would gain stamina during labor by drinking the mild stimulant tea. It has a long history of being used for hay fever and allergies. It is a diuretic and urinary tract astringent, and is also an absorbable source of calcium.

Brickelia, Hamula, Prodigiosa,
Brickellia grandiflora
Family: Compositacea

Brickellia is found in sandy areas in dry washes in the Southwestern United States. In Arizona there are over 26 species, which typically grow between 3 to 6 feet tall. This plant has been primarily used in Mexican and Native American herbal traditions.

Brickelia is used for combating high blood glucose levels, and is especially useful in type 2, insulin-resistant diabetes. It can also be used as a bitter tonic to boost digestion and stimulate bile production.

Ho Hoi'si, Cota, Navajo Tea, Hopi Tea
Thelesperma megapotamicum
Family: Asteracea

The characteristically golden yellow flowers create a glow around this little plant, which is common in Pinion-Juniper forests of the Southwest. The aerial parts are tied into bundles, which are then hung to dry and used throughout the year. It is used primarily as a beverage tea, a coffee substitute and a dye for basketry and textiles. As a dye it provides a beautiful reddish-brown hue.

Medicinally, it can be used to settle the stomach, often used in combination with spearmint and cinnamon. The Hopi use it for high blood pressure and water retention during pregnancy. It is one of the few plants that are particularly safe for use during pregnancy.

Snake Weed, Escoba de la Vibora
Gutierrezia sarothrae
Family: Asteraceae

This weed has ray flowers of a dull yellow hue, which are harvested and bundled into small bouquets. A perennial shrub that is common among the Pinion-Juniper forests and desert scrublands, its leaves have a waxy, resinous finish, and give off a slight piney scent when crushed. Traditionally, the flowering stems are clipped together into little bundles that are dried then used as a unit. It is most commonly used in a hot bath for arthritis, rheumatism, sore muscles, and hypertension. Navajos use Snake Weed, what they call "Beautiful Weed," for their ceremonies.

Monarda, Oregano de la Sierra, Wild Bergamot, Bee balm
Monarda fistulosa var. menthafolia
Family: Lamiaceae

Monarda is a perennial wildflower in the mint family, and is widespread and abundant in much of North America. It has whitish to purple flowers, with a delectable spicy-sweet fragrance that attracts both people and bees alike. It blooms in July and August in small patches along streams and in moist meadows of the Ponderosa Pine forest.

Medicinally, Native Americans of the Southwest use it in a similar fashion as the Oregano of Europe for fevers, colds, and flus. Standard infusions of the aerial parts are used as a mouthwash and gargle for sore throats, and a steam inhalation can be used to open up the sinus passages. It is used to treat urinary tract infections, and known for its properties as an emmenagogue and diaphoretic. Monarda can be made into a lovely medicinal honey as a cough and sore throat remedy.

Wild Rosemary Mint, Frosted Mint, Mo'ongtorshavu, Atza azee
Poliomintha incana
Family: Lamiacea

The branches of the Wild Rosemary mint are straight, slender and silvery colored, and can grow up to 3-4 feet. The flowers are pale, bluish-purple and are arranged in spikes at the tips of the branches. These strongly aromatic shrubs grow in mounds in sandy habitats of cold desert scrublands. The fragrant leaves are used as a flavoring for foods, and can be eaten both fresh and dry.

The Hopis collect the strong-smelling leaves in the spring and make delicious gravy used for scrambled eggs and other foods. The Navajos make a ceremonial tea of the leaves for washing eagle feathers that they use to make into fans. Both tribes use the leaves for food, as a fumigant, and mix it with their tobacco for flavoring.

It is used as a steam inhalation for cough, due to its antispasmodic properties. Wild Rosemary Mint tea is a wonderful carminative to aid in digestion when taken after meals, and will help combat gas and bloating. Due to its diaphoretic qualities, it is useful to help sweat out a fever. The tea is also an emmenagogue to help stimulate menstruation that may have been suppressed from stress or illness. For this reason, it is not safe to take during pregnancy.

References and Suggested Readings

Dedera, Jill and Hogan, Phyllis. Little Colorado Field School Plant and Field Guide.   Arizona Ethnobotanial Research Association. Flagstaff, Arizona 2005.

Epple, Anne Orth., and Lewis E. Epple. *A field guide to the Plants of Arizona*. Helena,   MT: Falcon Press, 1997. Print.

Hogan, Phyllis. "People and Plants in the Sierra Sinagua." Hisat'sinom. Ed. Christen E.   Downum. SAR Press, 2012. Print.

Kane, Charles W. *Medicinal plants of the American Southwest*. Oracle, AZ: Lincoln   Town Press, 2016. Print.

Moore, Michael. *Medicinal Plants of the Desert and Canyon West: a guide to identifying,
          preparing, and using traditional medicinal plants found in the deserts and canyons of the West and Southwest*. Santa Fe, NM: Museum of New Mexico   Press, 1989. Print.

Moore, Michael. *Medicinal Plants of the Mountain West*. Santa Fe: Museum of New   Mexico Press, 2003. Print.

Moore, Michael. *Medicinal Plants of the Pacific West*. Santa Fe: Museum of New   Mexico Press, 2011. Print.

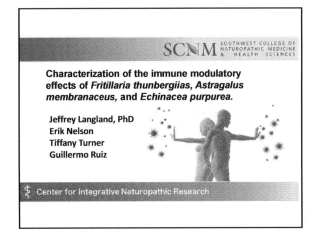

Characterization of the immune modulatory effects of *Fritillaria thunbergiias, Astragalus membranaceus,* and *Echinacea purpurea.*

Jeffrey Langland, PhD
Erik Nelson
Tiffany Turner
Guillermo Ruiz

$ Center for Integrative Naturopathic Research

Part I: Understanding the ancient Chinese (1023 AD) art of variolation (vaccination) for protection against smallpox

Jeffrey Langland, PhD

Ramesses V

Smallpox......
❖ *Present in human population for thousands of years*
❖ *Disease killed about 1 in 3*

Modern vaccination

Edward Jenner:
❖ Pioneer of smallpox vaccine
❖ Observed that cowpox would cause a less severe disease, but similar to smallpox
❖ Cowpox infection seemed to protect humans against smallpox

1796:
Material from cowpox pustules of a dairy maid was used as a vaccine

---

Last naturally-occurring case of smallpox in the world was contracted in October, 1977

Declared eradicated by World Health Assembly in 1980

The Art of Variolation for Protection Against Smallpox

Began during the reign of Emperor Jen Tsung (A.D. 1023-63) in the Song Dynasty of China

". . . instruction included implanting smallpox, which consisted in *selecting scabs from cases that had but few pustules*, and these pointed, round, red and glossy, full of greenish-yellow pus that became thick. The scabs to be used when a month old, or in *hot weather those that had fallen only 15 or 20 days might be used, while winter ones should be 40 or 50 days old before using*, which may be in spring or autumn. Take 8 grains of the desiccated scabs and 2 grains of *Uvularia grandiflora; pound the two together in a clean earthen mortar*. Employ for the operation a silver tube curved at the point; blow the prepared matter into the right nostril in the case of a boy, and into the left in girls; six days after there is slight fever, which on the following day increases greatly; in two or three days more an eruption appears, charged with matter, and then scabs. Not one in 10, not one in 100, that does not recover." (Needham, 1980)

Detective work…………

*Scabs from "cases that had but a few pustules"
   Hypothesis I: Mild infection. Likely a   weakened strain of smallpox.

*Use scabs from hot weather those that had fallen only 15 or 20 days or winter ones should be 40 or 50 days old.
   Hypothesis II: Storage/heat leads to   inactivation of the virus

*Combined with *Uvularia grandiflora*
   Hypothesis III: Botanical may act as an   adjuvant to induce immune response

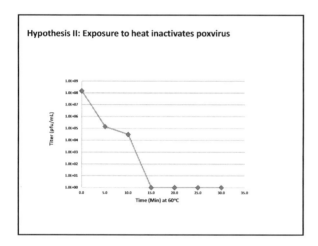

Hypothesis II: Exposure to heat inactivates poxvirus

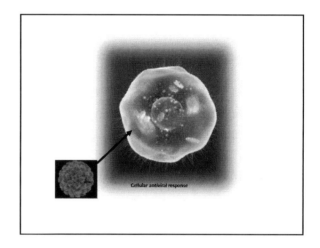

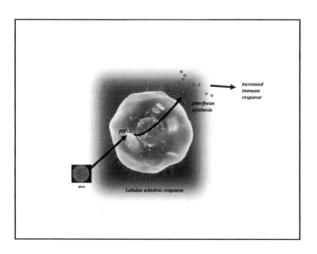

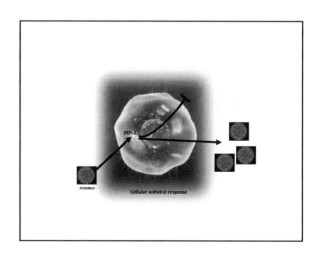

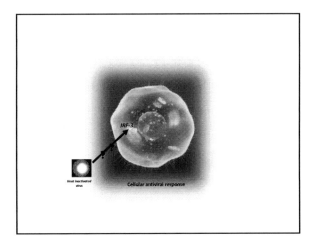

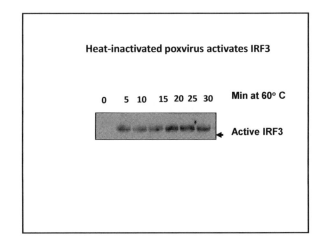

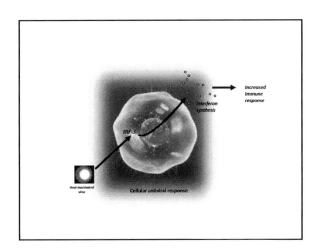

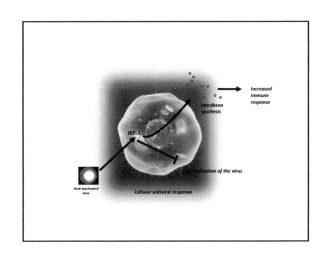

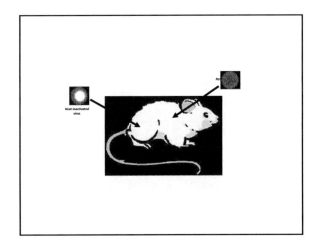

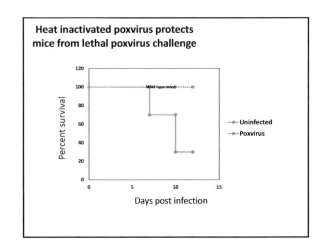

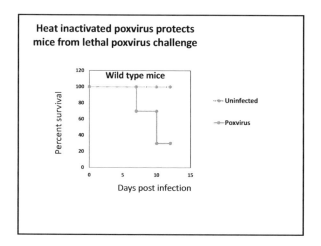

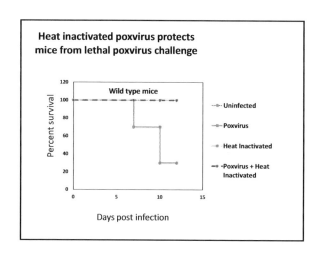

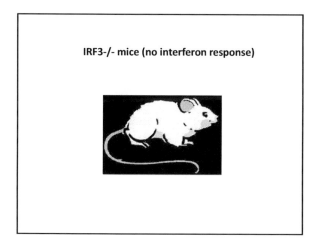

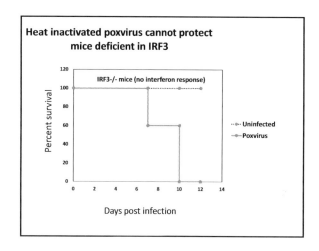

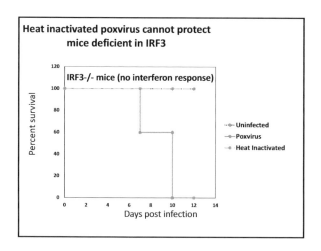

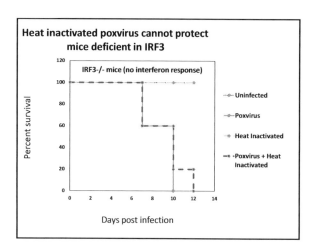

*Use scabs from hot weather those that had fallen only 15 or 20 days or winter ones should be 40 or 50 days old.
   Conclusion: Storage/heat leads to   inactivation of the virus, but is still able to induce a protective immune response

*Combined with *Uvularia grandiflora*
   Hypothesis III: Botanical may act as an   adjuvant to induce immune response

---

Role of *Uvularia grandiflora*

Original document translation:
   Uvularia grandiflora:
      Native to eastern North America :
      Did not exist in the China during Song
Dynasty and trade routes were not
established

Role of *Uvularia grandiflora*

Original document translation:
   Uvularia grandiflora:
      Native to eastern North America :
      Did not exist in the China during Song
      Dynasty and trade routes were not
      established

More likely candidate:

   Fritillaria thunbergii:
Similar appearance
Originally misidentified in Asia as *Uvularia*
      (KEW Bulletin, 66:2011)
Asian plant species native to Xinjiang Province
of western China.

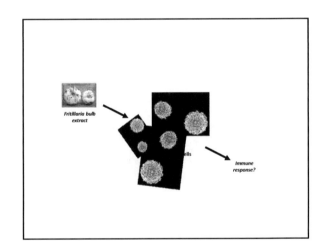

Fritillaria bulb extract → cells → Immune response?

Fritillaria induced cytokine synthesis in WBCs

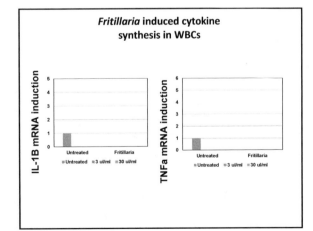

Fritillaria induced cytokine synthesis in WBCs

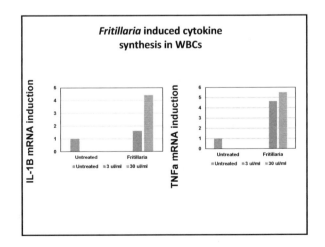

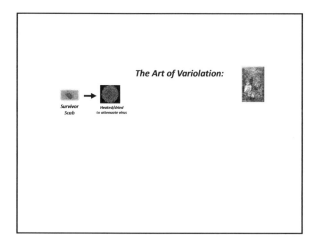

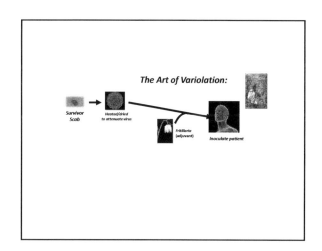

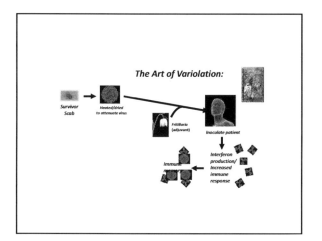

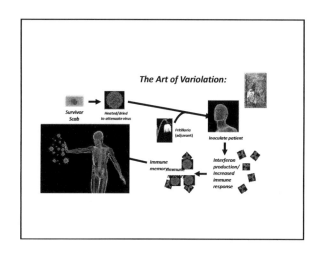

**Part IIA: The Immune Modulatory
Effects of Astragalus membranaceus:**
In vitro analysis

Erik Nelson

Astragalus membranaceus

- <u>Immune stimulatory</u>
- <u>Wound healing</u>
- <u>Blood circulation</u>
- <u>Pro-angiogenesis</u>
- <u>Antiviral</u>
- Adjunct cancer therapy
- Cardiovascular disease
- Diabetes
- Nephritis
- Male infertility
- and more....

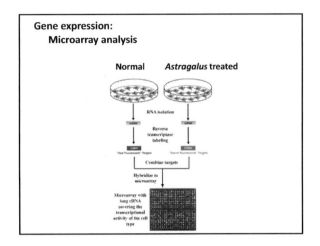

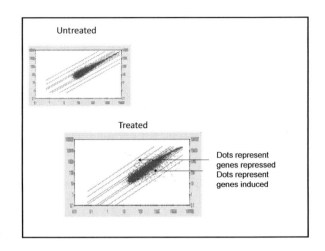

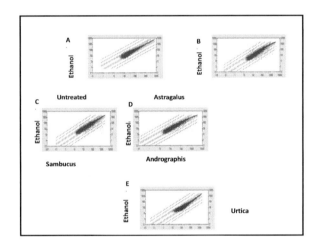

	3 HPT	8 HPT	18 HPT
Transcription/ RNA processing	18.2%	10.2%	8.9%
Translation/ Protein modification	9.5%	5.5%	8.1%
Signal transduction/ Protein transport	10.8%	2.8%	8.9%
Cell cycle/ DNA structure	5.8%	2.8%	4.9%
Metabolic processes	8.7%	4.8%	4.0%
Other	4.3%	7.4%	2.4%
Immune/Inflammation	26.6%	71.2%	62.6%

149 genes induced

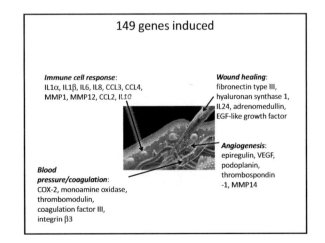

Immune cell response:
IL1α, IL1β, IL6, IL8, CCL3, CCL4, MMP1, MMP12, CCL2, IL10

Blood pressure/coagulation:
COX-2, monoamine oxidase, thrombomodulin, coagulation factor III, integrin β3

Wound healing:
fibronectin type III, hyaluronan synthase 1, IL24, adrenomedullin, EGF-like growth factor

Angiogenesis:
epiregulin, VEGF, podoplanin, thrombospondin-1, MMP14

What are the active constituents?

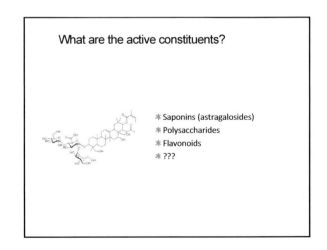

* Saponins (astragalosides)
* Polysaccharides
* Flavonoids
* ???

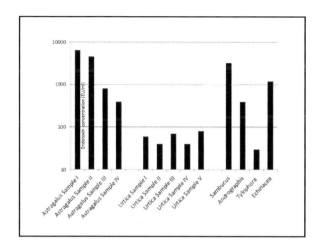

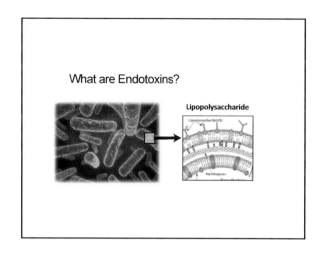

What are Endotoxins?

Lipopolysaccharide

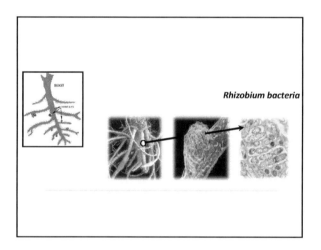

Rhizobium bacteria

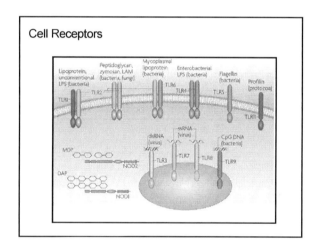

Cell Receptors

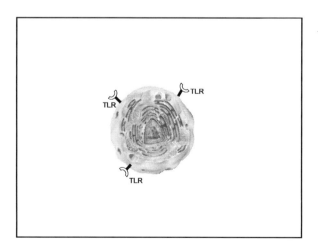

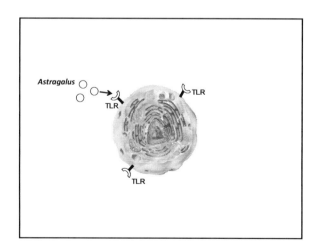

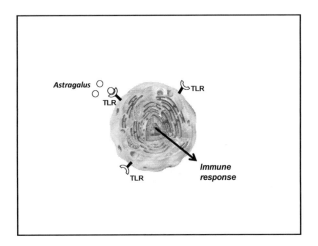

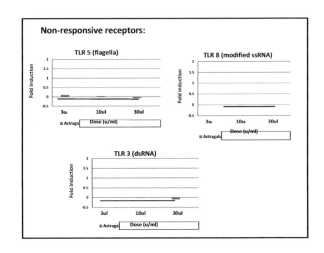

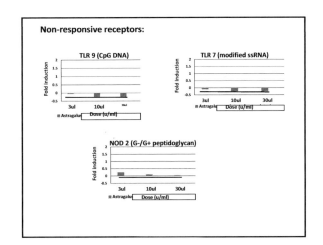

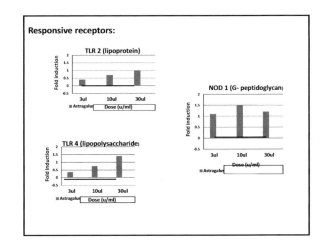

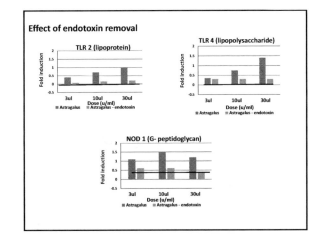

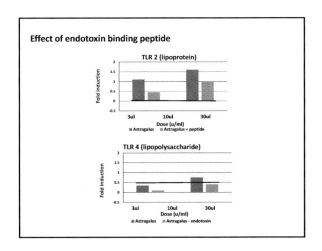

Effects on PBMC cells

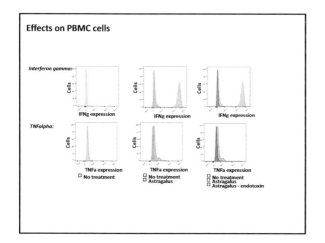

Conclusions:

- Immune gene induction was more generalized or preparative in the immune/inflammatory response

- Approximately 70% of the genes induced were immune/inflammatory related

- Putative genes involved in other activities of *Astragalus* were identified

- Lipopolysaccharide in *Astragalus* is likely an active component for the immunostimulatory response

- Potentially, the quality of herbal preparations may be related to the number of nodules present on the root

Part IIB:The Immune Modulatory Effects of Astragalus membranaceus:

In vivo analysis

Tiffany Turner

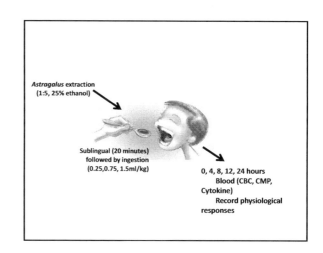

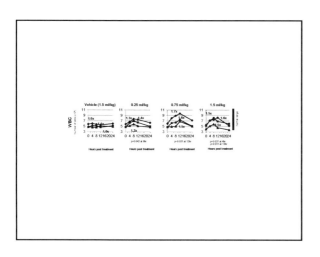

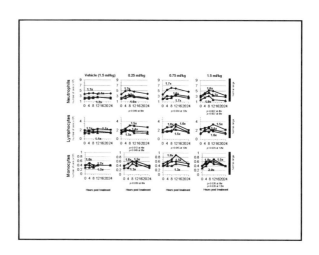

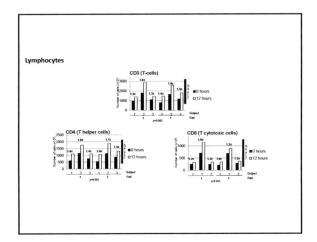

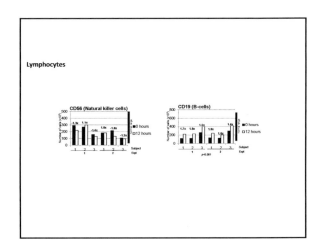

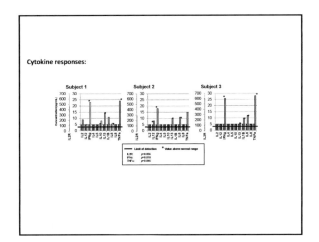

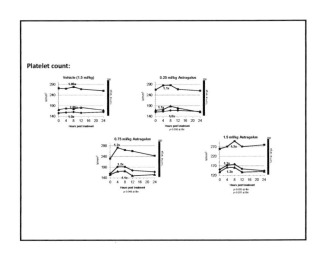

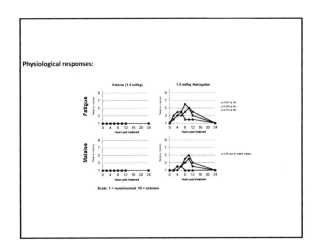

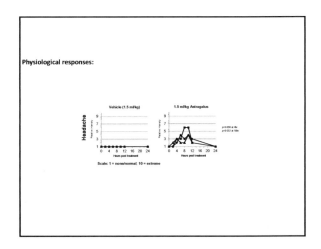

Physiological responses:

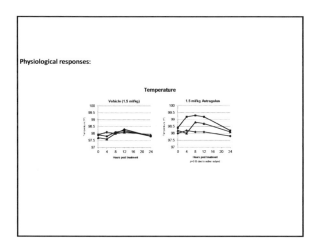

Physiological responses:

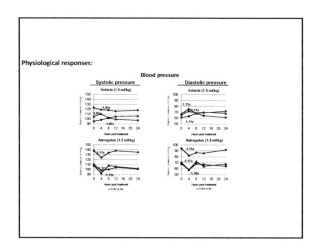

Conclusions:

- Increased white blood cells (monocytes, neutrophils, and lymphocytes) 8-12 hours after administration

- Dynamic changes in the levels of circulating cytokines:
  Th1 cytokines interferon-γ and tumor necrosis factor-α
  Th2 cytokine IL13
  Proinflammatory cytokine IL6 and soluble IL2-R

- Induced fatigue, malaise, and headache responses

- Supports the traditional use as an effective antiviral/antimicrobial agent

---

Part III: Understanding the effects of Echinacea purpurea during Rhinovirus (common cold) infections.

Guillermo Ruiz

Echinacea has been widely studied:
- **Common cold**
- **Influenza**
- **Immune stimulation**

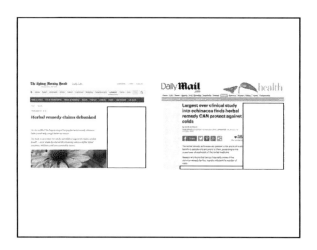

Rhinovirus

- Most commonly isolated virus from respiratory tract infections
- Discovered in the 1950's
- Rhino means "nose"
- It induces the production of IL-8

Interleukin - 8

- Interleukin 8 (IL-8) is a chemokine produced by macrophages and other cells such as the cells found in the lungs
- IL-8 has two primary functions
  - It induces chemotaxis in target cells causing them to migrate towards the cite of infection
  - It induces phagocytosis once those cells arrive
- **Interleukin-8 induces your "Cold like symptoms"**

mRNA as a Predictor of IL-8

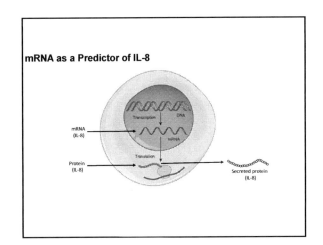

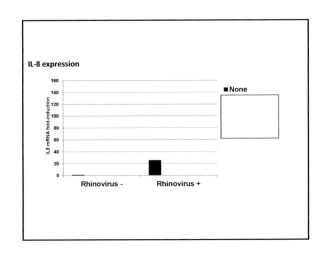

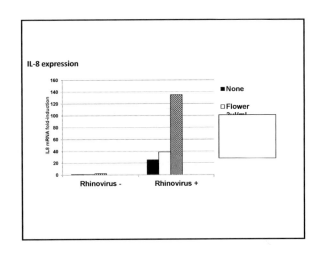

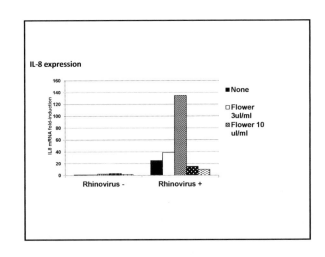

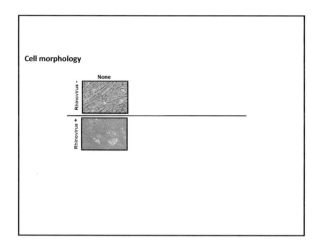

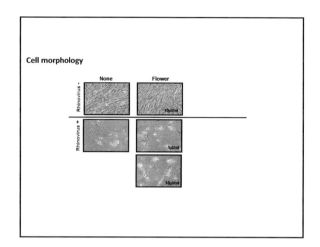

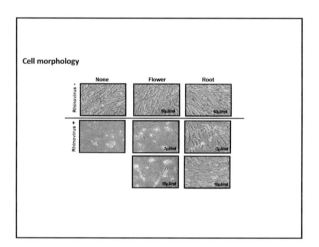

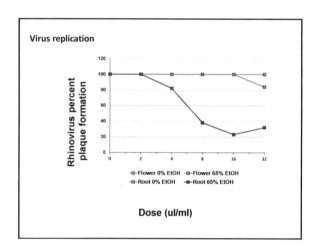

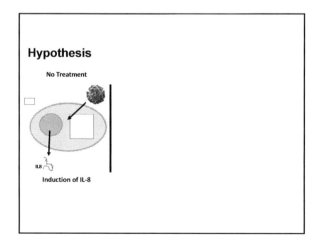

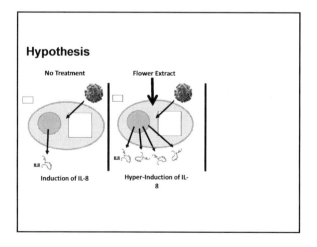

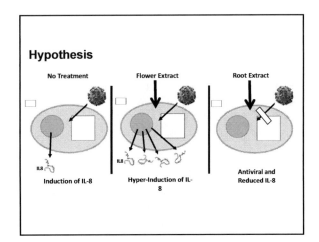

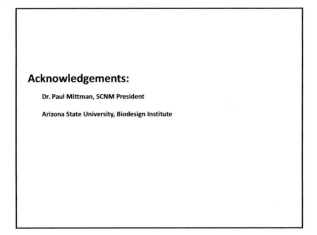

Flower Essences as BioAdaptogens
By Rhonda Mae PallasDowney

Living as Human Adaptors

Relaxing and reflecting on various herbs, flowers, trees, and plants, their uses and my relationship to them this past summer, touched a place inside of me that continues to guide my inquiry into the field of adaptogens. All the while, I was experiencing an adaptation of my own that included the awareness of my lifestyle and all that it encompasses. The mindfulness of the changing of the seasons and what each season requires of me, although familiar, is a new way to adapt.

For example, slipping in from spring to summer, especially changes my outdoor routine from walking and hiking most everyday to swimming. This includes getting up an hour earlier or so, and becoming accustomed with the timing of the sunrise, the sunset, and the Arizona heat. This timing change, then also affects everything else I do all day long and the time in which I do it in, affecting both my internal and external environments.

And as a plant enthusiast, I learn to readjust to the seasons changing within the season. Global warming, inconsistent weather conditions, the imbalance of drought vs. rain, etc. plays an enormous role in my life in the way that I gather plants and make essences, even if the flowers are just a few weeks or sometimes a month off of the normal blooming period.

Oh yeah, and then there's everyday living. There are some days that go smoothly and just require a general routine such as eating, sleeping, job, family, hobbies, etc. without any drama. Piece of cake, right? And then there are those other days, that may have various kinds of major dramas whether in the world (that is everyday, in the politics of our country and world-wide issues), in our communities, or at home. And the list goes on, suffering at many levels, sickness, recovery, death, birth, and the evolving re-birth (mind-body-spirit) of humankind.

Yes my friends, each and every day we live our lives navigating our way or not, planned and/or unplanned, looking for, grasping on, and letting go, being present, being mindful, over and over, while adapting to being "normal" and yet authentic in nature to who we are. Now that's a lot of energy we hold in our energy fields! We become used to it, familiar with it, and as long as we're feeling strong, usually we can hold the energy and get by without a collapse. However, if and when we have those weaker moments, perhaps of either physical or mental exhaustion or both, it then becomes more difficult to make adjustments throughout the day. Our relationship to the stress within our bodies, minds, and spirits along with the stresses created in our families or with our friends, and the stress in the world, then becomes elevated and expressed in many different ways. We lose the connection within ourselves and of the ways in which we adapt, and we begin to break down. However, that may be experienced with each of us and at any given time, expected or unexpected.

Moment to moment, we are faced with adapting to life, as life doesn't adapt to us! Learning to listen to ourselves from the deepest places within helps us to adapt to what our bodies-minds-spirits are telling us. The energetic field is pushing us to expand wider and wider, to push through those inner walls, and to adapt to the rhythm of the times.

We, as living beings, are human adaptive agents, uniting body-mind-spirit as a source of energy that surges through in the form of creating authentic expression, continuously transforming our energy fields to restore balance, grace, and harmony within ourselves, with others, mother earth, and the entire ecosystem. We strive to strengthen the vital essence we were born with, and to support that being moment to moment.

BioAdaptogens

The awareness of our ecological interrelatedness as One system that comprises all living organisms offers a unique opportunity to experience life as BioAdaptogenic, as I would like to refer to it. This to me, means adapting to life as life is and allowing life to unfold into its own natural expression of being, while holding a conscious path for its growth, restoring and harmonizing the vital force of all that is.

I choose the word "bio" as a reference to "life or a living organism", including any and all living organisms. With the awareness of living a bioadaptogenic life, we can begin to understand the synchronizing relationship of supporting the natural forces of nature. This relates to healthy conditions of life ranging from soil and organic farming and the foods we eat, to all the ways which are as naturally supporting to our environment as possible, which reinforce animal, plant, human health, and all the ways that we adapt to that, as well as all living organisms.

The word adaptogen originated from Dr. Nikolai Lazarev in 1947, who was a Russian pharmacologist. The awareness of adaptogens dates back thousands of years. Dr. Lazarev defined adaptogens as "agents which help an organism to counteract any adverse effects of a physical, chemical or biological stressor by generating nonspecific resistance."

The dictionary refers to adaptogen as "(in herbal medicine), a natural substance considered to help the body adapt to stress and to exert a normalizing effect upon bodily processes."

In his book, "Adaptogens in Medical Herbalism", Donald Yance describes adaptogen as "nonspecific, endocrine-regulating, immune-modulating effects of certain plants that increase a person's ability to maintain optimal balance in the face of physical or emotional stress. These botanical agents provide the perfect antidote for the life-robbing deficiencies in vitality created by the demands of modern life." (p.4)

To simplify this discussion, let's summarize adaptogens as natural substances that help improve the struggle with adverse effects on the body that are especially related to a multitude of stressors, which may be affected physically, chemically, or biologically, which offer a non-toxic normalizing effect with no specific responses indicated.

In today's world, there is not a true definition of adaptogens, however, they are considered to be of their own class as "natural, homeostatic metabolic regulators."
(Winston, David and Maimes, Steve, "*Adaptogens: Herbs for Strength, Stamina, and Stress Relief*, p.18.)

Adaptogenic herbs such as astragalus, Chinese/Korean ginseng, Siberian ginseng, ashwagandha, eleuthro, licorice, and others have been used in the treatment or as part of a treatment for various conditions including stress, anxiety and nervous disorders, chronic illnesses, chemotherapy and radiation therapy, cardiovascular health, liver and kidney disease, the immune system, and the endocrine systems.

Many of these adaptogenic herbs not only improve the body's defense mechanisms to hostile stresses, they also serve as a tonic and immune-stimulator while normalizing the inner environment, improving the vital force, and increasing a general sense of wellness and strength.

Using Flower and Tree Essences as BioAdaptogens

My personal inquiry into adaptogens guided me to explore flower and tree essences more deeply and how they may find their own place in the class of adaptogens, and what I now refer to as bioadaptogens. Before going any further on using flower essences as adaptogens, I contacted my dear friend and herbal mentor, JoAnnSanchez, for some feedback. I asked if she and other herbalists would think that flower essences could be considered adaptogens in their own form of use and overall constitutional make-up and preparation. JoAnn's response, "how exciting! Well, yes! Why wouldn't they be?" Her enthusiasm supported the journey of my inquiry…

Flower essences, including catkins from trees, are vibrational in design, and they are charged with a particular frequency and special quality of a flower's (or catkin's) subtle energetic life-force field. Flowers or catkins are picked and placed in a clear glass bowl filled with purified water. The bowl is then placed in direct sunlight or in some cases, moonlight, until the flowers or catkins have faded into the water, leaving their energetic imprint into the water. The energy of light and water transfers the energy of the blossoms or catkins, extracting a life-force pattern that embodies the character of the flower from the plant or tree that it is, or the character of the catkin from the tree that it is. This is called a flower essence infusion. The subtle energy pattern stored within the flower or catkin essence can be used for physical, emotional, mental, and spiritual healing.

As plant substances which offer a subtle energetic impact in the ways that people adapt to stress and anxiety, along with their relationship to themselves and the diseases in which they may incur, flower and tree essences are naturally adaptogenic. By nature these essences embody a living energy (bio), which can help a person bring awareness to the ways in which they adapt and connect to those places within that harmonize and calm, strengthen and restore, normalize and reinforce a healthy and vital inner and outer environment.

I love and appreciate the following quote written by Dr. Gladys Taylor McGarey, a founding member of the American Holistic Medical Association who wrote the foreword in one of my books, explaining the significance of living medicine. "The concept of living medicine is truly exciting because if we're alive, we're going to have illness, we're going to have pain, we're going to have all of the problems that go along with life, but we're going to be alive. Our focus needs to change from killing to helping enhance the life process within each individual. If we do this, we're going to need living materials, such as living air, living earth, living water, and living food."

…"with the *Healing Power of Flowers*, Rhonda brings a living healing method to our attention. This type of healing truly is working with living medicine. The plants and flowers have lived and they pass their living essence to the person who uses the naturally derived product. Life enhances life, and as we involve ourselves in the healing process, with its joys and sorrows, its good times and hard times, I know that nothing makes this truth more clear than flower essences." (PallasDowney, Rhonda, The Healing Power of Flowers, xv.xvi foreword written by Dr. GladysTaylor McGarey).

Through the development of conscious awareness of ourselves, others, the planet, and the ecosystem, we, as living organisms, can enhance our quality of living a bio-adaptogenic life, anchoring in the energy of restoration and harmony of all that is, from within to without.

Taking a flower essence as an alchemical stimulator can create a conversion of an emotional state, for example from anxiety and stress to calm and tranquility. By moving out of drama, and consciously letting the old patterns go, we enter into a more balanced state of homeostasis.

Flower essences help to create a fertile garden within our own inner environment that brings harmony to our natural landscape or our true self. They offer an invitation to start exercising and practicing the push to move beyond the walls and barriers, to open up the inner doorways, to feel into and to embrace living in a new world everyday. They help us to feel the world rather than just trying to understand it, to let the timeless be in charge of time, and to experience the mystery of our life's journey both naturally and consciously with the freedom for evolvement.

This being said, as each plant and each tree has its roots, each of us comes into our own life form with an innate primal force that encompasses an individualized spiritual and soul heritage along with a DNA energy which affects where we have come from and how we evolve the foundation of our authentic selves and well being. The root energy center located between the tailbone (the coccyx) and the pubic bone, includes the functions of the anus, rectum, circulatory system, lower extremities, legs, and entire pelvic area.   The root energy center or chakra of a person is governed by the adrenal glands of the endocrine system, which are located atop the kidneys and produce steroid hormones that regulate salt concentrates in the blood, hydrocortisone, which assists the body in its response to physical stress, and small amounts of sex hormones – both male (androgens) and female (estrogens)- that augment the hormones secreted by the gonad.

By connecting with our roots and grounding the energy of our beingness, going to the source or foundation of our health conditions, as well as understanding the integration of our human energy system as a whole, we have the ability to strengthen our vital force and heal our DNA origins.

Living Trees as Our Teachers and Friends

What better way to connect to and experience our own roots, than to study the species of trees including their root systems, doctrine of signatures, bark, leaves, catkins or flowers, and the ways in which they live and communicate? Experiencing the presence of where trees live and how they grow, and to take in their essence, their scents, their presence and vital force only heightens our awareness of these most powerful beings.

What we do know is that tree roots need water, oxygen, and certain soil and climate conditions, including proper drainage, that allow enough space for roots to penetrate and grow. Trees also join forces with many different kinds of fungi, depending on the location and conditions of the forests they live in. Fungi filaments find their way into the soft root hairs of the trees and both the trees and the fungi feed each other through photosynthesis, sugar, and carbohydrates. This exchange of energy opens spacious pathways for the fungi to expand into a forest web that helps the tree roots connect through electrical signals from nerve cells at the tip of the roots, thereby forming a huge network of nutrients, root systems, and information about pests, insects, animals, drought, and various dangers.

Tree roots spread out at least twice the size of its crown, creating a social network of family and environment. There are always those few trees that are isolated from the others, as hermits you may say, whose roots do not connect, and who tend to live a shorter life and are more susceptible to becoming diseased. I find this signature itself fascinating in comparison with people who live socially and those who may live a more isolated life.

Tree roots and trees bring an awareness of our own root system and of the physical ways in which we stay alive, such as the food we eat, the lifestyles we choose, where we live, how we survive in the world, our social networks, and the environments we choose to be in. Beneath the surface of who we are, as the tree roots grow inside the darkness of the earth finding nutrients for their survival, we are given opportunities to face the shadows within ourselves and experience the deep internal journey into the discovery of our human nature, giving us the space and growth needed to continue our evolvement with the support of friends and family.

Sure there are competitors, even with trees, as there's always competitors in our societies. How can trees not struggle with light and living conditions, especially in crowded areas with mixed species?

Trees communicate and survive through their roots and their electrical signals, sound waves, trunks and branches (wood), leaves, scent, catkins, flowers, seeds, and doctrine of signatures. Trees also mature in their own time and their own state of being. They are in no hurry, they have no place to go, they can take their time to extend their roots deeper into the earth as the tips of their branches begin to touch the tips of others. They serve as wonderful teachers to help us adapt, slow down, pace ourselves, ground and anchor, go to our roots and find the source of what we're looking for, to feel it, and to go deeper into it.

Trees generally are friends with their own species, of air, light, space, and in natural settings, avoiding taking away what is not theirs to take. They share their nutrients, they help each other grow, and they live as members in their communities. Trees heal the soul in so many ways. They teach us to breathe, to slow down, to take in the wonders of nature and its scents, to endure, to protect, to feel inspired, to stop and listen.

For generations and generations, trees, like animals, plants, human beings, and all of nature itself, are constantly adapting both in morphological adaptations (physical changes that occur over generations based on environmental conditions), and in physiological adaptations (how the internal system thrives and responds to external stimuli) to gain or maintain homeostasis.

My Search for Trees and making Essences

Growing up in a small town in the mid-west, with all the wonders of natural settings including family farms, creeks, woods, lakes and ponds, camping, and nature adventures, I became familiar with trees. My dad had a favorite hickory tree that lived an isolated life out in the middle of a bean field, that he would take me to. We would gather the fruit when they turned from green to brown, and when most of them had already fallen on the ground. We'd take them home, then put them in his vice to crack them. Cracking nuts was one of his favorite hobbies. We cracked many a walnut, pecan, and hickory.

As a child I became especially familiar with buckeyes, elms, walnuts, wild cherry, pines, chestnuts, spruces, birches, weeping willows, maples, oaks, and of course, many common fruit trees that my parents grew and which grew in our town of Bluffton, Ohio.

As a quest in my late 20's, I set up a campsite in the massive and rich forest of the Appalachian mountains of Southeastern Ohio. It was a three –four month initiation living alone in a forest, to a wealth of beautifully large hardwood trees such as sugar maples, ash, birch, oak, and flowering dogwoods. These trees became my guardians in which I gave many of them names, and got to know them on a very personal level. On the ridgeways lived the pines, spruces, and firs. I remember feeling the difference in the deciduous forests as being more of a rich, deep, grounding experience where plants such as goldenseal, American ginseng, black and blue cohosh live, to the coniferous forests with the higher elevations and the endless vistas of ridgeways and valleys before me, lifting my spirit, taking me soaring into their heights with their fresh, penetrating, and elevating scents.

And now, although familiar with trees, there was a lot about trees I knew that I needed educate myself further. Feeling overwhelmed by the time and energy it would take for me to find the location, explore, experience, learn, write about, and adapt to the idea of including tree essences in my brand stirred me to take a walk in nature.

On my walk, I stopped along the way to examine a tree's bark that I couldn't identify. Since it was winter, the tree was bare, and I hadn't remembered this particular tree from previous hikes. My intent however, was to familiarize myself with getting to know tree barks for better identification purposes, which would then allow me to take more time to experience and be with the trees.

Instead I went on to a familiar and older mesquite tree, placed my hands on the bark, and examined it closely. The bark was grayish brown, rough and thick, and it appeared ragged into long and narrow strips. I knew it was a strong and sturdy bark as we use it for firewood; some folks use it to smoke meats. Various parts of the tree, including the bark, offer a variety of herbal healing uses.

I placed my nose against the mesquite bark to take in its musty, sweet and earthy smell, with my arms wrapped around the tree. I stood alone, feeling trapped by my own thoughts and constrictions, and my awareness of my inability in that moment to think outside of the box. Deep inside I knew that I needed to shake off my attitude and move on to something new that would expand my entire energetic system from within to without.

As I moved deeper into the silent, grounding energy of the mesquite tree, it touched a place in me that brought a natural balance and harmony. It was as if a re-patterning from what appears to be old and musky, invited me into a new sense of invigoration and freshness. I felt gifted with an insight in what I wanted to achieve with the trees, knowing that one thing has to happen before another, and to allow the process of it to unfold naturally.

I made a connection with the mesquite tree that day which grounded and guided me to move forward and to trust the mystery of it all. Later on my hike, I was given the opportunity to step into myself, embody my power, and take charge of myself when I crossed paths with a mountain lion. Yes that is another story, and a big one by the way, that I will share another time.

The mountain lion, however, reminded me to gain a deeper and more expansive perspective, to widen my lense and senses, to stretch beyond my familiar comfort zone, and to step into the momentum of change that empowers the innate ability to respond and be in the moment.

The presence of the mountain lion liberated something in me that forced me to shift my consciousness, discover my stature, gain my power, and to look outside the circle through an ever expanding lens that required me to expand with it. It marked a new beginning of engaging in the world of trees from winter, spring, summer, and fall in 2016 that will be forever enduring in my heart.

My journey of adapting to new territories, both geographically and internally, led me to an exploration and an enriching multitude of experiences with various trees, forests, animals, and people this past year which has expanded my consciousness, relationship, and love for trees. The stories the trees shared with me, and the beautiful healing energies they have to offer, continue to be a source of wisdom and inspiration.

Featuring Six Trees as Bioadaptogenic Flower Essences

Aspen   CrabApple   Oak   Olive   Walnut   Willow

Aspen (*Populus tremuloides*)

Quality: Adaptability

Family: Willow (Salicaceae)

Other Names: Golden aspen, trembling poplar, quaking aspen, American aspen, trembling aspen, mountain aspen, alamillo, white poplar, whispering tree

Where Found: Grows in various regions with diversified climate environments, generally lower altitudes in the north and higher altitudes in the south, and in communities from Canada, Alaska, throughout the United States, and in Mexico.

Elevation: 6,500' to 10,000'

Height: Generally around 40' though can grow up to 80'

Trunk: Average 12" in diameter

Bark: Whitish gray to yellowish bark is smooth, thin, and appears waxy. Ridged black dots appear around the tree from bottom to top, with indented holes that look like a vulva or a mother's womb. Lower branches tend to droop down while higher limbs lift upward.

As the tree ages, bark becomes thicker and turns a darker gray, somewhat furrowed.

The bark layer of quaking aspens transmits photosynthesis, which is usually reserved for tree leaves. When most other deciduous trees are dormant in the winter, aspens continue to produce sugar for energy.

Sap is a deep rich amber orange that emerges from the inner core of the tree with an amber-like balsamic scent and a hint of fruitiness.

Roots: Aspens commonly propagate mostly through root sprouts, spreading out clonal colonies. Each colony then becomes its own clone in which every tree in the clone produces identical characteristics, sharing a single root structure. Above ground, the clonal colony may appear as separate trees, however, they are genetically identical. Clones may turn color at different times in the fall than other neighboring clones, which is a simple way of showing the different colonies, and then in the spring the synchrony continues when the colonies flower, form catkins, and re-grow their leaves.

Individual quaking aspen stems can live up to 50 or 60 years, however, since multiple stems sprout from the same root system, they are replaced with new growth, allowing a colony of aspens a life span of thousands of years.

Flowers: Very small, discreet flowers with white stamens/filaments that emerge from amber/orange colored buds before the leaves appear. They are firm yet soft on the outside and develop into a drooping cylindrical shape. The male catkins contain pollen, and female catkins, eggs, in which feathery tufts adorned with soft, tiny, cottony seeds try to find their way in the winds to germinate and reproduce. Reproduction of the aspens, however, takes place mostly through the root system. Male and female catkins appear on separate trees.

Bloom in early spring before leaves are formed.

Buds alternate, are a reddish amber color, similar to the aspen sap. Terminal buds are conical shaped, pointed, very aromatic and balsamic, waxy, and grow up to about ¼ - ½ inch long. They are fascinating to visit time after time to see how their growth evolves. In fact, the entire developmental process of the aspen is intriquing.

Leaves: Rounded and flat with a short point, very fine double teeth, shiny green on the outside, dull green on the underside. Leaf stalk is longer than the leaf blade (known as petioles). and are without glands. There is a pattern of 6 leaves growing from a central stem. The leaves are tender, delicate, and have a lemon or citrus like scent.

Branches appear scattered, thin, and flexible, however, they are sturdier than they look and expand outward and circular into the sky.

The leaves dance and move with the rhythm of the wind appearing to "quake" or "tremble" in even the slightest breeze. And when the winds are quiet, the aspen is still and centered, present, yet waiting for its next movement.

Fruits: Found in small capsules along the stem, each capsule contains floss and disk at the base, is thin walled and narrow.

National Wildlife Federation Fun Fact: A grove of quaking aspens in Utah is the largest known living thing on Earth. Nearly 50,000 stems protrude from a single root system. The entire organism covers over 100 acres and weighs 6,000 tons! **National Wildlife Federation, "Quaking Aspen", https://www.nwf.org/Wildlife/Wildlife-Library/Plants/Quaking-Aspen.aspx**

Properties: As a member of the Willow family, aspen trees offer compounds such as salicin and populin, both which contain properties similar to aspirin to reduce fevers, offer pain relief, used as a sedative, and anti-inflammation.

Traditional Use: Traditional uses include stomach and liver disorders, arthritis, cancer, common cold, cystitis, debility, diarrhea, dysentery, dyspepsia, fever, fibrositis, flatulence, inflammation, rheumatism, and rheumatoid arthritis.

Aspen is also considered a tonic, diuretic, stimulant, anodyne, antiseptic, astringent, bitter, and a cholagogue (promoting the flow of bile).

Leaves, bark, root bark, and buds are used.

Other uses include making a root bark tea for excess menstrual flow, making a poultice of the root for cuts and wounds, making a tea of the inner bark for urinary issues, venereal disease, worms, colds, gargle for sore throat, and fevers.

The aromatic and balsamic buds can also be made into a tea but are more known in their use as a salve to treat skin irritations and burns.

Homeopathic Use: Homeopathic remedy is made from a tincture of the inner bark to treat dyspepsia and catarrh of the bladder, particularly with the elderly. Also used to treat indigestion with flatulence and acidity, nausea and vomiting, and painful urination (urine containing mucus and pus). It is a good remedy for cystitis, fullness of head, and sensation of heat of the surfaces of the body. (Boericke, Clarke).

Doctrine of Signatures:

*The trembling and quaking of aspen leaves represent a kind of nervousness and anxiety, fearfulness, and fragility. Yet they also communicate a freedom of dance, movement, confidence, release, and song. They're rustling brings awareness to the sense of listening and hearing, from within to without. They help you to pay attention to your rhythms and movements, voice and sound, and how you express yourself through body, mind, emotions, and spirit in the ways you adapt to change in your life. Giving yourself the freedom to communicate helps you to trust the process, think through the steps, embrace the winds, feel protected, make peace with "distractions", bring balance into your life, move freely, and let go.

*Because the Aspens propagate mostly through their root sprouts, and spread out into clonal colonies, this is a signature of their strength of community and coming together for a certain cause or purpose. Although each colony becomes its own clone and every tree in the clone shares identical characteristics and a single root structure underground, above ground they look as if they are separate trees. The union the colonies represent all come from the same source below, however, their individual diversity shows above. This signature shows the commonality of our human race, and in our ability to work together for a higher purpose regardless of our differences such as age, religion, nationality, occupation, geographical location, etc.

*The strength of community, union, and diversity protects and sustains each of the individual appearing trees that are all united with the same root source. Aspen groves can be considered immortal in human standards as they live continuously for thousands of years, sprouting shoots from their roots, as human, animals, and plants continue to bear their offspring.

*Lime green aspen catkins appear firm, bold, and strong yet soft and fuzzy.
The tiny cottony seeds in the female catkins are lifted into the winds, a signature of letting go, be it fear or anxiety, and trusting that the journey will take you right where you need to be. If germination and reproduction doesn't occur from the seed, the connection made with the root sprouts is all that matters as the colony will always be together as one both above ground and underground.

Patterns of Balance:

*The ability to be adaptable, to pay attention to your own life cycles and rhythms, and how you choose to align with them.

*Taking time to think through and to act accordingly on the steps needed to bring about balance in the moment and in the ways to move forward.

*Bringing in new directions for new beginnings, letting go of fears of the unknown.

*Ability to listen to and be with the winds of change.

*Changing the direction of fear to one of protection, and looking outside the perimeters to see a larger picture.

*Recognizing the shimmer of confidence within yourself, and knowing that you can trust the moment and the future. By doing so, you naturally let go of anxiety, nervousness, and fear.

Patterns of Imbalance:

*Ongoing fears of the unknown and not understanding where these fears come from

*For those who feel anxious and nervous, especially about letting go of the old and the familiar

*For those afraid of facing the unforeseen and doing new things.

*Inability to let go and to trust the journey.

Affirmation:

 I consciously take each step along my journey in confidence and trust that my life is unfolding with my own natural rhythms, as I move forward and bring in new ways of being and living.

Chakras: 1st, 2nd, 3rd

CrabApple (*Malus spp.*)

Quality: Heart Wisdom

Family: Rosaceae

Other Names: Wild apple, Pomme d'Api, Lady's Finger, Wax Apple and Christmas Apple. Also known as "jewels of the landscape."

Malus is a genus of about 30–55 species of small deciduous apple **trees** or shrubs in the family

Where Found: Temperate zones of the Northern Hemisphere, throughout the USA, Canada, Russia, Asia, and Europe.

Wild crabapple habitats include woodlands, woodland openings and borders, grasslands, and thickets, and they grow both in upland and bottomland areas with other deciduous trees in moist, well drained, and slightly acidic soil. They can survive in adverse conditions with little water during dry weather. Crab apples also adapt to and have the ability to thrive in cold weather.

Elevation: 7,000 to 8,000'

Height: Average 15' to 25', though can grow up to 35' tall tat maturity, with a dense, twiggy yet canopy crown

Trunk: Short knotty, somewhat crooked trunk with large branches growing from it

Bark: Grayish-brown shaggy bark with a reddish hue, furrowed and rough, peels off. Longitudinal scales curve along the tree. Large branches are similar in color though smoother, and smaller thorny branches grow from the larger ones.

The trees grow in numerous shapes such as weeping or pendulous, rounded or canopy like, spreading horizontal, upright (more columnar), or the shape of a vase, or a shape of a pyramid.

Roots: Crabapple's root systems is mostly surface with just a few roots going deeper. The woody roots branch out, and they produce underground runners with clonal offspring.

Flowers: It's no wonder that Crabapple's are referred to as "jewels of the landscape" as they produce the most beautiful, elegant, and attractive showy fuschia and deep pink blossoms. The aromatic blossoms are filled with a fruity fragrance in the Spring that makes your heart sing!

Crabapple's flowers grow in a group or cluster that is arranged on a stem either from a larger main branch or from an irregular thorny branch. The cluster of flowers show a specific pattern in which the outer flowers grow on a longer though small stalk, and tend to bloom first so when the inner flowers of the cluster bloom, all are at the same common height.

The flower buds first appear as a small tight jaw (reminding me of a closed down heart), but when the flowers open, they appear in their cluster as a perfect floral arrangement with five symmetrical petals and a burst of stamens with golden yellow anthers that produce pollen. They have a half-interior ovary where the lower half is embedded in the stem, and the upper half is exposed.

Being in the presence of the flowering Crab Apple is a heart opening and heart awakening experience that lifts the soul.

Crabapples are cross-pollinated mostly by bees (and insects) which enjoy the flowers for both their nectar and their pollen. Crab Apple trees cannot self-pollinate.

Leaves: Ovate-like leaves average from about 1-2" wide to 2-3" long. They alternate along the stem and have a slightly saw-toothed margin.
The top of the leaf surface is yellowish to bright green in color and hairless. The underside surface of the leaf is a paler green and also hairless. The transition of the leaf from the stem (petiole) is about ¾-2" long, also hairless, and their color varies from a light green to a bright red.

Fruits: Crabapple fruits are similar to an apple, though they are much smaller and sour tasting. The colorful fruits appear in the Fall and often endure throughout the Winter.

The red fruit is referred to as a "globose pome" or ovoid shaped fruit that varies in size from about ½"-2" in diameter. There are five carpels arranged in a star-like shape in the center of the fruit, with each carpel containing 1-2 seeds.

The fruits are rarely eaten raw as they contain malic acid which causes the sour taste. However, there are some Asian cultures that make the fruit into a sour condiment, and eat the condiment with chili peppers or perhaps a shrimp paste.

Crabapples do contain pectin, and juiced or canned, can be made into jellies, preserves, and juices.

Properties: Astringent, Malic Acid

Traditional Use: The fruit can be used as an astringent and laxative.
Crushing the fruit and making a poultice from the fruit pulp can be used to treat inflammations, abrasions, and small flesh wounds. Bark, especially root bark can be used to destroy parasitic worms, to promote cooling, to induce drowsiness or sleep, and to treat intermittent fevers. Leaves can be dried and drank as a tea as they contain an antibacterial substance and are pleasantly tasting.

The seeds do produce an edible oil and can be extracted along with the pulp to make a cider or juiced drink.

Homeopathic Use: Unknown to Author

Doctrine of Signatures:
*Crabapple buds appear tight jawed, closed down, and due to the pink color you can't help but feel the presence of a closed down heart, confused in how to feel, speak, or just be. The opening of the flowers in their clusters yield an energetic presence and awareness of the heart field, offering a joyful, uplifting, and feeling of connection from deep within the heart. The flowers offer a power of divine mind and innocence, beauty and mystery of the soul. Residing in this power place of the heart, if we allow the flow of heart, mind, and emotions as one, we can activate that flow from a place of love rather than a place of control or fear. If in the mind we are letting go, we can truly freely expose the heart and soul by trusting the heart shield from within. Feeling replenished, we bring in wisdom and resources from the heart.

*Crabapple fruit is sour, and the signature for that resembles the crabby person or sour person we meet in our lives, or when that crabby nature comes out in ourselves. The fruit is a teacher of how to venture outside of the fence and to manage our boundaries when we feel exposed or controlled by others or conditions that make us feel vulnerable. This signature helps us to get out of our head, let go of our own toxicities, and trust the inner heart shield, feeling safe, loved, and supported depicted by the flower clusters.

Patterns of Balance:

*Ability to trust and surrender into the heart

*Making a conscious choice to activate love over fear and trusting the heart's flow

*Feeling replenished and cleansed, allowing and trusting the wisdom of what you feel inside your heart to guide you

*Letting go of what you consider as imperfections

*Feeling loved and supported as you cleanse old patterns and let go of the old

Patterns of Imbalance:

 *Stuck in the illusion of being in control

*Being and living out of touch of the flow of your heart.

*For those who live in fear, "the wounded child", and are blameful toward others

* For those who hold grief, unable or unwilling to let go and allow the heart to open

Affirmation:

"I love and support myself, trusting in my heart's wisdom."

Chakras: 1st and 4th

Crabapple Story:

I'd like to share a short story which is really a very long story about my experience with the Crabapple tree the day I made my first Crabapple flower essence in April 2016. I drove to Flagstaff to meet Phyliss Hogan and DeAnn Tracy at DeAnn's home where they live in a neighborhood prolific with Crabapples.
Upon determining which tree to be with, DeAnn, Mike (her husband), Bodhi (her son), Phyliss, and I all gathered around the abundantly flowered tree, feeling the energy of it, taking in its fragrance, and making an essence. It was definitely an experience of the heart, feeling the connection of family and friends, and including the intrigue of a youngster.

While the blossoms of the flowers were infusing in a bowl of water, DeAnn's dog somehow got out of the fenced in yard and ran away to the neighbors down the street, unbeknownst to us. When DeAnn saw her dog and hear an unknown woman walking across the street, she ran to go greet the woman and apologize for her dog. This interaction turned into quite a conflicting event as the woman was extremely upset and shouting her not so kind words that could be heard throughout the neighborhood including Bodhi and his friends.   It took all DeAnn had to stay in her heart centered power, hold her boundaries, and speak her truths to this unruly woman. It turned out, the woman was visiting from out of state, and her grandmother who lived down the street has just died.

The innocent and harmless dog wandered into the deceased grandmother's yard which triggered the woman to lash out at DeAnn. The woman verbally attacked DeAnn seemingly from a place of anger, grief, and emotional imbalance, and chose to vent her "crabbiness" and illusion of being in control onto DeAnn.

Stories and events that share the signatures of the flowers, plants, and trees seem to show up when I make flower essences. This story is quite profound in all the ways that Crabapple flower essence has to offer.

Oak (Quercus gambelii)

Quality: Enduring Strength

Family: Beech (Fagaceae)

Other Names: Rocky Mountain white oak, Live Oak, Gambel's Oak, Utah White Oak, Fendler's Oak, Encino

Where Found: Western North America in mountains, plateaus, foothills, and especially mountain ravines where there is runoff from above flourishing on rocky hillsides in alkaline soil with a heavy draw on soil moisture, and in full sun.

Elevation: 3,300' to 9,800' (though average is 5,000' to 8,000')

Height: Shrub to tree up to 50'

Trunk: Up to 2 ½' diameter though old trees can reach a larger girth, and often you will see them grow as multi trunks (more than one main trunk).

Bark: Is thick, rough and scaly, brownish-gray. Though the tree's wood is densely thick, branches are irregular and crooked.

Roots: The tree mainly spreads from its root sprouts, growing from an underground deep-feeding root system called lignotubers that have numerous scattered buds. Rhizomes interconnect clones that intervene with the lignotubers. Clones are generally uniform in their characteristics such as shape, color, and development. It is fascinating that the oak has the strength and ability to thrive under both morphological adaptations (physical changes that occur over generations based on environmental conditions such as water deficiency), and physiological adaptations (how the oak's internal response for survival responds to external stimuli, especially drought and moisture, to gain or maintain homeostasis). Its deep root system helps the tree to sustain soil stability and reduce erosion.

Oak trees in general, are known for their slow and steady growth, and the strength of their trunk and limbs.

Flowers: Small male and female flowers grow on the same tree, occurring in the Spring. Males appear as drooping fuzzy catkins that appear with the leaves, and the females in clusters with a ring of small leaves or bracts at the base and producing a short spike with a cup shaped growth and evolves into an acorn. The development and production of mature flowers and seeds is based on the availability of moisture. When there is a lot of moisture, both male and female flowers are produced abundantly.

Generally you will see the female flowers throughout the oak canopy, and the male flowers located more at the top of the tree.

Leaves: Upper leaves surface is a glossy dark green, while the undersurface is a paler green with soft hairs, velvety in touch. Leaves are oblong, growing up to 6" long and 2.5 " broad, with 7 to 11 rounded lobes. In the Fall, trees lace the mountainsides with leaves turning colors to orange, reds, and yellows.

Fruit: Acorns follow the catkins as a brownish, oval, bowl-like cup that grows under an inch long (.75" long and .63 " broad) and is enclosed by a cap or cup (called a cupule). As the acorns mature in the Fall, they turn from green to golden brown. Gambel oaks can reproduce from acorns as well as its root system.

The acorns are primarily scattered by rodents and birds, and sometimes, squirrels.

Properties: Astringent, Tannins, Tannic acid, Gallic acid, and Quercin
Oak is considered an ally to the Willow in which certain properties of Salacin and its compounds are similar to those of Quercin.

Traditional Use: As an astringent, a tea can be made from the bark as a wash to treat gum inflammations, a gargle for sore throats, and to drink as an intestinal tonic, and for diarrhea. (Michael Moore, *Medicinal Plants of the Mountain West*.

Michael Moore suggests that hikers and backpackers place the gambel oak in their list of native remedies for first aid intervention as it is easy to identify and easy to access. He also references all parts of the Oak as an antiseptic to treat inflammations, burns, abrasions, and cuts. Leaves can be chewed and used as a poultice for insect bites, and bark can be chewed to treat toothache pain.

Often you will see galls growing on the twigs or small branches of oak trees, known as 'oak apples' that are pale yellow-brownish in color and somewhat spongy. Larva hatches from the eggs laid by wasps on the twigs upon which they feed on, and secret an enzyme that forms the shape of a gall. The galls contain tannins/astringents that can also be used externally as a wash, either fresh or dried.

My first experience of taking time to examine galls was with David Holiday in our neighboring Sedona wilderness many years ago. Sure enough, upon opening several galls, we discovered that when fully developed, the gall-wasp enters a chrysalis state, bores a small hole into the side of the gall, and escapes into the air. If you break the gall open, you can see a tiny cavity that holds the remains of the larva. The gall itself has a slight and sweet astringent taste. Nature is so fascinating!

Acorns are generally considered indigestible for human consumption, however, dried and ground acorns can be made into a nourishing flour, as they are comprised of a starchy carbohydrate. Ground acorns have also been used as a coffee substitute.

Gambel oaks are a vital and ecological source of food, shelter, and habitat for many animals including deer, livestock, insects, squirrels, small animals and birds.

Homeopathic Use: Quercus robar (English Oak), made from a tincture of the peeled and crushed acorns, (Spiritus glandium quercus-Spirit distilled from the tincture), (Aqua glandium quercus – water extract with alcohol), are used to treat spleen, vertigo, deafness, reduce craving for alcoholics, constipation, diarrhea, gout, and intermittent fever. (Clarke and Boericke)

Doctrine of Signatures:

*Oak's ability to thrive and survive in various climate changes, soil and moisture conditions, and to pace itself slowly in its own growth cycles by depending on its deep root system, demonstrates the nature of Oak's strength and adaptability to gain, sustain, and maintain homeostasis. Oak's form a strong foundation, as their strength also comes from the inside, forming a structure of "strong bones", teaching us the importance of what it means to anchor and hold our energy from a place of strength and endurance.

* The rough appearance of Oak's trunk, irregular branches, bark, and its overall fortitude, shows a signature of its toughness and strength. The bark also represents a sturdy shield, guarding the boundary of our inner strength. By trusting the shield, we are reminded that we as humans, have choices in the ways we go about our life. There are times when we may have to get through something, to forge ahead, to be enduring and strong to accomplish our goals. Yet we can be enduring and strong in the ways we find balance in our lives, in our inner selves, and the ways we learn to adapt to our environment and situations, nourish ourselves, and be creative in allowing our life flow to unfold naturally.

*Oak's catkins/flowers are strong and fuzzy, they find their hold on the stem and don't seem to let go. Although letting go is certainly a needed life long process for each of us everyday, the catkins also show us when to grab on and to feed our own strength in those times of need to empower who we are. I like the signature and the meaning of the word "gall" as related to the galls that grow on the tree as sometimes it takes a lot of "gall" or nerve to stand up for ourselves, to speak our truths, and then through some amazing miracle or chrysalis state, we find a breath of fresh air, we transform and move forward in life, leaving only a slight imprint of the past behind.

* Acorns have intrigued me since I was a child. They have those tiny little hats and sturdy round bodies. You can create the most wonderful nature art with acorns, and also use them as buttons. As the fruit of the tree, acorns offer yet another creative endeavor, a developmental stage of true originality that sparks inspiration and encourages new ideas, as forward motion in something exciting to look forward to in moving on. Like the squirrel gathering acorns for the winter, it has food and sustenance to look forward to, that feeds its soul, body, and mind.

Patterns of Balance:

*Ability to anchor and protect your energy field while feeling grounded, balanced, and strong in who you are

*Ability to nourish your strength from deep inside

*Knowing who you are from a place of strength and fortitude, with the ability to adapt to life situations in ways that sustain and nourish you.

*Helps you to trust your foundation of self, allowing you to be inspired and creative from within to without as you move forward in your life.

Patterns of Imbalance:

*Feeling insecure and not connected to something stabilizing

*Lack of inner strength , endurance, and solid structure

*For those who are over-tired, fatigued, and overworked, looking for balance in their lives

*For those who feel hopelessness and despair

Affirmation:

"I am anchored in the power of my being and true to my own inner strength."

Chakras: 1st, 2nd, and 3rd

Olive (Oleo manzanillo)

Quality: Peace Tree

Family: Oleaceae

Other Names: Unknown to Author

Where Found: Originally from the Mediterranean (Spain), likes well drained soil and full sun, survives best in non-frost areas, and can tolerate cycles of drought. Loves living by the seacoast.

Is considered as an evergreen-deciduous tree, and known as the oldest cultivated tree dating back to more than 5,000 years.

Height: Ranges from 20' – 30'. It is a low spreading tree that makes it easier to manage and harvest.

Trunk: Known as a multi-trunk (more than one main trunk or stem), oval shaped tree, may grow cankers which are dead places on the trunk or bark on main branches, possibly by injury or bacteria, however these cankers do not seem to interrupt the growth or yield of the tree.

Bark: Gray, smooth, knotty at the base. Branches are smooth, slender, and firm, yet bending. Young stems shoot up straight into the sky, while older stems dangle/droop from branches. The stems are smooth, olive green, and firm yet flexible. There are numerous thin branches with smaller branchlets growing in opposites.

Roots: Root system is generally shallow, penetrating 3-4 feet deep into the soil, there are reports of roots in certain olive species found 49 feet from the tree trunk as well as living more than 1000 years.

Flowers: Creamy white flowers grow as a cylindrical flower cluster in a slender and drooping catkin. Flowers appear in pairs and are petalless with stamens fertile with pollen. Catkins are a lime green/pale green and grow in small clusters from a single leaf stem. They are bitter tasting, and offer a strong presence with a feeling of gentle grace. Infused with water, the catkins/blossoms carry a refreshing and aromatic taste and smell that invigorates and uplifts.

Leaves: Emerging from a short stalk on a branch, narrow pale green leaves with a silver lining and one central vein grow in opposites with single leaves in between. Darker shiny green on the topside, paler green and silvery on the underside. Lanceolate leaves appear sleek, elegant, strong, smooth, yet leathery.

Fruits: Develop from summer into fall into an ovoid or apple shape that begins light green in color and when mature, becomes black with a hint of purple, into a size of about an inch. It offers an excellent flesh-to-pit ratio, and the texture of the olive fruit is considered superb and also easy to remove the seed from the flesh. These attributes make it popular for processors of pitted and stuffed olives, and for pressing the fruit into oil, which produces into a rich green color with an abundant fruity flavor making it a fine grade oil. "Manzanillo" is one of the most common olive trees for commercial growing and shown to be one of the heaviest yields of fruit.

Properties: Rich in antioxidants, Oleic acid, (useful to protect the heart), polyphenols (reduces oxidative stress in the brain), iron, monounsaturated fats, various minerals and vitamins.

Traditional Use: The olive tree has an ancient history with great value not only for its fruit and oils as nutrition, or leaves for crowns, but also for its longevity and its recognition as a symbol of goodness and purity, happiness and peace.
The olive branch also represents a symbol of peace and even victory, and worn by brides and virgins form the customs of ancient Greece. The olive tree is culturally known to the West as well as to the Mediterranean basin.

Also, known as the tree of wisdom in various cultures, it is believed that the gods gifted the olive tree to the people. The symbol of the Goddess Athena holding an olive branch beside the owl, also represents peace.

The leaves of olive can be used as an extract, an herbal tea, and a powder, and are considered an astringent, antiseptic, anti-inflammatory, hypocholesterolemic, and also along with the bark and made into a tea, can help to reduce fevers.

Thus olive leaf treats viral, bacterial, infections relating to influenza, pneumonia, shingles, herpes, the common cold, ear and teeth infections, and even known to cure hepatitis B. Also good for high blood pressure, diabetes, hay fevers, diarrhea, and digestive issues.

The oil soothes and protects irritated tissue and is also a laxative. It can help relieve stings and burns, and is good to use for liniments. The wonderful healing and nourishing properties of olive oil can be made into a lubricant for the skin such as in lotions, salves, ointments, etc., to treat a variety of conditions (irritated skin, muscular, joint, chills, chest complaints, diaper rashes and more). Olive oil is known to prevent heart attacks and stroke, cardiovascular disease (lowering blood pressure), and to prevent breast cancer, rheumatoid arthritis and migraine headaches.

The oil is also used as a cleanser in liver or gall bladder detoxes or to boost bacteria in the gut.

Olives are filled with vitamins and minerals that include Vitamin E, copper, calcium, sodium, and other plant compounds that are particularly high in antioxidants. One serving of olives a day helps to improve memory and is a rich source of iron.

The curing process of olives includes the addition of vinegar which also helps to support good health. Low in calories, though high in healthy monounsaturated fats, Vitamin E, and antioxidant phytonutrients, including polyphenols, olives can also help a person lose weight and offer nutrient rich heart healthy support.

Olive oil is a delightful nutrient for cooking and salads.

Homeopathic Use: Unknown to Author

Doctrine of Signatures:
*Due to the symbolism of its history and the powerful energetic field that the olive tree demonstrates and emits, one can't help but feel a sense of deep wisdom, strength, and peace from being in the presence of this tree. The branches are strong and bending, yet yield an elegant and gentle grace. The tree itself seems to hold its ground, it leans toward the earth yet its branches reach toward the sky, anchoring a feeling of balance and rest while sitting under the tree.

*The presence of the olive tree also brings a feeling of being guided or directed from the inside, from a peaceful state of being in the moment, not looking behind or ahead.

*The natural flow of the tree, similar to the energy of willows, also shares a balance of giving and receiving, of trusting the flow, of allowing life to unfold on its own, of giving up control.

Patterns of Balance:

*Allowing yourself and your life experiences to unfold naturally rather than trying to be in control of them.

*"Trusting your inner guidance with a gentle presence."

*Conscious engagement of living life peacefully from within to without.

*Honoring your thoughts and feelings, as well as your lifestyle that brings you balance and flow."

Patterns of Imbalance:

*Struggling with being in control of yourself, others, and life situations

*Feeling overwhelmed and worn out in every way

*Feeling out of balance and lacking peace within yourself and your life's choices

*Inability to choose a direction, and to honor and allow it to unfold on its own

Affirmation:

 "With gentle grace, I live in peace, and allow my life to unfold naturally."

Chakras: 6th and 7th

*With gratitude to Rennie and Andrea Radoccia for sharing their most beautiful Manzanillo olive tree with me.

Walnut (*Juglans major*)

Primary Quality: New Directions

Family: Walnut

Other Names: Nogal, Black Walnut, "Nux" (Romans), "Wallnuss" (Germans), "Jupiter's nuts"

Where Found: Near streams, canyons in the higher desert, grasslands and meadows. woodlands

Elevation: 3,500' to 7,000"

Height: Can grow up to 40' to 60' tall with a crown of branches that spread out sporadically

Trunk: Up to 3' and sometimes larger in circumference, thick and massive

Bark: Grayish brown, rough and rugged as the tree matures. Young shoots are tender and smooth.

Roots: Extend up to 50 feet or more from the trunk and secrete a natural herbicide known as juglone that prevents other forms of plants from growing within their reach, including their own off-spring. Black walnuts need deep, fertile soil with a near-neutral or a touch of acidic pH. They live nearly disease-free with very few pests that threaten them.

Flowers: Both male and female flowers grow separately on the same tree.
Male flowers are a hanging catkin with a calyx of five or six scales encircled by stamens. The female flowers grow in an erect cluster and have a calyx that closely surrounds the ovary, bearing two or three fleshy stigmas.

Leaves: Pinnately compound, smooth and shiny and lime-green on top, duller green underneath, though young leaf shoots are reddish green and grow up to 4- 41/2 " long, 1 or so inches wide.
Mature leaves are coarsely toothed and lance-shaped, aromatic and spicy, and can grow up to 14" long. Walnut leaves are one of the first trees to loose their leaves in the fall and the last tree to leaf out in the spring.

Fruits: Are hard-shelled and round that generally produce nuts in a cycle with a more abundant crop about every 5-6 years that increasingly grow more with each year.

Properties: The active ingredient of the walnut tree, including all its parts - leaves, roots, husks, fruit (the epicarp), and bark and the nuts, is Nucin or Juglon which is harmful and growth-stunting to many other plants.

Traditional Use: Walnut wood is a valuable and unique species of hardwoods, used for cabinetry, furniture making, and many kinds of wooden objects and novelties.

Generally the bark and leaves are dried and contain properties as an alterative, laxative, astringent, and detergent used to treat various types of problems that may include tuberculosis, lymph nodes, eczema,

herpes,
internal ulcerations, inflammations, mucous and hemorrhagic discharges, diarrhea, tumors, cancers, abscesses, boils, skin itch and irritations, ringworms, shingles, as a purgative, and more. The husk, shell, and peel cause sweating especially when green for destroying all worms.

Juicing the green husks (and boiled with honey) is used for sore throats, and as a mouth gargle, and the water from the husks can be used externally for wounds.

Harvest time for walnuts is during the month of August. The thin cover on their green hull about the size of a baseball, but softer like a softball, starts to crack open and exposes the hard-shelled brownish nut inside which is about the size of a lemon. The actual walnut kernel consists of two ridged (bi-lobed), light brown lobes, characterizing the human brain and keeping their reputation from ancient days as a symbol of intellectualism. The lobes are covered with a papery thin skin, and the two lobes are attached together in the center.

Walnut kernals offer a rich source of nutritional benefits including minerals (**manganese, copper**, potassium, calcium, **iron,** magnesium, zinc, and selenium), antioxidants (*melatonin, ellagic acid, vitamin-E, carotenoids, and polyphenolic compounds* known to offer health benefits against cancer, aging, inflammation, and neurological diseases), vitamins (B-complex groups of vitamins such as riboflavin, niacin, thiamin, pantothenic acid, vitamin B-6, and folates), protein, and in particular, monounsaturated fatty acids such as oleic acid and omega-3 essential acids which support a healthy blood lipid profile.

A handful of walnuts daily may help to lower total cholesterol and LDL while improving HDL blood levels, thus diminishing chances for stroke and coronary artery disease, and protection from colon, breast, and prostate cancers.

Walnut oil can be used in skin care, as it helps the skin to preserve moisture and prevent dryness. The oil can also be used in cooking, and as a carrier oil in aroma and massage therapies, and in cosmetics.

Walnut oil and walnut butter both transmit a beautiful nutty and delicious flavor, gentle to the taste buds.

Homeopathic Use: A tincture of the whole plant may be useful of cutting the wisdom tooth. – "A Modern Herbal" Volume II – Editor p.842

Doctrine of Signatures:

* The outer green husk as a covering for the walnut offers a signature of the head, resembling the external skin of the skull (the Pericranium) and corresponds to the ability to know how to protect oneself from the outside world to prevent unnecessary hardships. It teaches us to learn how to adapt to and endure hardships if and when they do occur, and to step into new places while feeling shielded or protected.

*The fruit of the walnut or the smooth inner woody shell around the kernel demonstrates the signature of a human skull, offering yet another layer of protection for the actual kernel. This signature serves as a shield, allowing us to explore and trust the depths from deep within while feeling encircled with protection, allowing us to move forward as needed.

*The walnut kernel lies secure within its shell that is layered by the covering of the outer husk. Finding its place in the center, two halves joined as one, the kernel resembles the balance between the left and right atrium, left and right ventricles and corresponding tricuspid valve and mitral valve of the human heart. In addition, the walnut kernel's bi-lobed signature also characterizes the human brain and the true intellect of the brain which comes from living in the heart, being true to oneself in harmony with both the brain and the heart. This symbiotic relationship brings in a natural state of balance, inner strength, and inner stability reinforcing and supporting the journey of the soul.

*The natural property of juglon which is in every part of the walnut tree, offers a signature of strength, endurance, and protection that wards off predators, pests, and other plant life. This signature also refers to learning how to live dis-ease free, warding off the dangers that inhibit vitality.

* Male catkins are protected with a calyx of scales encircled by stamens, and female flowers are protected by a calyx that closely surrounds the ovary. The calyx has a sense of position, of strategy, of knowing its place. These signatures resemble that of knowing how to protect and guard your energies, while remaining true to yourself and living the path of your soul purpose.

* Catkins are plush, firm, and taste bitter. They offer a sense of vibrancy, of tenacity to stay true to oneself, to learn from the journey behind you, and to trust the journey that lies ahead.

*When the walnut hulls fall from the tree, those that bounce away from the tree stand a much better chance of surviving than those that fall into the soil of the parent tree that is spread with juglon. This is a signature depicting the the parents role to support the child to trust and move forward in life, allowing the child to find a new direction, yet offering guidance and support.
This signature symbolizes our ability to move forward yet to trust our roots and to feel grounded and anchored by the soul's journey.

Patterns of Balance:

*Ability to move forward yet being guided by your roots and anchored by your soul

*Ability to protect oneself from the outside world, and to know how to adapt to and endure hardships while staying strong and grounded especially in times of struggle

*Remaining true to yourself and your soul purpose

*Ability to explore and trust the depths of life's experiences and allowing them to unfold naturally

*Allowing your personal journey to trust from deep within, letting go of the past, living in the moment, and moving forward into the future, with strength and endurance, not looking back.

Patterns of Imbalance:

*For those who lack vitality and who feel insecure

*Inability to find ways to anchor yourself in order to have the strength and endurance needed to move forward in your life

*Inability to trust or tap into those places deep within that offer you guidance and strength.

*For those who give up easily and who have difficulty recognizing ways to empower themselves.

*For those who have difficulty letting go of the old

Affirmation:

"I trust that the core of my inner strength will carry me through life in a loving way."

Chakras: 1st, 2nd, 3rd, 4th, and 7th

Willow (Salix Goodingii)
Primary Quality: Forgiveness

Family: Willow (Salicaceae)

Other Names: Goodding Willow, Western Black Willow, Dudley Willow

Where Found: Along banks and streams in the western U.S. and river valleys in northern Mexico (Riparian areas from northern California to southern Utah, southeast through New Mexico to the Texas panhandle, and west to Arizona and southern California

Elevation: below 7,000'

Height: 20' – 60'

Trunk: Can grow up to 30 inches in diameter, and
usually has many branches growing from it. The branches are gray, thicker, and rougher toward the bottom, but light, slender, smoother, and yellowish toward the top. In fact, they are so light that they bend and sway gracefully in the wind

Bark: The grayish bark is thick and rough, with deep indentations
that have narrow ridges.

Roots: This willow species has a deep root system that helps stop stream erosion. Root depths grow up to 7 feet and have a deeper main root with small prolific surface roots.

Flowers: Green/white, grow in a small clustered spike that consists of tiny, unisexual, petalless flowers called "catkins." The tiny closed flowers alternate along the stem and are followed by white cottony seeds that bud open. The catkins are light and delicate, and grow up to 3 1/2 inches long.
Blooming Period: March through May

Leaves: The shiny leaves are bright green or lime green,
narrow, lanceolate, finely toothed, and long-pointed. The curved leaves are longer and larger toward the bottom of the stem and shorter and smaller toward the top of the stem. The leaves have one central vein and can grow up to 5 inches long and 3/4 inch wide.

Properties: The primary active ingredient is salicin extracted from the bark of the willow and is used to treat arthritis and rheumatism, and as a substitute for quinine.

Traditional Use: There are many species of willow. It is difficult to identify some species due to the variation of leaves and the cross-breeding of different species. Due to the complexity and numbers of willow trees, this section speaks to the general history and uses of a variety of willows. The willow has a fascinating history of uses and symbology. It was considered to be a symbol of death and/or immortality by several cultures. The Chinese viewed it as a symbol of immortality because a newtree can be grown from a small branch.

The willow was sacred to the Greek and Roman goddesses Circe, Hecate, and Persephone, all of whom are Mother Goddess death aspects. The plant has also been seen as a symbol of mourning in the form of the weeping willow. Ancient Greeks wore willow leaves around the neck after a heartbreaking love affair. Dioscorides prescribed willow for pain and inflammation, and the historically far-removed Hottentots used a willow concoction as a remedy for rheumatic fever.

The American Indians used the willow similarly and passed along this information to the white settlers. They also used branches as poles for tipis and to used to make sweat lodges, especially in the southwestern U.S., and they provide the structure for hoop weavings and dream catchers. They are known for their flexibility and strength.

Medicinally, willow bark has been used for centuries for its cooling actions to reduce pain and inflammation as well as to lower fevers. In the 1820s, the active ingredient salicin was isolated. In the late 1800s, a German chemist by the name of Felix Hoffman was looking for some relief for his father's arthritis. He formulated a drug now widely known as aspirin from salicin. Salicin extracted from the bark of the willow was also used as a substitute for quinine. Salicin is an active ingredient used to treat arthritis and rheumatism. Also, by steeping willow bark and twigs in water, you can make a bitter drink to relieve pains and chills.

Various willows have numerous other medicinal uses. They are used to make eye drops, as an astringent, as a sex depressant, for restoration of the stomach and liver, and to treat hay fever, chills, dandruff, diarrhea, earache, flu, heartburn, headache, impotence, chronic inflammation and infection, muscle soreness, night sweats, rheumatism, worms, dysentery, and disability of the digestive organs. Willow's antispasmodic qualities have been used to treat whooping cough and asthma. The willow herb has wonderful antiseptic qualities and can be used to treat infected wounds, ulcerations, or eczema. This makes it a useful first-aid herb for hikers to be familiar with.

Cosmetically, whole willow is found in face creams, detergents, lotions, and herbal baths due to its astringent properties. As an ornamental plant, willow is valued for its beauty. Willows offer practical landscaping solutions, especially in marshy areas and to stabilize stream banks.

Homeopathic Use: Salix nigra, or Black Willow, is a homeopathic remedy that regenerates the organs of both sexes, treats hysteria and nervousness, restrains genital irritability, and tempers sexual passion. It is used to treat conditions such as red and swollen face, sore and bloodshot eyes, nervousness before and after menses, painful menstruation, excessive menstrual discharge, pain associated with movement of the testicles, and back pain across sacral and lumbar areas.

Doctrine of Signatures:

*A significant signature of the willow is the strong, unique, bitter taste in the leaves and in the flower-essence water. The bitterness that the leaves and flower essence leaves in your mouth is similar to the bad feeling of bitterness toward an experience or person in your life. Emotional bitterness may cause resentment, biting criticism, slashing or snapping out, and a feeling of vengefulness.
It may also feed on the feeling of being a victim in an unjust
world. When injustice is experienced, an emotional bitterness
toward life may be carried over into other situations and relationships.
The lesson of this signature is to be aware of how bitterness thrives within each of us. Rather than falling into victim consciousness or vengeful consciousness, we need to find a way to
gather the power to come into our heart to let go of the bitterness and resentment. The acts of injustice done by others will sooner or later come back around to them, and these injustices will be taken care of in a natural way that is much bigger than us.

*The willow tree likes dampness and commonly grows along rivers and streams. Growing near water represents deep emotions which, if not allowed to flow with the waters, are kept inside where unhappiness, resentment, and bitterness can grow. The willow's deep root system holds the soil and stops streambank erosion. When the creek or stream rises, the willow holds the soil together to keep it from being eaten or worn away. This signature also relates to the one previously mentioned: When we are able to "keep it together," we can prevent ourselves from being worn out by the bitterness of others so that our own bitterness does not seep in. The positive willow will give a person the needed inner strength (related, again, to holding the soil together) to flow with the water or emotions and to release whatever bitterness, feelings of despair, or resentment a person is holding onto.

*The thick, rough ridges of the lower bark also symbolize our own rough emotional edges and our ability to deal with barriers in life that may appear to hold us back and drain our energy. Yet these barriers help us grow in our own inner strength. The upper branches are smooth, graceful, and flexible. They dance and move with the wind — with the ebb and flow of life's wisdom and grace. This signature relates to our ability to be flexible in the way we approach life and all living beings. Willow also demonstrates
flexibility and the flow of life in the way it grows along water and is nurtured by water. If you try to force the branches to bend, they
may snap; when they are moistened in water, they gain even more
strength, endurance, and ability to stretch and bend.

*The green tiny catkin flowers are petalless. They gently and humbly hang along the stem. They represent the fourth chakra, the heart. The opening of our hearts helps us let go of resentments and emotional wounds, past hurts, suffering, and bitterness. Slowly, tiny white cottony seeds emerge from the opening bud and expand into a soft cotton down covering the catkin, becoming exposed to the light. This signature relates to the seventh chakra, the expansion of consciousness, and the ability to seek and gain higher spiritual awareness in spite of our challenges. The passage from the closed, bitter, limiting catkin to the white cottony seed-bud opening is symbolic of reaching a broader understanding with ourselves and the Divine Power that is bigger than, yet inclusive of, the physical world and our experiences in it.

Patterns of Balance

* Helps us take our personal matters to their root cause, encouraging us to understand ourselves and any bitterness, resentment, or roughness

that we may feel.

* Teaches us to be flexible in the ways we approach life and all living things, and to move with the ebb and flow of life's wisdom and grace.

*Helps prevent ourselves from being worn out by the bitterness of others so that our own bitterness does not seep in.

*Helps us understand ourselves as a system of energy, guiding us to be mindful of the situations we find ourselves in and to expand our conscious awareness of our biological heritage.

*Helps us find compassion within ourselves, open our hearts toward others, and act accordingly.

Patterns of Imbalance: For those who:
* Feel resentment and emotional bitterness, especially related to unjust situations or people; symptoms of sleeplessness, restlessness, and impatience may develop
* Lash out blamefully, criticize others in a vengeful manner, and have closed down hearts
*Lack flexibility in how they approach life and carry grudges against others
*Feel victimized in an unjust world
*Are patient, understanding, and compassionate as long as they possibly can be in challenging situations until they are set off by people who are petty, who stretch boundaries, who take them to the edge where they snap when such injustices become blatant and unnerving, then impatience, restlessness, and bitterness seep in.

Affirmation: "As I am generous and forgiving of myself and others, resentments are released."

Chakras: 4th and 7th

* A special thanks to Rosemarie Brown and Sandi O'Connor for their friendship, inspirational conversations, and loving support on this journey.

References

"Biodynamic agriculture" from Wikipedia
"how tree roots grow"

"Malus", https://en.wikipedia.org/wiki/Malus
AUGUST 8, 2012 / LEDA MARRITZ deeproot.com Green Infrastructure For Your Community

Boericke, William, MD., "Homeopathic Materia Medica", B.Jain Publishers, Pvt.Ltd., 1995.

Clarke, John Henry, "A Dictionary of Practical Materia Medica", Volumes I, II, and III, B.Jain Publishers, Pvt.Ltd., 1994.

Grieve, Mrs. M, "A Modern Herbal" Volume I and II, Dover Publications, 1971.

Homesteader's PDC, Wheaton Labs Montana, "Quaking Aspen",

http://www.almanac.com/content/black-walnut-trees-roots-evil

http://www.medicinalplantsarchive.us/fruit-trees/pome-fruit.html

http://www.naturalmedicinalherbs.net/herbs/m/malus-sylvestris=crab-apple.php

http://www.smgrowers.com

https://authoritynutrition.com/foods/olives/

https://en.wikipedia.org/wiki/**Juglone**

https://en.wikipedia.org/wiki/Quercus_gambelii

https://permies.com/t/582/kitchen/Quaking-Aspen

https://www.fs.fed.us/database/feis/plants/tree/quegam/all.html

http://www.oplin.org/tree/fact%20pages/aspen_quaking/aspen_quaking.html

National Wildlife Federation, "Quaking Aspen", https://www.nwf.org/Wildlife/Wildlife-Library/Plants/Quaking-Aspen.aspx

Orth Epple, Anne, "Plants of Arizona", Falcon Press Publishing Co, 1995.
QuakingAspenTree,

PallasDowney, Rhonda, "The Healing Power of Flowers: Bridging Herbalism, Homeopathy, Flower Essences, and the Human Energy System,
Woodland Publishing, 2007.

Sanchez, JoAnn Castigliego, "Breaking Ground", 2016

Urban James, "How Deep Do Tree Roots Really Grow?" 2010 blog, FASLA

Winston, David and Maimes, Steve, "*Adaptogens: Herbs for Strength, Stamina, and Stress Relief*, Healing Arts Press, 2007.

Wohlleben, Peter, "The Hidden Life of Trees", Greystone Books, 2016.

Wood, Mathew, "The Book of Herbal Wisdom", North Atlantic Books, 1997.

Yance, Donald, CN, Mh, RH, "Adaptogens in Medical Herbalism", Healing Arts Press, 2013.

Eyes, Ears, Nose and Throat (EENT) Demonstration: Preparing and Applying Topically Applied EENT Preparations
Kenneth Proefrock, ND

This presentation demonstrates approaches to treating illness and disease at the interfaces of the body and the outside world. Specifically, we discuss common pathologies and topical approaches to treatment for eye diseases, external ear infections, nasal inflammation/sinusitis, tonsillitis, and cellulitis. Central to this discussion is the use of topical washes, poultices, drops and sprays. We discuss exactly how to go about making such items and will address the concepts of osmolarity, pH and temperature as they may pertain to therapeutic applications to the eyes, ears, nose, throat and skin.

We begin by talking about the physical and chemical properties of water as a medium for a therapeutic intervention, beginning with the relative density of any water based (aqueous) solution. Solutions that are iso-osmolar have roughly the same amount of dissolved solids as the blood stream—roughly 280-310 milliosmoles/ml. Solutions that are relatively hypo-osmolar, containing less than 280 mOsm/ml, tend to leave behind more of a water portion in the tissues, and can be relatively hydrating to those tissues. Solutions that are relatively hyper-osmolar, greater than 310 mOsm/ml, tend to pull more fluid from the tissues and leave them relatively more dehydrated, which can reduce tissue swelling. These are useful therapeutic qualities for topical solutions, for patients who have chronically dry eyes, a slightly hypo-osmolar solution can be a phenomenal way to hydrate the tissues while washing away irritating debris. A hyper-osmolar solution can be helpful in conditions of edema, in the throat, sinuses, eyes or skin by drawing fluid out of the interstitium, part of the rationale behind gargling with salt water for a sore throat. An iso-osmolar preparation that is commonly used in medicine is "normal saline", a preparation of 0.9% sodium chloride in water. 0.9 % means that there is 9 mg of salt in every ml of fluid, or 9000 mg of salt in a liter, this is roughly 1 1/4 -2 tsp, depending on the grind of the salt. The solution can be made more alkaline by trading ¼ tsp of salt for ¼ tsp (1.5 grms) potassium or sodium bicarbonate, because...

The pH of an aqueous solution is another therapeutically useful parameter to consider. Qualitatively, the most important of the pH buffering systems in the body is the bicarbonate buffer system, which involves the lungs and the kidneys. This system is unique in that it remains in equilibrium with atmospheric air through the respiratory system; thus, it is an open system with a much greater capacity to buffer body fluids than any closed system would be able to manage. The pH buffering impact of the bicarbonate system is based on an equilibration of CO_2 with carbonic acid, carbonic anhydrase activity, bicarbonate ion, hydrogen ions, the respiratory rate and the ability of the kidney to reabsorb and excrete bicarbonate and hydrogen ions into the urine.

$$CO_2 + H_2O <=> H_2CO_3 <=> H^+ + HCO_3^-$$

Increasing the reactants on the left has a tendency to push the reaction to the right, i.e. an accumulation of water and CO_2 in the tissues of the lungs tends to increase tissue production of carbonic acid and, ultimately, bicarbonate and protons. This is why breathing into a paper bag when one is hyperventilating can be helpful; the re-breathing of the CO_2 tends to make the system, initially, more alkaline, which tends to have a relaxing effect on the nervous system. Purposely increasing the bicarbonate levels in tissues by adding it to an aqueous solution tends to leave the tissues more alkaline and increases CO_2 and water movement out of the body through the lungs and kidneys, often a very beneficial effect for patients with restricted airways. While the lung plays a relatively acute role in managing pH, the kidney plays a similar and more long-term role by actively excreting acid, as H^+ or base, as HCO_3^- into the urine and making the urine either acidic or alkaline. An important consideration in this process is the role of adequate amounts of water in maintaining appropriate pH levels, where the water goes, so goes the electrolytes. Sufficient potassium in the system is also a critical factor in the way that the body is able to establish an effective buffer. Potassium has an alkalinizing effect by participating in the movement of H^+ (acid) through the body. Intracellular potassium can be exchanged for H^+ in the plasma, so the intracellular protein buffering system can have access to and neutralize the plasma increases in H^+ concentration. This exchange during metabolic acidosis often results in transient increases in plasma potassium levels with more long-term diminishment of the intracellular stores of potassium, where it was taken from, leading ultimately to a potassium deficiency. The reverse of this process is how the body deals effectively with metabolic alkalosis, that is, as the plasma levels of H^+ decline; potassium in the plasma is exchanged for intracellular hydrogen ions to compensate. Another point worth stating is that bronchodilators like Albuterol sulfate, often used chronically by asthma and COPD patients, has a known side effect of reducing the potassium stores of the body.

Mucus chemistry is a very fascinating aspect of membrane health that can be dramatically affected by shifting both osmolarity and pH. Mucus is a conglomeration of the secreted protein mucin and the numerous saccharides that glycosylate it. Some of the most critical of these saccharides are the family of sialic acids, and within this family, the compound neuraminic acid. Sialic acids contribute greatly to the viscosity of mucus, the more acidic the internal environment of the lung, the higher the viscosity or thickness of the mucus; alternately, the more alkaline the internal environment, the thinner the mucus. The acidic nature of the infectious process creates a thickening of the mucoid secretions, making them significantly more "sticky", a measure which helps impede further progression of the infection. Moreover, the acidic environment of the airways and other mucus membranes is conducive to tissue constriction through the neural reflex (acidity creates 'tension' in the tissues), inhibition of histamine breakdown, and is a contributor to tissue irritation. One of the reasons why the Influenza family of viruses is so virulent is that it has evolved a neuraminidase enzyme that allows the viral particles to cleave through the thickening and protective neuraminic acid component of the mucus and infect adjacent tissues to the primary site of infection. Neutralizing the acidity of mucus makes it a looser, thinner mucus, facilitating liquefaction of the harder secretions, promoting relaxation and improvement of blood flow into and out of affected tissues and inactivating histamines. Applying relatively alkaline solutions to the affected tissues represents a decided advantage in the treatment of patients with many congestive conditions of the mucus membranes. I find that using potassium bicarbonate, where reasonable, as a buffer to bring the pH of a topical solution into a slightly alkaline realm adds even more greatly to the therapeutic potential.

Closely related to the idea of mucus chemistry is the concept of biofilm. According to JW Costerton at the Center for Biofilm Engineering in Montana, a bacterial biofilm as "a structured community of bacterial cells enclosed in a self-produced polymeric matrix and adherent to an inert or living surface." In other words, bacteria can join together on essentially any surface and start to form a protective matrix around their colony. This matrix, or syncytium, has many of the same physical properties that mucus does and is made of similar polymers composed of molecules with repeating structural units that are connected by chemical bonds. These biofilms form when bacteria adhere to surfaces in aqueous environments and begin to excrete their slimy, glue-like polymeric substances that anchor them to some substrate material, which could be metals, plastics, soil particles, medical implant materials and, most significantly, human or animal tissue. The first bacterial colonists to adhere to a surface initially do so by inducing weak, reversible bonds called van der Waals forces. If the colonists are not immediately separated from the surface, they can anchor themselves more permanently using cell adhesion molecules. These bacteria facilitate and support the presence of other pathogens by providing more diverse adhesion sites. They also continue to build the matrix that holds the biofilm together, allowing an environment conducive to the presence of more and more micro-organisms, many that would not be able to survive in the host on their own. Several studies have shown that while a biofilm is being created, the pathogens inside it can communicate with each other via a phenomenon called quorum sensing which allows them to communicate their presence by emitting chemical messages that their fellow infectious agents are able to recognize. Although the mechanisms behind quorum sensing are not fully understood, the phenomenon allows a single-celled bacterium to perceive how many other bacteria are in close proximity. When a bacterium senses the presence of other microbes, it is more inclined to join them and contribute to the formation of a biofilm. When the messages grow strong enough, the bacteria respond en masse, behaving as a group. Quorum sensing can occur within a single bacterial species as well as between diverse species, and can regulate a host of different processes, essentially serving as a simple communication network that allows the biofilm community of organisms to act as a single organism.

As the biofilm grows through a combination of cell division and recruitment it allows the cells inside to become more resistant to antibiotics administered in a standard fashion. In fact, depending on the organism and type of antimicrobial, biofilm bacteria can be up to a thousand times more resistant to antimicrobial stress than free-swimming bacteria of the same species. Biofilms tend to grow slowly, in diverse locations, and biofilm infections are often slow to produce overt symptoms. However, biofilm bacteria can move in ways that allow them to insidiously expand and infect new tissues. Biofilms move collectively, by rippling or rolling across the surface, or by detaching in clumps. Sometimes, in a dispersal strategy referred to as "swarming/seeding", a biofilm colony differentiates to form an outer "wall" of stationary bacteria, while the inner region of the biofilm "liquefies", allowing planktonic cells to "swim" out of the biofilm and leave behind a hollow mound. Research on the molecular and genetic basis of biofilm development has made it clear that when cells switch from independent, planktonic to community mode, they also undergo a shift in behavior that involves alterations in the activity of numerous genes. There is evidence that specific genes must be transcribed during the attachment phase of biofilm development. In many cases, the activation of these genes is required for synthesis of the extracellular matrix that protects the pathogens inside. This represents an epigenetic phenomenon within the microorganisms themselves and speaks to how single organisms may have been able to consolidate and evolve into multi-cellular organisms.

According to Costerton, the genes that allow a biofilm to develop are activated after some critical mass number of cells attach to a solid surface. "Thus, it appears that attachment itself is what stimulates synthesis of the extracellular matrix in which the sessile bacteria are embedded," states the molecular biologist. "This notion that bacteria have a sense of touch that enables detection of a surface and the expression of specific genes, is, in itself, an exciting area of research." Biofilms can be broken down by topical application of hyperosmolar saline solutions, radical shifts of pH, and the judicious use of chelating agents like EDTA, DMSA and DMPS, sulfur products like Glutathione and N-Acetyl-Cysteine, mineral products like bismuth subnitrate and subgallate, proteolytic enzymes like serratiopeptidases as well as botanical agents like Achalypha Mexicana, Achillea, Allium sativa, Althea, Anemopsis, Arctostaphylos uva ursi, Baptisia, Boswellia, Bursera, Calendula, Commiphora myrrha, Echinacea, Hydrastis, Hypericum, Larrea, Myrica, Plantago, Propolis, and Thuja, among others. Most modern antibiotics are not effective against these biofilm communities; in fact, it is these types of communities that are direct contributors to the formation of antibiotic resistant strains of bacteria. It requires some physical as well as physiological/biochemical methods to break down and eradicate a biofilm community. We will discuss these strategies more in depth when we discuss specific conditions and where it will be more relevant.

We begin by discussing conditions of the eyes as they can be extremely debilitating to any patient and are very commonly seen in clinical practice, most of them can be effectively treated with botanical therapies. Conjunctivitis, cataracts and glaucoma are the most common conditions of the eye and respond very well to treatment with botanical agents.

Cataracts are primarily an oxidative disorder of the lens of the eye. Oxidation causes a disruption in the protein matrix of the lens, creating cross-linkages and making the lens more and more opaque as oxidation continues. This is the same phenomenon that occurs to the egg white proteins when they are fried or boiled. The treatment strategy is directed towards reducing oxidative damage both systemically and locally. Cataract risk is increased with obesity, hypertriglyceridemia, uncontrolled blood sugar, and poor circulation. A predominantly alkaline ash diet, low fat, moderate protein, with complex carbohydrate sources and strict avoidance of refined sugars and hydrogenated trans fats provides a good dietary foundation for treatment. Galactose and sorbitol can be a problem for some people—so reduction in dairy intake and avoiding processed sugar-free foods will often help. Generally abiding by a diet with a lot of anti-inflammatory foods and spices—fish, fresh fruits (at least one cup of previously frozen dark berries every day) and vegetables with spices like turmeric, cumin, ginger and garlic. Mixed carotenoids can be very helpful, my favorite sources are those from the algae Dunaliella Salinas, dosed at 150,000-300,000 units/day and mixed carotenoids from saffron, the flower pistils of Crocus sativa. Saffron is prescribed as a tea, 1-2 flower pistils in water twice a day, it can be added to other teas like green tea or bilberry tea. Saffron is the richest natural source of water-soluble carotenoids, a nice complement to the fat-soluble carotenoids in the Dunaliella sinensis. Vitamin E is another fat-soluble anti-oxidant that is essential for patients with cataracts, again, emphasizing a naturally occurring mix of tocopherols, dosed at 1400 mg (not IU's) twice a day. Hesperidin methyl chalcone is a flavonoid found in Uncaria gambir, which works similarly to the flavonoid Quercetin, reducing histamine release and inhibiting the activity of the aldose reductase enzyme, which is involved in the formation and accumulation of sorbitol inside the eye, another contributor to oxidative damage. No discussion regarding the botanical treatment of cataracts would be complete without mentioning the important role that bilberry, Vaccinium myrtillus, can play. It is generally regarded to be the proanthocyanidin content of the bilberry that makes it effective, my feeling is that by emphasizing the one cup of previously frozen dark berries, the proanthocyanidin facet of treatment is covered, some patients are still prescribed 500 mg of bilberry three times a day.

Eyewashes and eyedrops are the cornerstones of therapy; my personal favorite is an eyewash with succus of Cineraria maritima, Dusty Miller, 2-3 times/day. Cineraria has been shown to reduce and possibly reverse cataract formation, it acts to stimulate profound movement of lymph through the eye. It produces a burning sensation and redness when washed into the eye; I previously purchased the succus pre-made from Luytie's Homeopathic Pharmacy in Missouri. Other eyewash materials that I have used with more or less good effect include urine, rosewater, and salinated teas of green tea, triphala, chamomile, saffron and chrysanthemum. Eyedrops dosed at three times a day are very helpful for cataracts and consist of a calendula (1-2 tablespoons of finely ground flowers) and saffron (4-8 threads) water decoction with 1 ¼ tsps Sea salt and ¼ tsp potassium bicarbonate per liter of water. Acetyl-L-Carnosine can also be added at 1%. The drops are dosed at 2-3 drops three times a day, they act as a topical anti-oxidant, and inhibit the activity of the aldose reductase enzyme, reducing sorbitol accumulation in the eye.

Glaucoma is a major cause of blindness in adults, it is an insidious increase in intraocular pressure that may cause no symptoms whatsoever or may cause impaired vision and pain, ranging from slight vision loss to absolute blindness. The cause of glaucoma is often a derangement of collagen metabolism within the eye, there seems to be a genetic/anatomic component (narrow angle vs open angle duct), a diabetic component, and an allergy component. The therapeutic strategy is to create better flow of aqueous humor through the eye, improve collagen metabolism, and decrease accumulation of larger proteins and sugars within the aqueous humor of the eye.

Blood sugar plays a huge role in the etiology of glaucoma through the formation of sorbitol from excess glucose or fructose via the aldose reductase enzyme. Sorbitol does not diffuse through the cell membranes very well and accumulates within the aqueous humor, causing an osmotic increase inside the eye. Dietary treatment begins with a predominantly alkaline ash diet with moderate protein, low fat, moderate carbohydrates (as complex as possible) and no refined sugars or flours. You may need to rule out food sensitivities and allergies, avoid caffeine, and anything else that raises blood pressure, as there is a relationship between higher blood pressures and higher intra-ocular pressures. Bioflavonoids are an important consideration for the maintenance of proper connective tissue, my favorite prescription is one cup of previously frozen dark berries every day.

Supplemental considerations in the treatment of glaucoma include high vitamin C, 10-15 gms/day have been shown to reduce intraocular pressure by as much as 19 mm Hg! Quercetin as quercetin chalcone or hesperidin methyl chalcone from Uncaria gambir at a dosage of 500-1500 mg/day stabilizes mast cell activity, reducing allergy mediated histamine release and also significantly reduces the activity of the enzyme aldose reductase. Liposomal preparations of R-Alpha-Lipoic Acid at dosages of 150-300 mg/day has been shown to help stabilize blood sugars, reduce oxidation throughout the body, and has been shown to reduce internal pressure.

Topical measures in the treatment of glaucoma include eyedrops and eyewashes containing mast cell stabilizers like quercetin, cromolyn, Albizia, and Scute, as well as agents that promote better flow of fluid through the vitreal humor like Coleus and Pilocarpus dosed three times a day. A 1% solution of the Ayurvedic herb Coleus forskohlii, and Pilocarpus jaborandi into the eye drops works as well as prescription eyedrops for some patients. I make the coleus and pilocarpus addition in the office from a tincture, evaporating the alcohol and replacing it with normal saline and adding them to an eyedrop base that is 01% hyaluronic acid (for moisture), and 2% cromolyn sodium, or a lactated ringers solution or saline. The 1% solution of Coleus has abundant research supporting its use, it is tolerable and the majority of the time it works as well as the prescription drops at a dosage of 2-3 drops three times a day.

Eye exercises can have a dramatic impact on the progression of glaucoma, one of the most important eye exercises is purposeful crying everyday. Crying has a cleansing effect on the eyes and the spirit, it also helps cleanse the nerves, the liver and the blood according to Ayurveda. Suppression of emotion and crying causes a build up of subtle toxins. Crying can be stimulated by onion juice from a fresh cut onion or by old "Little House on the Prairie" reruns. Range of motion exercises are also helpful to promote better drainage through the eye, going outside so that a distant horizon can be peered at, is often an overlooked, pardon the pun, activity that urban life has all but eliminated. Remember that focusing the eyes to accommodate different distances requires an actual conformational change to the eyeball itself, which is physically helpful in removing accumulated debris.

Conjunctivitis or pinkeye is, very simply, inflammation of the conjunctiva, the mucus membrane that lines the eye. It is most often due to infection from a virus or bacteria or from allergy, it can also come from irritation due to overexposure to sun, wind, pollution, chlorine or contact lens solution. The first thing that has to be established in developing a strategy for the treatment of pinkeye is whether or not there is a foreign object or organism present. If the tissue is simply irritated, treatment is different than if there is something that has to be removed or eliminated. Allergy is a major contributor to conjunctivitis and will be addressed in the next section.

When a foreign object is present, dust, dirt, ash, or other environmental debris of a non-infective origin, the single best remedy is a series of eyewashes. The agents chosen would ideally be astringent agents and demulcent agents in an isotonic base. An isotonic base can be created by placing 1 ½ tsps of sea salt and ¼ tsp of baking soda in each quart of your final product. A wonderful, refreshing mixture that I have used many times myself and with my children is 1 tbsp calendula flowers, Calendula officinalis, 1 tsp of triphala powder and 1 tbsp of comfrey leaves, Symphytum officinale, steeped in 1 quart of pure water, taking care not to let any large particulate matter escape into the decoction, finally adding the salt and baking soda once the herbs have been sufficiently decocted. The calendula acts as an anti-inflammatory, antiseptic and promotes wound healing, the high amount of flavonoids and carotenoids in the flowers accounts for these activities. Triphala is an Ayurvedic combination of three myrobalan fruits, haritaki (Terminalia chebula), amalaki (Emblica officinalis), and bibhitaki (Terminalia belerica), it is very astringent and strengthening to the tissues of the eye. Comfrey acts as a wonderful demulcent, soothing the irritated membranes of the conjunctiva, it also has an anti-inflammatory action and a long, consistent history of use as a topical agent for healing wounds. Mucilage and allantoin are two major constituents that contribute to its healing nature, water extracts of comfrey have been shown to modify prostaglandin production, altering blood flow through the membrane, decreasing swelling. This eye wash can be used several times a day without any fear of toxicity or side effects, I usually prescribe it as a copious wash 4 times a day, often, a single application is sufficient. Warming compresses are also very helpful in these cases to improve blood flow into and out of the affected tissues as well as to impart a drawing effect to pull debris from the superficial tissues. A used black tea bag is often an easy and effective compress material, the idea is to put the bag on the eye cold, let it warm up, make it cold again and reapply. A series of 4-5 applications like this is often effective at resolving much of the swelling and tissue irritation, the tannins in the tea tend to have an astringent effect on the tissues as well as imparting some anti-microbial activity.

When you suspect an infecting organism is present, the strategy alters slightly. One of the most overlooked aspects of infectious disease management is the role that the patient's internal terrain plays in establishing susceptibility to a particular disease. Western medicine has created a militaristic approach to infectious disease, "They are the enemy and must be eradicated". An important alternative perspective is that the existing terrain supports the presence of an opportunistic organism to the point that it is allowed to create disease. "We have met the enemy and he is us", seems a more apt description of the situation. The task then becomes one of radically altering the terrain so that the organism is not supported and cannot survive. Infectious conjunctivitis usually does not require antibiotic intervention, it is, however, the responsibility of every health practitioner to evaluate every case individually and be able to determine when overgrowth of an organism has reached the point where antibiotic intervention may be necessary. Antibiotic intervention should never be the "last stand" therapy, what you resort to when all else has failed; it is not 100% effective, contrary to popular opinion. It is only a part of a greater therapeutic strategy, by anticipating the growth potential of any infectious organism; one can create a strategy from the beginning of treatment that will preclude the need for antibiotics.

Eyewashes are a very effective way of altering the terrain around the eye, the addition of antimicrobial botanicals to the above saline recipe are a great place to begin. One of my favorites is a combination of Coptis chinensis, *huang lian*, and Scutellaria baicalensis, *scute*, because they have long been used for their anti-inflammatory, antiviral, antibacterial, and antifungal activities, making them nicely broad spectrum for conjunctivitis when you don't know exactly what is causing it. It is probably the berberine in coptis that gives it its astringent anti-microbial effect, as such, other berberine containing plants like Mahonia, Berberis, Algerita, and Hydrastis Canadensis, are probably similarly effective. Coptis has been studied and used as an ophthalmological agent for many years in China; a 5-10% solution is effective for both acute conjunctivitis as well as superficial keratitis. From a Chinese medicine perspective, Coptis clears heat topically, relieves toxicity and drains dampness, making it an ideal agent for conjunctivitis. It is also very inexpensive compared to other berberine containing herbs and isn't as endangered as goldenseal. An effective recipe would include 35 gms of whole root herb or 1-2 tbsps of powdered herb per quart of saline with 2 tbsps of calendula and 1 tbsp of comfrey. This solution is very yellow! It should be used as a wash, over a sink with water running, 4 times a day. Between washes, eyedrops should be used, a 1% berberine sulfate equivalent eyedrop in a base of 0.1% hyaluronic acid and 2% cromolyn is helpfully soothing and stabilizing of mast cells that might release histamine, these are dosed at 2-3 drops in each eye three times a day in between eye washes.

Lysozymes are enzymes that damage bacteria by catalyzing hydrolysis of 1,4-beta-linkages in the cell wall. They are naturally abundant in human secretions, such as tears, saliva, human milk, and mucus. They are also present in cytoplasmic granules of the macrophages and the neutrophils and play a significant role in non-specific immune response. Lysozymes are commercially prepared from egg whites, we purchase 100 gms at a time and mix them into eyedrops, nasal sprays, nebulizer solutions, and for wound healing poultices and compresses at a 1mg/ml dilution in saline or lactated ringer's solution. Lactated ringers solution is a broader electrolyte solution, which is made isotonic and contains, in addition to sodium chloride, sodium lactate, potassium chloride, and calcium chloride in water. Ringer's lactate has an osmolarity of 273 mOsm/L, and is inherently alkalinizing, making it helpful in correcting regional metabolic acidosis. The solution is formulated to have concentrations of potassium and calcium that are similar to the ionized concentrations found in normal blood plasma. To maintain electrical neutrality, the solution has a lower level of sodium than that found in blood plasma or normal saline. I find it helpful as the base for eyedrops, nasal washes, and for wetting warming compresses for wound healing.

Systemically, we need to alter the secretions of the eye so that they are less supportive of microbial growth. N-Acetyl-Cysteine is a sulfur containing amino acid that can be found in any health food store. It is very mucolytic, thins the secretions of the mucus membranes, and its sulfur content extends to the mucus it becomes a component of and provides a bacteriostatic quality to the mucus secretions. The dosage is 1200 mg three times a day for 1 week (it seldom takes more than a three or four days to clear up conjunctivitis). Sulfur containing botanicals with an expectorating, mucolytic effect can also be helpful; I have used Symplocarpus, skunk cabbage, Ferula foetida, asafeotida, garlic and onions to good effect in the past. Garlic and onions are dietary and at the patient's discretion—the more the better. Asafoetida and skunk cabbage as tinctures—30 drops 3 times a day. The more you reek, the less susceptible you become, is the general idea.

A point should be made that the vast majority of pinkeye patients that I see are children. Children are inherently non-compliant if a treatment tastes really bad or hurts. The eyewash is not painful, or shouldn't be, I try it on myself or have the parent try it to make sure, it is just "weird", I emphasize its importance to the kids and tell them to expect the "weirdness" of it, they are usually alright with that, the same is true of the eyedrops. I have not met the child, yet, who is willing to take asafoetida or skunk cabbage as a tincture, I usually emphasize dietary garlic, lots of it, especially in soups.

Relatively speaking, allergic conjunctivitis is a pretty straight-forward condition to treat, it requires compliance on the part of the patient and that is often the hardest part. So much of the time our role as a health care practitioner is to educate our patients about their condition and explain how the strategy you employ is going to resolve this problem. As the patient understands their role, they want to participate, as they participate, they get better, as they see improvement, they want to participate even more. A lot of our responsibility, in the meantime, is to act as their teacher, their coach, their motivational speaker and their friend.

Allergy is a condition that begins with the mucus membranes. The role of the mucus membrane is to secrete a mucus layer that serves to protect the inside of the body from the outside world. As the mucus lining performs its function it collects all of the pollen, dust, dirt and other debris in the air, ideally keeping it from the actual tissues and allowing a person to cough, blow, sneeze or secrete the foreign material out of the body. Allergic problems arise when the mucus no longer protects the membrane, either from a patchy distribution resulting from local dehydration or mucus that has acquired a globular consistency rather than a planar one. Mucus is a protein/sugar complex, under normal, ideal circumstances this complex has a planar structure, dietary proteins can have an effect on the structure of the mucus. Dairy, wheat and corn tend to create a more globular, less planar mucus. This globular mucus tends to stick together and it is not as effective at protecting the membranes, in fact, it has a tendency to accumulate in the smaller sinus and bronchial passageways. Once environmental debris reaches the tissue level, the body often responds to it as though it were a foreign invader, part of this response is the formation of antibodies or immunoglobulins specific to the invader. There are two kinds of immunoglobulins to be found in the mucus membranes, IgA and IgE. IgA binds to the offending agent and allows it to enter the body where it is dealt with by the immune system. These are typically substances that the body has not developed an overly rigorous response towards, as they are allowed to enter the body proper before they are dealt with. IgE presents a more rigorous response to offending agents, as the agent and the antibody pass through the membrane, IgE causes a destabilization of mast cells. The mast cells release histamine and a host of other substances which increase the permeability of the blood vessels, incite aggressive immune activity locally, and trigger the complement cascade to begin breaking down larger proteins in the area. In essence, IgE "walls off" the area of the potential invader, allowing it to be dealt with immunologically before it enters the body proper. This is what creates the swelling and itching associated with allergy.

An effective strategy consists of making more planar, protective mucus, stabilizing mast cells so that they are less likely to release histamine and keeping the mucus membranes clean so that a build up of debris doesn't trigger the same response again. Desensitization through avoidance of the offending allergen is the hallmark of conventional allergy treatment; the flaw in this strategy is that unless you move to a desert island, there is little chance that you are going to be able to avoid the offenders in your environment. The best way of avoiding the offending allergen is to create better membrane protection so that the offender doesn't reach the tissue level regardless of its presence in your world. Creating more planar, protective mucus begins with sulfur containing agents, the presence of sulfur in protein structures allow for the formation of disulfide bridges between polypeptide chains of proteins. The disulfide bridges provide a lateral stability within the protein promoting a more planar behavior to the protein molecule. N-Acetyl-Cysteine (NAC) accomplishes this objective nicely and is widely available and inexpensive, it has a dependable mucolytic effect, imparts a bacteriostatic quality to the mucus, and has been shown to increase the relative amount of IgA secreted through mucus membranes. As described earlier, the dosage that I prescribe most frequently is 1200 mg 3 times a day for the first week, then 1200 mg twice a day for the second two weeks and then 600 mg twice a day thereafter. An expectorating, mucolytic tincture is also beneficial at this point, a combination of 2 parts licorice, Glycyrrhiza glabra, 2 parts hyssop, Hyssopus officinalis, and 2 parts asafeotida, Ferula foetida, dosed at 60 drops three times a day is helpful. Hyssop can be traded for bloodroot, Sanguinaria Canadensis, or Symplocarpus foetida, skunk cabbage.

Stabilizing mast cells so that they are more resistant to IgE mediated degranulation is a helpful measure that gives the quickest relief. If you can keep the histamine from being released, the patient won't have the symptoms of allergy. My favorite tool for this is a solution of 0.1% hyaluronic acid and 2% cromolyn sodium that I use as a base for eyewashes, eyedrops, and nasal sprays. The drops are dosed at 2-3 drops three times a day and work very quickly. An eyewash used twice a day is an effective way of keeping the membranes clear of accumulated debris. The ideal agents in such an eyewash would have an additional effect of stabilizing mast cells. Scutellaria baicalensis is an excellent source of quercetin and Uncaria gambir is a good source of hesperidin, which also stabilize mast cells, and these herbs can be made into a tea pretty easily. The tea is then prepared as an isotonic solution by placing 1 ½ tsps of sea salt and ¼ tsp of baking soda in each quart of your final product. Most patients respond very quickly to this type of a strategy, occasionally we will add in a nasal lavage through a neti-pot to further stabilize mast cells in the sinus passageways. If the sinuses have become swollen and boggy due to chronic allergies, or if the patient is forming polyps in their nasal passages, we will employ a hypertonic solution for the nasal lavage. A typical recipe would be two tbsp of sea salt, ½ tsp baking soda in 1 quart of licorice root tea or green tea, and this solution is poured through the nasal passages two to three times a day.

Chronic rhinosinusitis is one of the most common complaints in North American medical visits, and one of the main reasons for antibiotic prescriptions. About 135 in 1,000 persons – 31 million people - are affected yearly in the US. The general classification of rhinosinusitis is according to the length of the condition, acute cases last less than 12 weeks and chronic case are those lasting over 12 weeks. Chronic rhinosinusitis sufferers may present with nasal polyps, associated with neutrophilic presence and a likely fungal infection where those without polyps are largely associated with allergic eosinophilic infiltration. Biofilm expression in rhinosinusitis cases has been studied since 2001 when scanning electron microscopy (SEM) was initially used to identify biofilms in Eustachian tubes, sinus passageways, ventilation tubes, and associated with chronic otitis media. Biofilms have also been demonstrated in cholesteatomas, chronic tonsillitis, adenoids of patients with chronic sinusitis, and infections associated with biomaterials such as voice prostheses and myringotomy tubes.

There are several agents that I have used quite extensively in a nasal spray form for patients with rhinosinusitis. The first of these agents is reduced L-glutathione, made as a nebulizer solution of 100 mg/ml or 200 mg/ml in sterile saline. Gutathione is a tripeptide of the amino acids glycine, glutamine and N-acetyl-cysteine; it is heavily involved in tissue detoxification reactions, requires selenium as a cofactor. Glutathione is one of the most versatile and important anti-oxidants that are produced by our bodies. It has a specific affinity for liver and mucus membrane tissues where it has been shown to inhibit angiogenesis, facilitate the repair of DNA, scavenge free radicals, have anti-tumor activity and is required for optimal activation of T-lymphocytes. It is generally well tolerated in eyedrops, nasal sprays, nebulizers and is dosed 4 times a day. I generally augment it with NAC, in half the concentration of the glutathione, as an agent that helps keep the glutathione in a reduced form. By itself, it is often used in asthma and COPD patients as a mucolytic agent, helping to make mucus have a less globular and more planar structure, making it more protective and less likely to get stuck in the smaller bronchioles of the lungs. NAC is also a very strong free radical scavenger, inhibits angiogenesis, facilitates the repair of DNA as well as being a major component of glutathione. Other systemic considerations that are often helpful include 1/8-1/2 tsp of local bee pollen consumed daily (start small and work up to the higher doses) to create an oral desensitization to commonly occurring pollens in your area. N-Acetyl-Glutamine, orally dosed at 5-10 grams per day is often very helpful in repairing damaged membranes as well as creating newer membranes that are more durable.

Herbal teas can be quite effective when applied as nasal washes, sprays, eyewashes/drops. I generally make the tea, then try to get it to an iso-osmolar concentration by creating a 0.9% solution of sodium chloride and potassium bicarbonate (as mentioned previously, 1 measured teaspoon of finely ground salt is approximately 7.5 grams and ¼ teaspoon of potassium bicarbonate=1.5 grams). The best course of action in initiating this type of therapy is to start with dilute, weak teas and then make them stronger as the need might present. Green and black teas exert an astringent effect in the nasal passageway, which is helpful in boggy, swollen, polypoid conditions, 2 tbsps colloidal silver in a quart of nasal wash can be nicely anti-microbial, Licorice tea is nicely demulcent, soothing and anti-inflammatory in a nasal wash. Berberis, Mahonia, Hydrastis, and Achalypha have been shown to be helpful in breaking down biofilms. Twice a day application of 30-50 ml of nasal wash through a neti-pot can be wildly effective.

Otitis media, inner ear infections, often respond to the same measures as rhinosinusitis. Often they result from clogged Eustachian tubes that don't allow proper drainage from the inner ear into the throat. This can be caused by allergy, thick chunky mucus from certain foods, or acute infectious processes like staph, strep or haemophilus influenza. Generally, the inner ear becomes an anaerobic environment which allows a micro-organismal overgrowth that produces a pressurized compartment of the inner ear, which presses against the eardrum and hurts like crazy. It is self-limiting in that once the membrane ruptures, the bacterial overgrowth resolves in the now aerobic environment. If the environment remains susceptible, as soon as that tympanic membrane knits and recreates an anaerobic environment, pressure will build again and re-rupture the freshly knitted and not quite cured membrane and the ensuing scar tissue can compromise the ability of the eardrum to properly transmit sound and hearing loss can occur. This is a great source of consternation for parents of small children and a major reason why parents visit emergency rooms at all times of the day and night. It is one of the most common reasons why children are given antibiotic prescriptions that then disrupt the intestinal microbiome, facilitate fungal overgrowths and start cycles of ecological and immune dysfunction. We have answers!! Avoiding sugar and dairy helps a majority of children with this issue...as does limiting wheat, soy and eggs. Lean proteins and fresh fruits and vegetables are practically foreign to families that start their days with cold cereal and milk, toast, or eggs, engage in fast food burger/chicken nugget lunches, with macaroni and cheese or cheese crisp snacks and pizza for dinner. Judicious application of normal sleep cycles, lots of loving touch, soothing language, apples, pears, plums, blueberries, blackberries, avocados, lean meats and nuts and seeds through the days of small children's lives is practically miraculous. Herbal teas with a small amount of agave syrup through crazy straws are fun and therapeutic. Hydrotherapy techniques like alternating hot and cold, wet sheet packs, and wet socks are amazingly effective in resolving the inevitable upper respiratory infections of childhood. The classic herbs, Echinacea, Thyme, Anemopsis, Baptisia, Licorice, Ginger, even Datura and Lobelia can be extremely helpful in stimulating immune responses, opening up Eustachian tubes and sinus passageways and resolving infectious conditions. N-acetyl-cysteine as a powder smells like a fart but tastes a little sour and can be mixed in applesauce at 300 mg 2-3 times a day and works well for otitis media resolution. Swollen lymph nodes in the head and neck respond to small amounts of Iris and Phytolacca. Swollen, indurated tonsils and sore throats respond to throat sprays of Spilanthes, Zanthoxylum and Echinacea, with tinctures of Baptisia, Sambucus, Elecampane and Salvia apania.

Otitis externa or 'Swimmer's Ear' is most often responsive to a mixture of eternally applied ear drops. Prevention can be achieved by prophylactic use of Lobelia acetract mixed with tincture of Thyme mixed half and half and 5 drops applied after swimming or bathing. The same preparation can be used in cases of infection but can be painful, we often add a drop or two of aconite tincture or procaine to the solution. Ear oils, like garlic and mullein can be soothing in some cases but mostly cause more problems for people and should definitely be avoided if you suspect that there is a chance of membrane rupture. Occasionally we will see patients with a chronic otitis externa and the following paragraph on topical would healing is appropriate in most of those cases.

Topical application of botanical agents in the treatment of wounds is a very ancient approach. One of the earliest recipes for a topical wound application comes to use from ancient Egypt where a recorded treatment for a crocodile bite was to mix goose fat with wood ash and rinse the wound in the Nile. Mixing ash with goose fat makes soap, and was probably a pretty effective method of keeping the wound clean and avoiding infection in a time when such an infection would be life threatening. Water itself is therapeutic for topical wound healing, as we have discussed, adjusting the pH and osmolarity of the water can make a huge difference. One of the historic mainstays in Naturopathic medical interventions is hydrotherapy, intentionally using the temperature of the water application to effect physiologic changes. We are all familiar with the idea that putting ice on an acute burn or injury can reduce the swelling associated with the injury, the relative effectiveness of such an intervention is dependent on the application of cold causing a constriction of regional blood vessels, reducing the amount of blood coming into the area. The idea of applying heat to a spastic muscle or areas of soreness is to cause a relative vasodilation into a region and improve blood flow that may have been restricted by inflammation and swelling. These are the extremes of this type of therapy, more apropos to healing wounds of the skin or the sense organs, is the warming compress, which is applied to the wound cool and allowed to warm up by an increase in circulation to the area under the compress. Once the compress is warm, cool it with fresh liquid and allow the body to warm it again, repeated application can dramatically improve blood flow into and out of poorly healing tissue. When the application is done with botanical agents infused into the water, we often achieve an accelerated healing response.

It is not uncommon in our practice to see patients who have been diagnosed with a resistant Staph infection somewhere on their body; we have seen this in 3 year olds up to 90+ year olds. The rampant overuse of antibiotic drugs over the past five decades has created an environment where even relatively healthy patients can develop these antibiotic resistant cellulitis conditions. Effective treatment requires dramatically changing the terrain at the site, and immediately reducing the bacterial load. An antibacterial soap, like Dr. Bronner's Lavender Castille soap, to wash the area three times a day, followed by an antibacterial rinse, a strong decoction of Hydrastis, Mahonia or Berberis usually works well. Unpasteurized honey can be placed directly on the lesion with a band-aid or other covering; the sugar in the honey has a desiccating effect on the bacteria and presents some anti-microbial action of its own. I also like conifer resin, straight or in a salve base to keep the wound moist (when that is appropriate) and to impart an anti-bacterial effect. Propolis applied to acute lesions is a good preventive, and also a decent adjunct for chronic wounds that might need to be kept dry. Simple lesions usually resolve within 5-7 days without complication. In more complex situations, the invading bacteria, or the normal flora present on the skin in response to biofilm directives, produces streptokinase, DNAse, and hyaluronidase each of which digest the cellular architecture of the body that would normally keep the infection contained to one area. This condition usually begins with some break in the skin, scratching or other trauma, in order for the bacteria to be able to descend deep enough into the tissue to cause a resistant cellulitis. Increased susceptibility to this condition is recognized in alcoholics, patients with nephrotic edema, stasis dermatitis, lymphedema and malnutrition. We also see it quite often in young adults with body piercings. The manifestation of cellulitis begins with redness, swelling, heat and tenderness, occasionally there will be blistering or an infiltrated surface that looks like the skin of an orange. Treatment should be rather aggressive; a rotation of topically applied cooling and astringent herbs applied as compresses or fomentations several times a day, keeping the area clean and if it is wet, try to keep it dry, if it is dry, keep it moist. A moist environment more easily fosters bacterial growth, but allows wound edges to migrate together more quickly. Dryness in a wound tends to promote the formation of granulomas (termed 'proud flesh' in horses), which take far longer to heal and leave scarring in their wake. It is important to stay flexible and shift one's approach as needed while the wound heals and changes its character.

Topical demulcents can be very helpful in promoting wound healing, especially when moisture is deemed to be helpful. Plantain (Plantago spp), Calendula, Aloe (or other cacti) and Althea are widely available and topically anti-inflammatory and antiseptic, they can be used as poultices (spit poultice for lysozymes), the teas for compresses, the powders as drawing agents. Better drawing agents are typically bentonite clay and charcoal, which can be added to the powdered herbs and applied topically. Astringent anti-inflammatory herbs like Achillea millefolium, Hypericum perforatum, Hydrastis spp, Berberis spp, Mahonia, Echinacea, Commiphora, etc can be applied as strong infusions to bandage material several times a day. Lysozymes can be applied topically in a similar manner, H2Ocean is a commercial product that contains lysozymes in saline and is used in the body piercing industry with decent effect. Historically, for painful cellulitis, Veratrum viride, false hellebore, in a strong decoction as an external treatment is suggested by Ellingwood in his *American Materia Medica, Therapeutics and Pharmacognosy*. I have had opportunity to use it with good effect as the moistening agent in a warming compress applied directly to the infected area, mixed half and half with a strong Echinacea decoction (which looks like a handful of Echinacea root, cut and sifted, steeped in a quart of boiled water). Internally, a tincture of Echinacea (4 parts), Phytolacca (3 parts), Mahonia (3 parts), and Baptisia (1 part) can be quite effective in stimulating better host response, especially when used in tandem with alternating hot/cold or warming compress application to the area. Sunlight is essential and drawing poultices made from ground flax, bentonite clay or slippery elm can also be helpful in suppurating, purulent discharge wounds.

Non-healing wounds that are associated with biofilm formation can be treated as described above and most will resolve. Occasionally, we have to do something more in order to facilitate breakdown of the biofilm more specifically. In cases where a drawing poultice of charcoal or bentonite clay seems warranted, I will add Bismuth subnitrate powder to the other powder at 25% of the weight, EDTA powder can be purchased online and also added on the order of 5% of the poultice material, adding essential oils like Melissa, Commiphora, Lemon, Tangerine or Grapefruit on the order of 5-20 drops in a handful of poultice powder are also helpful...especially because many of these wounds have an odor...especially if pseudomonas is present...and it often is. Systemic antibiotics seldom work for these patients. Sometimes topical antibiotics work, but, most often I am using a pinon resin salve in between 2-3 times a day wound washing with a gentle lavender or tea tree castile soap, herbal soaks with cotton bandages soaked in Echinacea, Thyme, Oregano, Mahonia, Hydrastis, Berberis, and/or Andrographis decoctions. Rotating the agents as often as is reasonable, to avoid resistance. With strategic alternating hot/cold and warming compress application. In cases of diabetic foot ulcers, topical application of ozone can preserve foot tissue and toes. Debridement of dead and dying tissue is a must, it is icky and gross and needs to be done daily at first. This is the place where medicine is a service to one's fellow human and that level of humility is a healing expression of love that every practitioner of the healing arts should be obligated to perform at least weekly.

"Helping, fixing and serving represent three different ways of seeing life.

When you help, you see life as weak. When you fix, you see life as broken.
When you serve, you see life as whole.
Fixing and helping may be the work of the ego, and service the work of the soul.

Service rests on the premise that the nature of life is sacred, that life is a holy mystery which has
an unknown purpose.
When we serve, we know that we belong to life and to that purpose.
From the perspective of service, we are
all connected:
All suffering is like my
suffering and all joy is like my joy.
The impulse to serve emerges
naturally and inevitably from this
way of seeing. "

Rachel Naomi Remen

Functional Genetic Mutations and Herbal/Dietary Therapies to Mitigate Their Impact
Kenneth Proefrock, ND

Summary: We discuss supportive nutritional and botanical therapies for those with cystic fibrosis, autism spectrum disorders, Fragile X, Klinefelter, Marfan and Down syndromes. These genetic conditions are not necessarily pathological in themselves, but they create different pathological predispositions. This is a good place to have a conversation about such things as neurodiversity; the importance of individualized health care and understanding the far-reaching impact that something like a genetic anomaly can have on a person's life, family and community.

I have been immensely fortunate to find myself in the practice of Naturopathic Medicine for over 20 years now. As a profession, we are truly in an unprecedented place in the modern medical industry. The understanding of biochemistry, physiology and pathology that provides the basis for a modern medical practice often leaves physicians in the smug position of declaring that condition x is to be treated this way, condition y that way and condition z is incurable, so don't even try. The great joy of being involved in a Naturopathic medical practice is that we are coming from the same basis of basic science understanding, but, the intervention toolbox is much larger than that which other physicians are able to draw from. It is phenomenal to be able to engage my occupation on a daily basis knowing that there will always be something that can be done for someone. It is even more phenomenal to be in the position of helping people achieve states of health that the modern medical paradigm says are impossible given their original diagnosis. I am presenting several cases in this lecture, each of which involved a diagnosis/prognosis with an outcome that would have been considered impossible by the conventional medical establishment. The most interesting aspects of these cases might be that our approach to intervention was predicated on basic Nature Cure strategies that have been around for hundreds of years. I will present the specifics of each patient's case during the lecture, here in the proceedings notes, I intend to simply give an overview of therapeutic strategies that might be employed under certain circumstances. Please don't mistake this information for protocols; I don't really have many that I use in my practice. Sometimes I laughingly joke that it isn't about protocols, it is about wake-up calls. What I prefer to rely on are strategies, how to get from point A to point B, how to engage the patient in the process of their own healing and how to explain what it is that we are trying to accomplish. I am a firm believer that our minds are the most powerful healing tools that we possess, if our mind can understand what we are trying to accomplish, it will help us in ways we could have never anticipated. I am committed to maintaining the therapeutic relationship between doctor and patient as a partnership, it is as we work together, with everybody on the same page, that miraculous things can happen. I remember, during our senior year of medical school, Dr. Mitchell taught a class called "Advanced Naturopathic Therapeutics", in that class he expressed the view that the most effective interaction that one can have with another human being is to connect at a soul level; to have some part of that essence of your being in contact with the essence of their being. It is out of such a connection that the deepest level of healing can unfold. I say this to emphasize that substances, natural or synthetic, don't "fix" people. I believe that people are able to resolve the pathological portions of even genetic condition states by acquiring shifts in their perspective regarding who they are as a mental and emotional individual, as a physical organism, as members of their respective communities, and as a participant in their own Spiritual unfolding. We have a growing field of epigenetics that describes the ways in which genetic conditions end up manifesting in a human.

Cystic fibrosis (CF) is a recessive genetic disorder that is the most prevalent in North American and Northern European people. It affects 1 in 2500 infants and is caused by mutation of the genes coding for CFTR (cystic fibrosis transmembrane regulator protein), which is a cAMP regulated chloride transporter. CF typically manifests as an exocrine pancreatic insufficiency, an increase in the concentration of chloride ions is sweat, infertility in males and chronic respiratory disease. The progressive lung dysfunction from repeated infectious processes is the major cause of morbidity and mortality in cystic fibrosis patients. Clinically, our goal is to keep these patients from getting sick. The essential problem is that their secretions, mucus, sweat, saliva and digestive fluids are thicker than might be ideal. Thinning those secretions requires an understanding of the chemistry involved in their production and activity. We will discuss the role of acid vs alkaline physiology in mucus chemistry, the role of digestive enzymes in impacting the viscosity of secretions as well as the ability of a body to digest food, and the far reaching role that sulfur containing amino acids and peptides, like N-Acetyl-Cysteine, methionine, glutathione, and selenomethionine play in the formation and activity of mucus. We will also discuss the critical role that botanical interventions can play in maintaining a healthy environment despite thickened secretions, including Ligusticum, Allium, Symplocarpus, Lobelia, Datura, Alpinia, and Anemopsis.

Autism— I believe that it is a mistake to 'blame' the development of autism on any single factor like genetics, epigenetics, vaccines or antibiotics. I also believe that it is a mistake to call it anything but a complex and multi-factorial neurologic manifestation that has a number of diverse contributors and predispositions. I believe that we have a far ranging spectrum of neurodiversity in the modern human condition and not every non-neurotypical manifestation is pathological. Some of these patients are intelligent beyond any normal human level of comprehension; they don't always express themselves efficiently. Some of them are lost within themselves and desperately trying to find a way out...others are quite content to stay right where they are. There are some interesting presumptions that modern understanding makes about the mind, the brain and spirit that may not be correct or appropriate presumptions. A good example is how easily we could lose ourselves in a conversation about whether the mind of a human being is housed within their brain, or somewhere else in the body, or outside of the physical body. Many people who have been diagnosed as being on the autistic spectrum early in their development find themselves, at some point in their lives, better able to communicate effectively with the world around them and they tell us that they were conscious while they were 'deeply autistic', they remember intimate details of what happened to them during that time, how they thought about things, how they were treated, what seemed to make them feel better or worse. Where were they? Where was their mind? Was it trapped inside their physical form? Some cultures do not believe that a spirit or mind is solely housed within the braincase, they may have recognized that some part of a person's spirit resides in the heart, another part in the liver, and yet another part somewhere distant from the physical self; other cultures fail to see any difference between physical placement of mind and body, that these two are one in the same. The modern medical model contends that neurotransmitters and neural circuitry are the primary determiners of behavior and, therefore, presupposes that the mind is housed within the nervous system. Spirit, in some sense, resides in some kind of interaction between dopamine, serotonin and acetylcholine as they pass across a vast array of neurons and synapses. When that system breaks down or becomes dysfunctional, neurological/mental illness manifests, so the theory goes. Of course, it is overly simplistic to reduce the richness of human experience down to a series of chemical reactions within the nervous system. Each of us is certainly more than the sum of our parts.

Autism is a tricky arena because there are fuzzy margins around what is truly pathological and what is a valid, but different, way of conducting one's life. Autism is considered a "spectrum disorder," meaning you can be anywhere in between a little autistic or very autistic. Until May, 2013, there were five "official" autism spectrum diagnoses, but the diagnoses within the autism spectrum weren't clearly named, nor were the symptoms always the same even within the same diagnosis. What's worse, terms like "severe autism," "mild autism" and "high functioning autism" aren't true diagnoses at all - they're just descriptive terms to help parents and teachers better understand a child's status on the autism spectrum. Today, with the DSM-5, there is just one "autism spectrum disorder" -- and everyone is lumped under that single diagnosis.

This "autism spectrum" describes a set of developmental delays and disorders, which affect social and communication skills and, to a greater or lesser degree, motor and language skills. It is such a broad diagnosis that it can include people with high IQ's as well as those with mental retardation - and people with autism can be chatty or silent, affectionate or cold, methodical or disorganized. It can include, for example, from poorly integrated verbal and nonverbal communication; to abnormalities in eye contact and body language or deficits in understanding and use of gestures; to a total lack of facial expressions and nonverbal communication. The diagnosis officially includes deficits in developing, maintaining, and understanding relationships, ranging from difficulties adapting behavior to suit various social contexts; to difficulties in sharing imaginative play or in making friends; to a complete absence of interest in peers.

These are people who tend toward self-restrictive, repetitive patterns of behavior, interests, or activities that could include stereotyped or repetitive motor movements, ritualized use of objects, or speech (e.g., simple motor stereotypes, lining up toys or flipping objects, echolalia, idiosyncratic phrases that have lost context or have an unknown context). They are often insistent on sameness; predictability and consistency seem to bring a sense of safety and security. Often, these patients have a sensory integration component to their condition that makes them hyper or hypo-reactive to certain kinds of sensory input. They may have an apparent indifference to pain or temperature changes, an adverse response to specific sounds or textures, they may smell everything around them or touch objects with a fascination toward textures or sounds or have a visual fascination with lights or movement. The barest inkling of these tendencies may be present early on in development but may not become fully manifest until social demands exceed their capacities and the individual resorts to self-soothing, comforting behaviors and turning more inward.

In sorting out what might be a pathological manifestation vs. simply a manifestion of neurodiversity, and how we may best help this population of people find their way to a place of peace and self-reliance, it might make sense to start with a brief and admittedly, oversimplified, overview of the major neurotransmitters and what their functions are, so that we can discuss what sorts of methods and agents are able to impact them in the developing mind-field. The major players are recognized to be the monoamines; dopamine, serotonin, and norepinephrine. Serotonin, of course, has practically become a household name since the advent of Prozac, the original Selective Serotonin Reuptake Inhibitor (SSRI). When serotonin levels are good, a person is able to socialize well, they are able to take on leadership roles and interact with other people in a positive and meaningful way. When serotonin levels fall too low, a person can become depressed and anti-social and when they are too high, a person can develop autistic tendencies and be anti-social, or, at least, easily over-stimulated by the social arena. Norepinephrine is made from dopamine and was the second neurotransmitter ever to be discovered (after acetylcholine). When it is present in appropriate amounts, it allows a person to drive a decent stress response such as increasing heart rate and blood vessel tone, it provides a certain "get up and go", and it largely stimulates emotional responsiveness. When it is too low, this can cause depression and fatigue, when it is too high, anxiety and panic attacks. Dopamine is the major neurotransmitter in the corpus striatum of the brain and is heavily involved in motor function and emotional responsiveness. When dopamine levels are right and its receptors appropriate, dopamine allows a sense of euphoria, it allows a mind to learn, problem-solve, and have spiritual epiphanies, it also allows for pattern recognition, abstract thought processes, executive behaviors and the appropriate development of learning strategies. When Dopamine levels are too low in the body, this can cause tremors and memory loss, levels that are too high can trigger schizophrenic and psychotic experiences. Dopamine and norepinephrine are considered to be the seat of addiction as well as the central pivot point for obsessive-compulsive conditions; a lot of the agents that have addictive properties are recreational because they are able to create a euphoric state through modulation of the emotional responsiveness of the limbic system. Other factors that affect the ability of a neurotransmitter to function predictably is the state and levels of its respective receptors. Serotonin, for example, has seven classes of receptor types, with some of these classes also containing several subtypes each of which performs a subtly different role than the others in its class. Dopamine has five families of receptors, and norepinephrine has two families (alpha and beta) with several subtypes within each family. It is not enough to talk about a neurotransmitter being too high or low, we also have to take into account the relative responsiveness of the receptors and the genetic/epigenetic basis for creating more of one type of receptor and less of another. Some part of this genetic basis creates the predisposition for autistic tendencies in an individual. We are coming into a greater understanding of epigenetics and mutations in the genes for enzymes like the methyltetrahydrofolate reductases. What happens if a system is unable to adequately process the necessary components for the formation of a particular neurotransmitter? It develops anyway and finds ways around the deficit, for better or for worse. It is clear that a certain amount of normal human neurodiversity is related to this kind of phenomenon. There are thousands, if not millions, of subtle biochemistries that affect the way that we experience everyday life, the beautiful redundancy of the human organism is such that many of our building blocks can play roles outside those that are originally assigned to them. Using the amino acids serine, glycine and threonine, as an example, for a neurobiological role that is not usual for them, potentially allows for the formation of a brand new perspective in a nervous system. It may allow this individual to suddenly see their world in a wholly new way. We might consider that it was a 'wrong' event because we think serine should have played the role that glycine played, perhaps we could fix that glitch and that person's physiology could better match what current medical thinking says it should look like. We have to ask ourselves, what kind of difference would that make? Is there a net gain or a net loss in bringing 'dysfunctional' neurochemistry into a more neuro-typical pattern? I would present that the next levels of human neuro-evolution may well resemble autism, and this question of neurodiversity vs pathology may have bigger consequences at stake than any of us currently realize.

Fragile X—The incidence of mental developmental delays and retardation is well established to be higher in males than in females. In 1943, Martin and Bell reported a genetically based mental retardation consistent with x-linked inheritance. In 1969, Lubs described a marker X, which consisted of a constriction in the distal long arm of the X chromosome that was present in affected males and non-affected carrier females of a family with X-linked inherited mental retardation. In 1977, Sutherland established the best medium for culturing and determining what was then termed 'fragile X syndrome'. The syndrome is not terribly common, occurring in approximately 1 in 1250 males and 1 in 2500 females and accounts for 20% of all inherited cases of mental retardation. Typical post-pubertal males physically manifest the "Martin-Bell" syndrome-global mental development delays, long face and everted ears and macro-orchidism (abnormally large testes). Other cranial features include a prominent jaw, large forehead, and relative macrocephaly.

Other features that are related to connective tissue dysplasia include hyper-mobile joints, mitral valve prolapse, and dilatation of the ascending aorta. Developmental delay and mental retardation are the most significant and prominent symptoms of Fragile X syndrome. Most male patients will have an IQ in the 20-60 range and exhibit some characteristic behaviors, which include hyperactivity, short attention span, emotional instability, hand mannerisms and autistic features. The physical and behavioral features of the condition differs a bit in females, it is generally milder, the somatic features may be absent or mild, the intelligence deficit in female patients is far less severe with mild-to-borderline mental impairment. There is an increase in psychological and psychiatric problems in female patients.

Conventional medicine offers no specific treatment for patients suffering from Fragile X. For the most part, there is no real pathology other than anxiety and hyperactivity. Unfortunately, these patients are identified as mentally retarded, they certainly have a lower IQ, but they also aren't necessarily great at taking standardized tests, so a true evaluation of their intelligence potential is unable to be adequately conducted. Patients with Fragile X tend to have more difficulty with auditory processing than with visual processing, which tends to correlate to their attentional problems, impulsivity and distractibility. Calming techniques, such as deep breathing, meditation, relaxation and music therapy are helpful in avoiding emotional upsets and outbursts in new situations or confusing circumstances. Botanical medicine and appropriate nutritional support can be tremendously supportive for these patients in their pursuit of a good quality of life. We discuss strategies for mitigating anxiety and improving cognitive functioning through consistent dietary interventions and creative botanical medicine preparations using such agents as Leonotis leonurus, Sceletium tortuosom, Albizia lebbeck, Scutellaria baicalensis, Valeriana spp, Nardostachys, Schisandra and Leonurus cardiaca. Nutritionally supportive agents like Phenibut, theanine, threonine, glycine phosphatidylserine, and other phospholipids will also be discussed.

Klinefelter syndrome is a genetic condition that results when a male is born with an extra X chromosome. It is a relatively common genetic condition and it often isn't diagnosed until after puberty because its most dramatic impact is on testicular growth, resulting in smaller than normal testicles, which can lead to lower production of testosterone. The syndrome may ultimately cause reduced muscle mass, reduced body and facial hair, and enlarged breast tissue. However, signs and symptoms of Klinefelter syndrome are present at all ages, often recognized retrospectively.

Infants and toddlers may present with weak muscles, delayed motor development (taking longer than average to sit up, crawl and walk), delay in speaking, quiet, docile personality and mono or cryptorchidism (failure of the testes to descend).

At pubertal age, the signs and symptoms often include taller than average stature with longer legs, shorter torso and broader hips compared with other boys their age, absent, delayed or incomplete puberty, less muscle, facial and body hair compared with peers, small genitals, enlarged breast tissue, weak bones, lowered energy levels, tendency to introversion, social awkwardness with difficulty expressing thoughts and feelings, cognitive delays in reading, writing, spelling or math.

Adults tend to present with tall stature, small genitals, lowered sex drive and sperm count, weak bones and teeth, reduced muscle and tone, decreased facial and body hair, and enlarged breast tissue.

The vast majority of the complications caused by Klinefelter syndrome are related to low testosterone and low thyroid function. Testosterone and thyroid replacement therapy reduces the risk of certain health problems, especially when therapy is started at the beginning of puberty. Modifications of testosterone receptors and regulation of metabolic enzymes with botanical medicines can be very helpful. These are patients who present with infertility and sexual dysfunction alongside anxiety and depression. Osteoporosis, cardiovascular disease, breast cancer, diabetes, autoimmune tendencies toward lupus and RA, and dental issues from poor calcification of bone are also common in this population of patients. We will discuss botanical and nutritional interventions that impact testosterone production and utilization, including testosterone precursors like androstenedione, and androstenediol, and 6-OXO, as well as botanicals which impact receptor sensitivity like Cissus quadrangularis, Tribulus terrestris, Panax spp, elutherococcus, Withania somnifera, Pfaffia paniculata, and animal derived substances like deer and elk antler velvet.

Marfan's Syndrome is autosomal dominant genetic disorder that impacts the 15th chromosome and affects 1 in 10,000 live births; it carries a wide range of expressions in those affected. It primarily presents as a connective tissue disorder involving the production of the fibrillin needed to make connective tissue. Fibrillin is a glycoprotein, which is secreted into the extracellular matrix by fibroblasts and becomes incorporated into the tissue microfibrils to provide a scaffold for the deposition of elastin. It is essential for the formation of elastic fibers found in all connective tissue, without it, the tissue becomes too elastic and stretches beyond the norm. This condition creates a triad of musculoskeletal, ocular and cardiac diseases. These patients tend to be tall with a very slender build, have a tendency toward scoliosis, an armspan that exceeds height and leg length that exceeds trunk length. They tend to be hyperflexible in their joints, possess arachnodactyly (Spider fingers), Pectus deformity (Pigeon Breast or Funnel Breast), and a high narrow palate.

Cardiovascular concerns are variable and may consist of mitral valve prolapse, aortic root dilatation, myocardial infarction, aortic insufficiency, congestive heart failure, subacute bacterial endocarditis, aneurysm and aortic dissection. Epigenetically, these patients don't methylate appropriately and tend to have high homocysteine levels. Ocular signs and conditions are related to improper deposition of elastin and dysfunctional protein shape and include upward ectopia lentis, myopia, iridodonesis, glaucoma and retinal detachment. We will discuss epigenetic factors like methylation processes, connective tissue considerations like the roles of lysine, proline and ascorbic acid in the formation of the collagen triple braid, preservation of connective tissue through anabolic methods driven by some of the botanical agents discussed with Klinefelter's syndrome. As well as some of the cardiovascular botanicals that are extremely helpful for these patients like Terminali arjuna, Convallaria majalis, Urginea, Selenocereus and Leonurus.

Down syndrome (DS) is the most common genetic cause of intellectual disability, affecting 1 in 650-1000 live births. In 1866, the condition was initially described by British physician John Langdon Down. Over 95% of DS cases are a result of a whole chromosome trisomy due to a failed separation of one pair of the 21st chromosome. The three copies of the chromosome 21 lead to a characteristic facial appearance, intellectual disability defined by impaired language skills, diminished learning and memory capacities. They also experience accelerated aging, and early onset alzheimer's disease. DS is characterized by extensive individual variability, the triplet of chromosome 21 alone would be expected to produce a predictable and consistent set of pathologies, which is not the case. Conceivably, epigenetic mechanisms play a crucial role in the physical manifestations of Down's syndrome. Although most of the role of epigenetics in DS is currently far from being completely understood, and increasing body of evidence suggests the involvement of DNA methylation processes, post-translational histone modifications and histone core variants in these physical manifestations. This is an important consideration because epigenetic mechanisms are often reversible, and offer therapeutic potential to prevent or improve the cognitive symptoms of DS. Included in these interventions are such disparate approaches as low dose thyroid hormone replacement therapy, supplementation of methyl donors like methylcobalamin, trimethylglycine, MTH-Folate, Pyridoxal-5-phosphate, and the histone modifiers NAD+, EGCG and SAMe.

These are some of the sweetest, kindest patients we will ever see in clinical practice. Some of them have savant capabilities, most of them are just bright lights in a cynical and tumultuous world. There is no real 'management' of their condition, many of them tend to be low thyroid, they can be easily sucked into the world of electronics and tend to thrive more when they are exposed to the outside world. I try to encourage families to engage socially with other families who have a member with Down syndrome as appropriate socialization really makes a difference in all of our sense of well-being. Any of us who find ourselves different than the norm depicted on the television or on advertising billboards are going to tend to feel somewhat alone and alienated. Being a part of a community of people that look and act like us can be truly liberating and encouraging on a very deep level. Thriving is dependent on the individual and what literally feeds them intellectually.

Epigenetics and Mental Health: Botanical and Dietary Influences
Kenneth Proefrock, ND

Summary: We discuss the biochemical specifics of neurotransmitter production, receptor sensitivity and activity, and neurotransmitter metabolism. We cover the complex subject of human mental activity, emotional responsiveness and this vague idea of a sense of self, a sense of accomplishment and the impact that early life events have on full grown adults. We will cover the interaction of certain hormones and their impact on neurotransmitter activity—especially cortisol, testosterone, estrogen and progesterone and the epigenetics that impact production and activity of those factors. Most importantly, we discuss therapeutic strategies that are helpful…and the fact that narrowly acting pharmaceuticals seldom effect long-term and beneficial change, whereas shifting the ecology makeup of the microbiome, and the subtleties of botanical medicine and dietary interventions are better suited to long term beneficial impact.

Mental illness is an uncomfortable and mysterious subject for many of us; at one time it was all chalked up to demonic possession and blamed on spiritual factors. It would be convenient to maintain the position that if you get right with your Gods, all of this pathology drops away and sanity persists. Clearly, this is not the case; in fact, in some corners of society religiosity can be the last refuge of the insane. Mental disorders are the leading cause of disability in North America for people aged 15-44. About 1 in 4 adults over the age of 18 suffer from a diagnosable mental disorder. We have this kind of data from the relatively privileged lives inhabiting industrialized nations; in Third World countries these numbers are simply not available. The Global Forum for Health Research tells us that more than 90% of the global budget for health research is spent on less than 10% of the world's health problems. For the Third World, this means that many diseases that could be treated effectively simply are not. Is the mother in Uganda whose 11 year old was killed after being inducted into a Holy War militia depressed? What about the family in Somalia whose house was turned into rubble overnight, do they have a diagnosable anxiety disorder? How many children die every year from something as simple as dehydration from diarrhea—the answer is 2 million. Are their parents depressed, anxious, neurotic or psychotic? What can they tell us about panic disorders, what do they have to say about the conditions of life, and how the environment they call home impacts their sense of well being? We are not separate from our neighbors, the collective consciousness of humanity may well be disgruntled at this moment in time, that disgruntlement will find itself manifested where it is able, and we can measure and perhaps better understand some of the physical ramifications of that disgruntlement by looking through the lens of epigenetics.

Epigenetics, literally, "above" or "in addition to" genetics, includes a multitude of mechanisms that regulate and control genetic expression. These molecular mechanisms include processes like DNA methylation, histone modification and RNA-mediated regulation. It is an arena of cellular understanding that is garnering a more significant amount of attention from the medical community because it provides an explanation for the relationship between an individual's genetic background, their environment, aging and disease and their ability to function and maintain a sense of well-being through life. There are some technically oriented explanations within this realm that go beyond the scope of this discussion. However, as a brief introduction, consider that every cell in your body has the same 23 chromosomes with the exact same encoded DNA. A liver cell has to look and act differently than a nerve cell, yet they contain the same genetic material. Epigenetics describes the process by which any particular cell takes on the necessary characteristics for it to be different enough to perform a unique set of functions. Everything begins with a primordial stem cell, a cell that has the potential to become any cell in the body. Within the nucleus of that cell, which has a diameter of a few microns, those 23 pairs of chromosomes are encoding so much information that if you were to stretch them out, end-to-end, they would be several meters long. The bundling process involves winding the double-stranded DNA filaments around basic (alkaline) protein bundles called histones. Literally, each histone bundle has eight parts (it is an octamer) with four core histone types that affect the way that DNA can be replicated. Each histone octamer, and the DNA filaments wound around it, are called a nucleosome. The histones are integrally involved in how the DNA is replicated and they can be modified in 6 different ways: acetylation, methylation, phosphorylation, ADP-ribosylation, mono-ubiquitylation, and sumoylation. As the histones are modified, they dictate which genes and how much of them can be replicated at any portion of the DNA. These 6 primary epigenetic changes influence a broad range of effects on everything from gene transcription, DNA replication/repair, to gene silencing and chromosomal assembly and condensation. There are four core types of histones and they interact with one another very specifically. H2A and H2B form a dimer with one another, (H2A-H2B), two H3 and two H4 histones link up to form a tetramer $(H3-H4)_2$. The histone octamer consists of one $(H3-H4)_2$ tetramer and two (H2A-H2B) dimers, $(H3-H4)_2-(H2A-H2B)_2$. Associated with each nucleosome are the enzymes and other proteins (including some RNA) that are involved in DNA replication. Nucleosomes are bound together by the DNA that winds around them like beads on a string. Bundled nucleosomes become chromatin, the building block of the chromosome.

Mental disorders are vague conditions for many people and are roughly categorized by abnormalities in cognition, emotion or mood, or the higher integrative aspects of behavior, such as social interactions or planning of future activities. These mental functions are currently believed to be mediated by the brain. However, throughout ancient history, the world over, and up until the middle ages, humans have associated aspects of our mental lives with organs other than the brain, such as the heart, the liver or the spleen. The concept of 'nervous diseases', which included psychiatric and neurological conditions together resulting from dysfunction of the brain, didn't become consolidated and strengthened until the 18th century. In the 19th century, we see these two realms diverging into separate areas of study. Disorders accompanied by a structural abnormality of the brain tended to be called neurological disorders. Disorders of the 'psychic apparatus' of the brain tend to be called psychiatric disorders, and were thought, by some, to be neurology without the physical signs. For much of the 20th century, these two disciplines were separated by divergent philosophical foundations, which impacted the research and therapeutic approaches toward them. The triumph of neuropathology and the clinico-pathologic methodology led to neurology becoming refined as a structurally based discipline. The advent of psychoanalysis in the US during the 1930's reinforced the concept of psychodynamic psychiatry within a conceptual framework of a psychic apparatus that began to be seen as no longer separated from the physical brain, but only loosely linked by circumstance. Medical understanding has now melded these two worlds so completely that the core tenet of modern science is that the neurotransmitters and circuitry of the nervous system are the primary determiners of behavior. The current presupposition is that the "mind" is housed somewhere within this nervous system. That Spirit, in some physically tangible sense, resides in some kind of interaction between the neurotransmitters dopamine, serotonin and acetylcholine within the limbic system.

We might agree that it is a mistake to reduce the richness of human experience down to a series of chemical reactions. We certainly seem to be more than the sum of these parts. Even so, the graspable portion of this mystery that is life is often the solid, concrete, and measurable aspect of this state. As we discuss these concrete and relatively objective aspects, we don't want to fall into the trap of thinking that this is all there is. What separates you and I from other medical arts is a fundamental philosophy towards life and the preservation of it. In discussing the subject matter of neurotransmitters and their relationship to mental illness, epigenetics ensures that we don't reduce the richness of the human experience down to so many molecules.

Neuropsychiatric epigenetics represents the progressive edge of understanding the nuts and bolts of how the psychosocial, environmental and, even spiritual factors impact biological unfolding and modification of DNA and RNA in the constantly remodeling expression of this physical form. The brain is the most complex and complicated organ in the body; it is comprised of 100 billion neurons connected in a vast network of circuitry. The whole human genome only contains 20,000-24,000 genes; it is highly improbable that such a relatively small number of genes could have encoded enough information to specify such a high level of complexity that is the human brain. Epigenetic regulation of gene expression represents a critical facet of human biochemistry that is subject to environmental feedback and offers an avenue to more completely encode the development and functioning of the human brain. Epigenetics provides as much a 'why' as a 'how' with environmental factors affecting gene expression as the human experience unfolds. Molecular epigenetic mechanisms literally inscribe early life experiences into the DNA and chromatin of neural cells and thus act as a mediator between one's environment and reflexive adaptation strategies.

The nuts and bolts of the six types of epigenetic changes described above consist of a wide range of effects that include, post-translational modifications of core histones, structure of chromatin, nucleosome positioning, and RNA translation. Originally, DNA methylation represented the core concept of molecular epigenetics. The methylenetetrahydrofolate reductase (MTHFR) mutation was one of the first epigenetic changes to be tested in patients. It is involved in folate metabolism and in the formation of cellular reserves of the methyl donor S-adenosyl-methionine (SAMe). MTHFR deficiency interferes with the conversion of homocysteine to methionine and allows high levels of homocysteine to accumulate. This causes a predisposition to inflammation in the blood vessels, leading to an increased risk for stroke and cardiovascular disease. Specific MTHFR polymorphisms (C677T and A1298C) are associated with types of depression. If the issue is a reduction in methylation, perhaps we should blanket the population with DNA methylators like methylcobalamin, methyltetrahydrofolate (MTHF), Pyridoxal-5-Phosphate and S-Adenosyl-methionine (SAMe)? No, we tried that in the early days of epigenetic understanding and we made some people far worse. It turns out that a balance has to be created that involves both methylation and de-methylation, in appropriate balance. In fact, DNA methylation has become defined as an all purpose repressive mechanism in gene regulation…too much and we inhibit too much genetic expression, too little and the system is unable to control gene over-expression. To get a little technical…DNA methylation describes the addition of a methyl group the fifth carbon of the nucleotide base cytosine that takes place primarily in somatic cells. The existence of DNA methylation was hypothesized as early as 1925 and its function was believed to produce inactivation of X-chromosome activity and play a role in cancer development and progression. Current understanding suggests that the effect of DNA methylation is dependent on genomic composition, sequence composition, and transcriptional status…and can contribute to gene activation or suppression.

Recall from earlier in this work that core histones represent highly basic proteins that serve to tightly package DNA so that it fits within the nucleus of the cell. This compressed state, chromatin, provides a platform on which gene regulation is carried out and modification of the histone proteins represents a common mechanism for epigenetically impacting genomic translation. These histone modifications can be related to methylation processes or be completely independent of them. The nucleus of the cell contains 23 pairs of DNA wound around histone octamers composed of two copies of each core histone to generate a nucleosome, the building block of chromatin. As the nucleosomes become further contained into higher order structures in the presence of linking histones and other non-histone proteins, they become less available to the transcriptional machinery. Epigenetic modifications of the chromatin play an important role in DNA packaging, gene transcription, cross-talk between DNA methylation and chromatin configuration, and ultimately, integration of intrinsic and environmental signals into the epigenome.

During neurological development, neural stem cells differentiate into brain tissue, neurons and glial cells (astrocytes and oligodendrocytes). Remaining neural stem cells serve as a reservoir of dormant undifferentiated material throughout life and have the ability to self-renew and differentiate into new tissues on an as needed basis, a process that is driven and regulated by epigenetic factors that are, in turn, driven by environmental cues and feedback. Epigenetics governs the unfolding of brain functions like synaptic transmission, memory storage and retrieval, neuronal plasticity, cognition, behavior, neuroendocrinology, neuroimmunology and neuroinflammation. As epigenetic mechanisms of gene expression play a major role in the proper development and functioning of the brain, they are also heavily involved in the development of disorders of the brain and neural tissue, and are triggered by environmental cues. The ultimate objective in any arena of medical understanding is to improve the clinical management and quality of life of the affected patients in terms of diagnosis, prevention and treatment. This requires a translation of theoretically oriented research into the practical world of patient care, a process that, unfortunately, is currently funded by large corporations with a vested interest in creating pharmaceutical interventions for these conditions. Interestingly, most abnormal epigenetic patterns of gene expression are potentially reversible by changes in the environmental triggers that created them in the first place. The human body is constantly in a state of remodeling, most cells of the body have a finite life and as newer tissue is formed to replace dead and dying tissues, the epigenetic influence of the environment either supports a continued dysfunctional operation or helps improve functionality. Botanical medicines, with their broader base of activity and richer array of constituents than prescribed drugs, as well as dietary modification, psychotherapy, and physical exercise are able to help correct abnormal epigenetic mechanisms of gene expression most effectively. There are currently no pharmaceutical drugs that can accomplish this objective to the same degree.

In order to continue this conversation into neurotransmitter production, we have to include sharing some concepts and language, beginning with a brief overview of the major neurotransmitters and associated neural architecture and how we currently understand their function. The concept of neurodiversity has a home here; it is the idea that human consciousness is a complex and multi-factorial neurologic manifestation that has a number of diverse contributors and predispositions. Humans enjoy a far ranging spectrum of neurodiversity and not every non-neurotypical manifestation is pathological. Every stage of human development allows our psyche a set of choices, the first is to either expand into that level of development and embrace everything that is associated with it or contract certain aspects of our unfolding and create a defensive psychological position at that level of development. The relative degree of safeness vs. unsafeness in a person's perception of their world is often the primary driver for whether they are expanding or contracting at any particular stage of their developmental process. An important consideration is that every stage provides the foundation of development for the next stage, if a patient starts contracting and defending at 6 years old, that is far more significant when they are 30 than if they started that process at 25 years of age.

Early life adversity (ELA) also known as adverse childhood experiences (ACEs) play a far more significant role than ever before realized in the manifestation of psychiatric diseases like major depressive disorder (MDD), PTSD, schizophrenia and borderline personality disorder. ELA is defined by a number of conditions comprising parental maladjustment (mental illness, substance abuse, violence, criminal tendencies), interpersonal loss (separation from parents or caregivers through death or estrangement), life threatening childhood physical illness, severe poverty, and maltreatment (sexual and physical abuse, neglect). There were 668,000 child victims of abuse and neglect in the US reported in 2012. Childhood neglect is the most common form of mistreatment, representing 78.3% of reported abuse; physical abuse represented 18.3% and sexual abuse/molestation 9.3%. Maternal mood disorders represent a major risk factor for the developing fetus and are associated with premature delivery and restricted growth during the neonatal period of life. Offspring of depressed mothers are more likely to manifest impairments in mental, emotional, and motor development and are at greater risk for developing adolescent depression and anxiety. Maternal under-nutrition during gestation is associated with increased risk for metabolic abnormalities later in life such as obesity, diabetes, elevated lipid levels and cardiovascular disease. Early under-nutrition in in humans most commonly occurs in the context of severe socioeconomic distress or parental misbehavior, it is impossible to dissect the effects of under-nutrition on general brain development vs specific mental dysfunctions, nonetheless, it is strongly associated with lasting impairments in cognitive and social behaviors.

As we go deeper and discuss the reasons why these associations are believed to exist, we should discuss the primary affected players in the processes of adaptation, appropriate mental functioning and emotional responsiveness. The major players in this process are the monoamines neurotransmitters; dopamine, serotonin, and norepinephrine. Serotonin, of course, has practically become a household name since the advent of Prozac, the original Selective Serotonin Reuptake Inhibitor (SSRI). When serotonin levels are good, a person is able to socialize well, they are able to take on leadership roles and interact with other people in a positive and meaningful way. When serotonin levels fall too low, a person can become depressed and anti-social and when they are too high, a person can develop autistic tendencies, and become anti-social. The amino acids tryptophan and 5-hydroxytryptophan are precursors in serotonin production; S-Adenosyl-methionine (SAMe) is a necessary cofactor in the process. Norepinephrine is the next big player; it is made from dopamine and was the second neurotransmitter to be discovered. When it is present in appropriate amounts, it allows a person to drive a decent stress response such as increasing heart rate and blood vessel tone, it provides a certain "get up and go", and it largely regulates emotional responsiveness. When it is too low, this can cause depression and fatigue, when it is too high, anxiety and panic attacks. Dopamine is the major neurotransmitter in the corpus striatum of the brain and is heavily involved in motor function and, with norepinephrine, emotional responsiveness. It is made form L-Tyrosine and/or Phenylalanine and requires Vitamin B6 as a cofactor. When dopamine levels are right and its receptors appropriate, dopamine allows a sense of euphoria, it allows a mind to learn, problem-solve, and have spiritual epiphanies. When Dopamine levels are too low in the body, this can cause tremors and memory loss, levels that are too high can trigger schizophrenia and psychosis. Dopamine and norepinephrine are considered to be the seat of addiction; a lot of the agents that have addictive properties are recreational because they are able to create a euphoric state through modulation of the emotional responsiveness of the limbic system.

Of course, what I have just presented is a gross oversimplification; it is just a starting point. One other major factor that affects the ability of a neurotransmitter to function is the state and levels of its respective receptors. Serotonin, for example, has seven classes of receptor types, with some of these classes also containing several subtypes, each of which performs a subtly different role than the others in its class, and epigenetics serve to improve or reduce their relative sensitivity. Dopamine has five families of receptors, and norepinephrine has two families (alpha and beta) with several subtypes within each family. It is not enough to talk about a neurotransmitter being too high or low, we also have to take into account the relative responsiveness of the receptors and the epigenetic basis for creating more of one type of receptor and less of another. It is a natural response to high levels of a particular receptor to down-regulate the receptors for that neurotransmitter, the other side of the coin is that chronically low levels of a particular neurotransmitter tend to up-regulate the activity of its respective receptors. Modern pharmacology utilizes re-uptake inhibition as a way of keeping a neurotransmitter around for longer, the idea is that if low neurotransmitter production is "causing" the depressed state; let's increase the available amount of that neurotransmitter by inhibiting its breakdown. The problem with this approach is that it typically takes 3-4 weeks to see any appreciable affect, and last week's neurotransmitters still in use this week may contribute to what a lot of patients refer to as stagnant thought processes and lack of creativity while on these agents. There are certainly many botanical agents that possess a similar mechanism of action, Peganum harmala, Syrian Rue and Terrestris terribilis, Gokshura, contain the alkaloids, harmine and harmaline which are Mono-amine oxidase inhibitors, they tend to keep all of the mono-amines around for longer. Most of the botanical agents that are currently in clinical use aren't that specific, many of them seem to have an amphipathic effect on the neurotransmitter receptor. There are constituents within these plant medicines that have a particular affinity for the different neurotransmitter receptors. That affinity is typically much less than the affinity that the neurotransmitter itself possesses, when the plant constituent binds to the receptor it can temporarily interfere with the binding of the neurotransmitter if it is present in abundance or it can replace the binding of the neurotransmitter when it is deficient.

Acetylcholine was the first neurotransmitter to be identified. It was originally found in the heart and is the neurotransmitter at nerve-muscle connections for all of the voluntary muscles of the body as well as at many of the involuntary nervous system synapses. It serves as the neurotransmitter for 10-15 percent of all of the neurons of the body. It plays a crucial role in memory and reflective thinking. Acetylcholine has two distinct families of receptors, nicotinic and muscarinic. It is the nicotinic receptor that the alkaloids nicotine and lobeline, from tobacco and Lobelia, respectively, bind. It is the muscarinic receptor that binds the tropane alkaloids from Belladonna, Datura, and Hyoscyamus.

GABA is the most prevalent neurotransmitter in the brain, serving as the transmitter for 25-40% of all synapses in the brain. It is an inhibitory neurotransmitter; it slows the firing rate of a nerve. Research in the early 1960's showed that these inhibitory effects were potentiated by alcohol, barbiturates, and benzodiazepines. GABA plays a major role in inducing a normal sleep/wake cycle, inhibiting norepinephrine output and reducing anxiety. If GABA levels are too high, or if the receptor is over-stimulated, depression from low norepinephrine can result, this is one of the side effects of the benzodiazepine class of medications, this includes valium, xanax, klonopin, and restoril. Valeriana spp. are the botanical agents that are used in a similar manner, these contain constituents, like valerianic acid which bind to the GABA receptor with significantly less affinity than either GABA or the benzodiazepines. Valerian can be extremely helpful for some instances of anxiety and insomnia. Glycine is the simplest amino acid and has an inhibitory effect on the locus ceruleus, inhibiting norepinephrine output and augmenting the effect of Valerian, a typical and effective dosage is 2.5-5 gms 3-4 times per day.

Histamine is usually considered when we talk about allergy or stomach acid secretion. It also acts as a stimulating neurotransmitter, enhancing wakefulness and perception of "unsafeness" and an increase in "vigilance". This is one of the reasons why antihistamines often leave people feeling drowsy. It is also the reason why people can become "addicted" to the things that they are allergic to, histamine creates a certain type of "buzz" that seems more pronounced in some people more than others. Many flavonoids, like Quercetin, have a stabilizing quality on mast cells and help prevent excess histamine output.

Glutamic acid is the principle excitatory neurotransmitter in the nervous system; it stimulates neurons to fire. It is the neurotransmitter of the major neuronal pathway that connects the cerebral cortex and the corpus striatum. In vascular stroke, a massive amount of glutamic acid is released and accounts for much of the stroke associated neuronal damage. This is the pathway by which monosodium glutamate and aspartame are considered to be acting when a person has an adverse reaction to those agents. Over-stimulation of the glutamate receptors results in irritability, agitation, and headaches. Vinca spp. and Ginkgo biloba are helpful in many cases of excess glutamate output by helping to remove the excess neurotransmitter from the nervous system more quickly, vitamin B-6 is also extremely helpful in such situations at dosages of 100-300 mg/day.

The central endocrine axis of the body is the hypothalamic-pituitary-adrenal axis or HPA axis. The name is pretty self-descriptive, as some generic stressor is perceived in one's environment neurologically (sensorially), this triggers a response on the part of the hypothalamus, which, in turn, triggers a response within the anterior pituitary gland, which then stimulates an adrenal response. We should emphasize that stress is not what happens to an organism, but rather, how they respond to what has happened to them, which is also directed by epigenetic expectations and personal history of stress and nutrition status. This is a critical distinction, we may have no control over what happens to us, b ut, to some degree, we can control how we respond to that event. This distinction can be incredibly empowering to an overwhelmed patient who feels that their world is falling down around them. No substance in the world can ever keep their world from continuing to fall apart, but, a well placed physical agent and a change in perception can help trigger a different response towards their situation and make all the difference in their ability to handle it. Perception then, becomes the first important area to understand at a fundamental level. Deep in your brain stem dwells an area called your reticular activating system (RAS), this is the area of your nervous system that helps you become more aware of some aspect of your environment. If you buy a blue car, suddenly you notice all of the other blue cars on the road. A more important function of this area of the brain from an anthropological perspective is that if your village is being stalked by some large predator, you are noticing every shadow, every movement, as a potential attacker. Epigenetically induced hypervigilance makes one begin treating unimportant stimuli as if it were novel and potentially threatening. The RAS affects and is affected by an area just a little further upstream anatomically, the locus ceruleus. The locus ceruleus is a blue (cerulean blue) streak of tissue located in the pons of the brain and contains the highest concentration of catecholamine releasing neurons in the body. It can rightly be looked at as the vigilance center of the brain, as a person's world is perceived as being "unsafe", the locus ceruleus increases its output of norepinephrine. As norepinephrine levels increase in the brain, the hypothalamus increases output of corticotropin releasing factor (CRF), which, in turn, stimulates the release by the anterior pituitary gland of adrenocorticotropic hormone (ACTH). ACTH stimulates the adrenal glands to increase their output of the cortisol, the primary glucocorticoid stress hormone which provides most of the impetus for physiological shunting throughout the body allowing the person to better survive whatever stressor has been presented to them. You should get the idea that there is a complex series of events at play here, allowing for several different metabolic sites for regulation of the process.

The function of the anterior pituitary gland is absolutely critical at this point in the process. The anterior pituitary gland releases "releasing" hormones, agents that allow for the release of other hormones. This is important because it plays the role of master gland for the other glands of the body, regulating their function. There are six releasing hormones; adrenocorticotropic hormone (ACTH), thyroid stimulating hormone (TSH), follicle stimulating hormone (FSH), luteinizing hormone (LH), growth hormone (GH), and prolactin. The release of these agents follows somewhat of a hierarchy, such that, if one of the releasing hormones is being produced at an increased rate, it suppresses the output of other releasing hormones. A perfect example of this phenomenon is prolactin-mediated suppression of FSH and LH output in lactating women, preventing initiation of a menstrual cycle and helping to avoid another pregnancy while the woman is breastfeeding. Another example is the role that ACTH plays to suppress output of FSH, LH, and TSH in order to slow metabolism and suspend the menstrual cycle or sperm formation under periods of greater stress. This is the level that most neuroenodcrine dysfunction begins to develop.

Cortisol is a glucocorticoid, as its name suggests, it has a profound role in maintaining appropriate blood glucose levels. Cortisol causes an increase in the mobilization of amino acids, stimulates gluconeogenesis and causes a decrease in glucose utilization by the tissues. As the primary stress hormone produced in the body, it also has profound anti-inflammatory effects, decreases immune responses and allergy, and increases red blood cell production. Sustained levels of glucocorticoids epigenetically alter the HPA axis such that perception and subsequent response to various stressors predisposes the individual to stress-related diseases later in life. Long-term stress and its epigenetic impact yields shrinkage and less branching of dendrites with a reduced synaptic input. A very important point to bear in mind is that cortisol shifts the whole system in order to better respond to stress. If a person has donuts and a soda for breakfast and then experiences a blood sugar slump at 10:30, which creates a need for cortisol to raise blood sugars, the whole system has had to respond to that need as if their world were suddenly an unsafe place. If such a thing takes place every day, several times a day, their world is perceived as a progressively less safe place—which may not necessarily be true, but the body begins responding that way. What happens when that person experiences a real stressor? Like any other hormone in the body, if you are exposed to increasingly higher amounts over a long period of time, you become less sensitive to the hormone. This process is driven by receptors becoming fewer in number as the cell is exposed to increased amounts of the hormone as well as by epigenetic changes in the DNA encoding for hormone production. If a person is already putting out 3-5 times the amount of cortisol that is normally needed in a day, then any additional stress is going to require either a tremendously greater amount of cortisol to get the job done, or a stronger hormone. Epinephrine, or adrenalin, becomes that stronger hormone and usually brings some panic and anxiety along with it. Can extreme fluctuations in blood sugar over a long period of time contribute to the development of panic and anxiety disorder? You bet it can! The challenge is to instruct the patient about better dietary habits and then to progressively decrease their need for cortisol by helping them shift their adaptation strategies away from needing cortisol.

The locus ceruleus is one of the most remarkable structures in the brain. In humans, it is an area that contains only about three thousand neurons—a small number of neurons when one considers that there are several billion neuronal cells that comprise the cerebral cortex. These three thousand cells have axons that are incredibly long and branched in multiple places so that these cells are estimated to directly interact with as many as a third to a half of all the cells in the brain. The majority of the norepinephrine neurons in the brain have their origin in the locus ceruleus. As mentioned above, the norepinephrine system, with its myriad branching connections is thought to regulate emotional responses to the environment. It, in fact, is the center of vigilance within the nervous system, that is, it responds to the relative degree of "safeness vs. unsafeness" that might be present in a person's world.

The Reticular Activating System (RAS), mentioned earlier, is a structure in the brain stem that is primarily responsible for arousal and sleep. All sensory input is routed through the RAS, and any change in the environment that is detected by the sensory nerves is registered as such, and any change in the internal environment is registered as such. It is a complex collection of neurons that serve as a point of convergence for signals from the outside of the body and from inside. It is the place where external stimuli and internal thoughts and feelings meet. It plays a significant role in processing and learning information, and paying attention to what is important in one's world, what one should watch out for to stay safe. It essentially, establishes the "need" for vigilance based on a synthesis of internally derived and externally perceived information. An increase in the need for vigilance is responded to in the locus ceruleus by an increase in norepinephrine output. Increasing the norepinephrine output from the locus ceruleus has the effect in the hypothalamus of increasing output of Corticotropin Releasing Factor (CRF). This, in turn, causes an increase in pituitary output of Adrenocorticotropic hormone (ACTH) and this, in its turn, causes an increase in adrenal output of cortisol, the primary somatic stress hormone. This increase in cortisol provides a feedback loop through the RAS that things are better and the locus ceruleus can quiet down.

It is important to realize that an entire chain of events is generated by the output of ACTH and cortisol. A chain of events that affect pituitary output of other releasing hormones, inappropriate conversion of thyroid hormone, reproductive issues, and depression. Lifestyle habits can be huge contributors—coffee and doughnuts for breakfast—blood sugar highs and lows, hyperinsulinemia, catabolic vs. anabolic states, membrane neglect, allergy, IgE histamine and craving the foods that you are allergic to. The point is that simply manipulating neurotransmitters is seldom enough of an intervention to resolve a person's emotional issues, which is why the drug model has an estimated 60% failure rate.

Building on the foundation of a rudimentary understanding of the presumed principle players in the drama of life, let's take a look at some of the more common categories of dysfunction that we are likely to see in a clinical setting. With each condition, we will discuss the epigenetic components and attempt to set up a reasonable intervention strategy, not cook-book recipes, but specific interventions for specific situations drawn from a more global understanding of the condition.

The diagnosis of mental disorders is often more difficult than diagnosis of other general medical disorders; there is typically no definitive lesion, laboratory test, or abnormality in brain tissue that can identify the illness. The diagnosis of mental disorders must rest with the patients' reports of the intensity and duration of symptoms, signs from their mental status examination, and clinical observation of their behavior including functional impairment. These clues are grouped together by the clinician into recognizable patterns, or syndromes. When the syndrome meets all the criteria for a diagnosis, it constitutes a mental disorder. Most mental health conditions are referred to as disorders, rather than as diseases, because diagnosis rests on clinical criteria. The term "disease" generally is reserved for conditions with known pathology (detectable physical change). The term "disorder," on the other hand, is reserved for clusters of symptoms and signs associated with distress and disability (i.e., impairment of functioning), yet whose pathology and etiology may remain unknown. In this discussion, we use the term dis-ease to imply that there is a spectrum of "normal" human experience and when things are working properly and well, a person's body and mind are at "ease". When things are not going well, for any reason at all, we experience a sense of "dis-ease", my intention with presenting this term is to emphasize that the full expression of human emotion is essential for a healthy existence. In the same way that it isn't healthy to be sad or angry or depressed all of the time, it isn't healthy to be manically happy, either. The spontaneous arising of emotion in response to one's perceptions of the world is a beautiful response that should be honored, the full spectrum, the comfortable as well as the uncomfortable is essential to a healthy being.

The standard manual used for diagnosis of mental disorders in the United States is the *Diagnostic and Statistical Manual of Mental Disorders*. The first edition was published in 1952 by the American Psychiatric Association; subsequent revisions, which were made on the basis of field trials, analysis of data sets, and systematic reviews of the research literature, have sought to gain greater objectivity, diagnostic precision, and reliability. DSM-IV organizes mental disorders into 16 major diagnostic classes. For each disorder within a diagnostic class, DSM-IV enumerates specific criteria for making the diagnosis. DSM-IV also lists diagnostic "subtypes" for some disorders. A subtype is a subgroup within a diagnosis that confers greater specificity. DSM-IV is descriptive in its listing of symptoms and does not take a position about underlying causation.

Anxiety may be one of the most universal manifestations of mental dis-ease. Each of us encounters some form of anxiety throughout the course of our lives. It may often take the concrete form of intense fear experienced in response to an immediately threatening experience such as narrowly avoiding a traffic accident. Experiences like this are typically accompanied by strong emotional responses of fear and dread as well as physical signs of anxiety such as rapid heart beat and increased perspiration. Appropriate anxiety should be a normal part of how we deal with immediate threats to one's safety; this is norepinephrine, the limbic system, the locus ceruleus, and the Reticular Activiating System working the way that they should to protect the system. Inappropriate anxiety pervades one's daily existence and robs a person of their quality of life, often triggered by situations that one can only vaguely imagine or anticipate, often triggered by nothing in particular.

Specific examples of anxiety disorders include phobias, panic attacks, and generalized anxiety. In phobias, high-level anxiety is aroused by specific situations or objects that may range from concrete entities such as snakes, to complex circumstances such as social interactions or public speaking. Panic attacks are brief and very intense episodes of anxiety that often occur without a precipitating event or stimulus. Generalized anxiety represents a more diffuse and nonspecific kind of anxiety that is most often experienced as excessive worrying, restlessness, and tension occurring with a chronic and sustained pattern. In each case, an anxiety disorder may be said to exist if the anxiety experienced is disproportionate to the circumstance, is difficult for the individual to control, or interferes with normal functioning. Epigenetic programming can be heavily involved in anxiety conditions, early undernutrition and the conception that one's world is a relatively unsafe place are prime drivers of long-term anxiety. Epigenetic modifications involve methylation processes in DNA, Histone modification and alteration of RNA transcription and post-translational modification. Specifically, early life under-nutrition generally yields under-methylation of DNA and distorted neural development with receptors inappropriately insensitive to GABA and overly sensitive to Norepinephrine. Metabolism can be likewise distorted in adults with epigenetically programmed anxiety conditions, the message of an 'unsafe' world tends to reinforce processes that inhibit conversion of thyroid hormones, T4 to T3, as well as enhance storage of incoming resources rather than burning them as if more will come in the near future.

A high fiber, protein rich, omnivorous diet is often very helpful for these patients. I emphasize starting their day with 25-30 grams of good quality protein. I like to add a combination of Glycine/L-Threonine/Phosphatidylserine 2-3 times per day to inhibit the release of norepinephrine from the locus ceruleus, as well as to support better myelination of neurons. Dosages look like 1.5 gms glycine and L-Threonine and 100-200 mg phosphatidylserine, depending on sedating vs relieving anxiety effects. Daily aerobic exercise and meditation are game changers for most of these patients. Desensitization therapies like EMDR, neurofeedback and EFT can be immeasurably helpful, as time passes and the world around them can take on the characteristics of a safer place (avoid the media), the epigenome takes account and shifts to accommodate.

Obsessive-compulsive disorder (OCD) and post-traumatic stress disorder (PTSD) are related to anxiety disorders. In the case of obsessive-compulsive disorders, individuals experience a high level of anxiety that drives their obsessional thinking or compulsive behaviors. When such an individual fails to carry out a repetitive behavior such as hand washing or checking, there is an experience of severe anxiety. There appears to be a strong component of abnormal regulation of dopamine and norepinephrine in this situation, the ritualized behaviour brings relief, described by some of my patients like a "high". This may be related to a relative increase in dopamine within the limbic system. Unrealized or non-acted upon compulsions tend to build and cause an increase in anxiety that is quite similar to the withdrawal symptoms in addiction patients. Post-traumatic stress disorder is produced by an intense and overwhelmingly fearful event that is often perceived as life-threatening in nature. Originally it was a diagnosis that was used to help explain the difficulties that many Vietnam veterans were experiencing in the early 1970's reintegrating back into society after being in the war. The characteristic symptoms that result from such a traumatic event include the persistent re-experience of the event in dreams and memories; persistent avoidance of stimuli associated with the event, and increased arousal. Consider that here is a situation where the nervous system increased conversion of dopamine to norepinephrine to ensure its own survival. The definition of an effective survival adaptation is that you survived the circumstance; there may be little motivation for a system to revert back to a baseline "normal", after all, the subconscious mind might say, if the circumstances presented once, they are likely to present again.

Measures that can prove effective for these patients involve helping to reduce conversion of dopamine to norepinephrine, there are hundreds of ways that this can be accomplished. I have found that cognitive therapy combined with the right homeopathic remedies (selected for the individual) and botanical agents can be quite effective for people who suffer from anxiety disorders. There are over 360 different kinds of psychotherapy that are recognized by the American Psychological Association, they all work as long as they are able to provide a structure whereby the patient is able to objectify and the transcend their situation. Objectification involves creating a narrative of one's experiences and the feelings that those experiences evoke, the creation of a narrative allows the person to momentarily step outside of themselves in order to describe the circumstances, this allows some reprieve and a readjustment of their perception, the readjustment of perception often is what allows the transcendence. Guided imagery, visualization and hypnosis can be very effective measures to help the individual access buried memories and repressed emotions. Homeopathic remedies are chosen to help facilitate the readjustment of perception, they are often chosen for the individual based on a repertorization of their symptoms and as an archetypal anchoring tool. Botanical agents that are often effective include Valeriana spp., Scutellaria spp., Avena spp., Leonurus spp., Passiflora spp., Melissa, and neurological adaptogens like Aralia and Oplopanax. Cannabis and Psilocybin have also shown great promise in allowing the nervous system to 'reset' itself. Cannabinoids like THC and CBD can act as a primary messenger across synapses between nerves and allow for an unprecedented retrograde feedback control that modulates the flow of other neurotransmitters, keeping the nervous system running smoothly and not as subject to reflexive, reactive responses to normal triggers. Their role in neurological signaling has led to a hypothesis that endogenous cannabinoids may be responsible for the baseline level of neural sensitivity to particular triggers for pain and anxiety in the body. In fact, there is a growing understanding that the constant release of endocannabinoids could have a tonic effect on muscle tightness in multiple sclerosis, neuropathic pain, inflammation and appetite. The term 'endocannabinoid tone' is becoming used more frequently and appears to play a significant role in a general sense of one's well-being and has an epigenetic impact that is yet to be elucidated completely.

The cannabinoid 1 (CB1) receptor is expressed primarily in the central nervous system where endocannabinoids bind to CB1 receptors and act as a 'circuit breaker', modulating the release of other neurotransmitters. The brain functions that are modified by CB1 binding are quite enormous and include: decision-making, cognition, emotional responsiveness, learning and memory as well as regulation of body movement, anxiety, stress and fear responsiveness, appetite and motor control. Activation of the CB1 receptor is responsible for the psychoactive effects of Cannabis and results in the psychological and physical effects associated with recreational use. CB2 receptors are primarily found in blood cells, tonsils and the spleen (both of which are lymph organs), and present with none of the psychological or physical effects of CB1 activation. CB2 receptors control the release of cytokines linked to inflammation and refine immune response throughout the body. The far reaching impact that this plant and other psychotropic botanicals can have on the nervous system and epigenetic processes is just beginning to be understood.

The concept of psychosis, as we know it, dates only from the late 19th century. It was formed out of the remnants of three ancient categories: insanity, alienation and dementia. Psychoses are vaguely defined as disturbances of perception and thought processes. The threshold for determining whether one's perceptions and thoughts are appropriate or impaired varies tremendously with one's cultural context. Like anxiety, psychotic symptoms may occur in a wide variety of mental dis-eases. They are most characteristically associated with schizophrenia, but psychotic symptoms can also occur in severe mood disorders. One of the most commonly considered groups of symptoms that result from disordered processing and interpretation of sensory information are hallucinations and delusions. Hallucinations are presumed to occur when an individual experiences a sensory impression that has no counterpart in another individual in the same situation. This impression could involve any of the sensory modalities. Thus hallucinations may be auditory, olfactory, gustatory, kinesthetic, tactile, or visual. In contrast, a delusion is a false belief that an individual holds despite evidence to the contrary. A common example is paranoia, in which a person has delusional beliefs that others are trying to harm him or her. Attempts to persuade the person that these beliefs are unfounded typically fail and may even result in the further entrenchment of the beliefs. An important element that I feel deserves to be said regarding both hallucinations and delusions is that the inappropriateness of these experiences is established by people outside the person experiencing the hallucination or delusion. Often, when one engages in an interactive dialog with these patients, when that is possible, there is a clear logic that presents itself and makes one realize that given their perception of the world, any one of us might share their delusions. Consider that we depend on an appropriate kind of sensory information in order to make sense of the world around us, if we suddenly found ourselves receiving more information than any one else due to an increased sensitivity of a receptor or amount of neurotransmitter, we might derive significantly different conclusions about our reality. Who is to say that the shared reality that is dependent on a limited input of sensory information is the truest reality? Anyone who has experienced the relative psychosis that is evoked by the consumption of psychedelic substances may well understand the relative state of accepted reality.

The symptoms of schizophrenia are divided into two broad classes, *positive* symptoms and *negative* symptoms. Positive symptoms generally involve the experience of something in consciousness that would not normally be present. For example, hallucinations and delusions represent perceptions or beliefs that not everyone is experiencing; consider the interesting position of spirituality, prophecy, divination and other psychic phenomena in this paradigm. Major deficits in motivation and spontaneity are referred to as negative symptoms. While positive symptoms represent the presence of something not normally experienced, negative symptoms reflect the absence of thoughts and behaviors that would otherwise be expected. Concreteness of thought represents impairment in the ability to think abstractly. Blunting of affect refers to a general reduction in the ability to express emotion. Motivational failure and inability to initiate activities represent a major source of long-term disability in schizophrenic patients. Anhedonia reflects a deficit in the ability to experience pleasure and to react appropriately to pleasurable situations. Positive symptoms such as hallucinations are responsible for much of the acute distress associated with schizophrenia, but negative symptoms appear to be responsible for the long term destruction of quality of life associated with the condition. These are people who aren't being heard, mostly because they come across as crazy, and without the signposts of the collective consciousness to guide them in their journey through life, they become lost. I believe that, for many of these patients, the spectacular spiritual epiphanies that characterize their hallucinations are discounted as the crazy rantings of a lunatic, in another time and another place, who is to say that these wouldn't have been the spiritual leaders of great movements? Moses, John the Baptist, Jesus Christ, and Mohammed seem very psychotic when viewed through the lens of modern psychiatry. The complete discounting of powerful spiritual experience can be a very depressing event in a person's life. I am not proposing that the dominant spiritual/religious movements of our time are psychotic shadows of the past, nor am I suggesting that within every psychotic lies a messiah, just that it is too easy to institutionalize these individuals or drug them into complacency without seriously considering that they have something more to offer.

     Treatment of patients with psychosis is a dicey affair. One has to determine whether this is an individual that might present a risk to those around them or themselves. One has to also determine whether the medication the person is on is appropriate for their condition and that they have reached a stable point. Some people who suffer from psychoses have so lost their way that they may have to be over-medicated in order to objectify where they are and recover their perspective, unfortunately, these individuals are kept on that regimen indefinitely, mostly out of fear for their own safety and that of others. No single area of alternative medicine is fraught with the medico-legal issues that treatment of psychoses presents. I am happy to say that I have been successful with many of these patients—success determined by a reduction or elimination of their medication needs, and a restoration of a good quality of life with relatively normal relationships with those around them. The most important element, I believe is a re-empowerment of these individuals and conferring an understanding that they are perhaps receiving more information from the cosmos than the rest of us and it frankly freaks the rest of us out when they go off on some of those tangents. Journaling, when it can be engaged, is often a safer method of relating the significance of their perspective and a useful tool to realize when they may be becoming less rational and more delusional. It is imperative that these individuals maintain a long-term relationship with an understanding healthcare practitioner who can help them determine when they might be slipping into a more delusional state. I have relied on Rauwolfia serpentina and Rauwolfia vomitoria in many of these cases with very good resolution of the delusional states. Diet, exercise, amino acid supplementation and cognitive therapy are hugely important aspects of long term maintenance for these patients.

     The goal in using Rauwolfia as a an intervention is to bring the patient's dopamine levels down into a more normal range, so that they don't hear voices in their head anymore and can stay sane enough to hold down a job. There are more than 50 alkaloids isolated from Rauwolfia serpentina, reserpine is the most widely researched and understood. It has been the parent compound for a wide array of anti-hypertensive and anti-psychotic compounds that now proliferate modern medicine. Reserpine causes an alteration of the permeability of the membrane around pre-synaptic neurotransmitter storage vesicles so that the mono-amines leaks out and are degraded by monoamine oxidase before they ever reach the synaptic cleft between neurons. This effectively reduces the amount of available neurotransmitter and "blunts" the message that would have, ordinarily, been sent to the next neuron. This mechanism has been inappropriately attributed to the whole plant extract of Rauwolfia, but there are many other alkaloids present in this plant that serve to buffer its effects. The problem with reserpine is that too much of it can cause too great of a depletion of neurotransmitters like dopamine, serotonin and norepinephrine, causing depression, or Parkinson's symptoms. Many of the patients that I have treated for schizophrenia and bipolar developed their psychosis as a direct or indirect result of drug abuse, primarily methamphetamines and/or LSD. These are the patients that will use dosages high enough to experience side effects; we start these patients on a moderate dosage (1.5 mg equivalent of reserpine 3x/day) and gradually increase in 1-2 week intervals until they are reasonably stable. It usually takes two weeks to get them to a stable place with their dosage, then we decide whether or not to increase the dose, based on their symptoms. Most of these patients present with agitation, restlessness, voices in their head, paranoia and anxiety, some are on other medications while they undergo treatment at my clinic and others are just using our therapies. Rauwolfia consistently makes a marked difference in their subjective symptoms.

The most common side effects of Rauwolfia with a small to moderate dosage are diarrhea and nasal congestion. Less common side effects are inappetence, drowsiness, slowed reflexes and bradycardia. In the larger doses used for the treatment of psychosis, mental depression and parkinson-like symptoms can develop, both are reversible but may take 4-6 weeks to reverse. Alcohol and other central nervous system depressants should be avoided with Rauwolfia, as their effect may well be amplified. Care should be used with patients on digoxin as concomitant use can cause bradycardia, angina, and arrhythmias.

Most of us have an immediate and intuitive understanding of the notion of mood. We readily comprehend what it means to feel sad or happy. These concepts are nonetheless very difficult to formulate in a scientifically precise and quantifiable way; the challenge is greater given the cultural differences that are associated with the expression of mood. In turn, disorders that impact on the regulation of mood are relatively difficult to define and to approach in a quantitative manner. Nevertheless, dysregulation of mood and the expression of mood, or affect, represent a major category among mental dis-eases.

Disturbances of mood characteristically manifest themselves as a sustained feeling of sadness or sustained elevation of mood. The diagnosis most closely associated with persistent sadness is major depression disorder (MDD), while that associated with sustained elevation of mood is mania and extreme fluctuation of mood is bipolar disorder (BD). Along with the prevailing feelings of sadness or elation, disorders of mood are associated with a host of related symptoms that include disturbances in appetite, sleep patterns, energy level, impulsiveness, concentration, and memory.

The state of one's mood represents a complex group of behaviors and responses that are precisely and tightly controlled and subject to a large amount of epigenetic modification. Any organism that must adapt to a changing environment has to be able to control the basic functions of sleep, appetite, sex, and physical activity. This regulation must allow appropriate adaptation to diurnal and seasonal changes in the environment. More complex behaviors such as exploration, aggression, and social interaction must also undergo a similar, perhaps closely linked, regulation. In humans, these complex behaviors and their regulation are believed to be associated with the expression of mood. A depressed mood appears to reflect a kind of global damping of these functions, while a manic state may result from an excessive activation of these same functions. Humans are among the most adaptable creatures on the planet, not only can we reflexively and subconsciously, epigenetically, respond to external stimuli like touching a hot stove or being in the presence of a large predator, we can consciously alter our behavior to avoid such situations, we can turn off a stove, avoid the Tiger's waterhole or create a rifle. We have an unprecedented ability to alter our environment, create hovels or skyscrapers, stockpile food, and domesticate animals. There is a fundamental empowerment that comes from engaging in even the simplest activities that remind us of our own self-reliance. Too often, the disturbance of mood that presents in an individual is due to a certain dis-empowerment that can stem from circumstances where something of importance is taken from someone, accidentally or forcefully. Alternatively, dis-empowerment can stem from not having the opportunity to cultivate those self-reliant skills, the old "silver spoon" adage; there is a simple and profound enjoyment that one experiences when they have created something functional or beautiful, there is a place within each of us that revels at our ability to positively affect the world around us. We have, ironically, created a culture where we don't have to engage in such activity, and we have unprecedented numbers of people with mood disturbances who are consuming psychotropic substances to find relief.

References on following pages..

References for Epigenetics and Mental Health

Allis, Caparros, Jenuwen, Reinberg. **Epigenetics, 2nd Ed**, Cold Spring Harbor Laboratory Press, New York, 2015.

Carey, Nessa. **The Epigenetics Revolution**, Columbia University Press, New York, 2012

Francis, Richard. **Epigenetics: How Environment Shapes Our Genes,** Norton and Co., New York, 2011.

Glew and Rosenthal, **Clinical Studies in Medical Biochemistry, 3rd ed,** Oxford University Press, New York, 2007.

Kane, Charles. **Herbal Medicine of the American Southwest**, Lincoln Town Press, Tucson, AZ, 2006.

Lende and Downey. **The Encultured Brain: An Introduction to Neuroanthropology**, MIT Press, Boston, MA, 2012

McGowan, Sasaki, D'Alessio, et al. Epigenetic Regulation of the Glucocorticoid Receptor in Human Brain Associated with Childhood Abuse. Nat Neurosci 2009;12(3):342-8.

Moalem, Sharon. **Survival of the Sickest,** William Morrow Publishers, New York, 2007.

Rodwell, Bender, Botham, Kennelly, Weil. **Harper's Illustrated Biochemistry, 30th ed.** McGraw-Hill, New York, 2015

Ross, Julia, **The Mood Cure**, Penguin Books, New York, 2002.

Silberman, Steve, **Neurotribes: The Legacy of Autism and the Future of Neurodiversity,** Penguin Books, New York, 2015.

Tollesfbol, Trygve. **Handbook of Epigenetics**, Elsevier Academic Press, San Diego, 2011.

Weaver, Cervoni, Champagne, et al. Epigenetic Programming by Maternal Behavior. Nat Neurosci 2004;7(8):847-854.

Yasui, Peedicayil, Grayson, **Neuropsychiatric Disorders and Epigenetics,** Elsevier Academic Press, San Diego, CA, 2017.

Neurohacking: Cognitive and Performance Enhancing Therapies
© Katie Stagem ND, RH (AHG)

Introduction

Humans, for millennia, have been driven to improve themselves, whether by changing their appearance through clothing, their physique through athletic training, or their perception through stimulants such as coffee or entheogens. A logical next step might be to use substances to alter mental performance with the goal of increasing the speed and accuracy of cognition. High school and college students are increasingly utilizing such substances to facilitate better grades on tests and papers; in 2009, an estimated 25% of college students used cognition-enhancing drugs (Cadik, 2009), and incidence continues to rise. Additionally, there are those, particularly in high profile jobs, including the highly competitive and well-compensated atmosphere of Silicon Valley, who feel that increasing their cognitive output is not just desirable, but a necessity. Computer programmers, who already create much of modern reality, easily identified with the concept of hacking into one's own mental hardware to improve it. Hence **neurohacking**: biological interventions to optimize cognition, mental acuity, and mental performance.

The Romanian psychologist and chemist **Corneliu E. Giurgea** coined the term "nootropic" in 1972 from *noos* (mind) and *tropos* (turn), meaning substances that enhance cognition. He stated that nootropics should have the following characteristics (Gouliaev and Senning, 1994):

* Enhancement of learning and memory;
* Facilitation of the flow of information between the cerebral hemispheres;
* Enhanced resistance to chemical (drug-induced) and physical (such as electroconvulsive shock) injuries;
* Lack of the typical psychological and physiological side effects associated with drugs (stimulation, sedation) and minimal toxicity.

As the use of nootropic substances becomes increasingly common, new terms have emerged: "smart drugs", "lifestyle drugs", "cosmetic neurology", and "academic doping". This presentation will explore the biology of cognition, the mechanism of action, efficacy, and safety of nootropic drugs and herbs, and other therapies that can increase mental performance. Finally, we will consider the ethics of neurohacking.

Of note, the focus here is on improving cognition in the *healthy*, although there are, of course, applications for these therapies in cases of dementia and other types of cognitive decline. As nootropics must, by definition, enhance resistance to chemical injuries, another application of these substances is in attenuating the side effects of medications that adversely affect cognition, such as phenytoin, colchicine, and benzodiazepines (Aguiar & Borowski, 2013).

The Biology of Cognition

Acetylcholine (ACh) transmission was the first identified physiological mechanism of cognition. Disrupted ACh was seen in Alzheimer's disease, although other deficits have also been identified, such as oxidative and inflammatory damage to neurons and beta-amyloid formation (Kennedy & Scholey, 2006). Thus, using agents that enhance ACh transmission, or block acetylcholinesterase (AChE, which breaks down ACh), should support memory and cognition.

Other factors involved in cognition include transmission of neurotransmitters serotonin, epinephrine, norepinephrine (NE), dopamine, glutamate, and GABA. Alterations to serotonin levels, in those with suboptimal endogenous levels, affect long-term memory, cognitive flexibility, focused attention, and task vigilance without modifying mood. Normalizing serotonin levels in those with depression (for whom serotonin tends to be low) seems to increase cognition (Schmidt, Wingen, Ramaekers, Evers, & Riedel, 2006), although further studies are needed in this area.

NE and epinephrine play complex roles in cognition, and alterations in levels have been shown to both increase and decrease cognition and memory. Both neurotransmitters are released under stressful conditions; NE appears to affect the prefrontal cortex by influencing different adrenergic receptor subtypes (α1, α2, and β1). α2 receptors modulate working memory during non-stressful moments, whereas α1 or β1 are engaged during stress to impair prefrontal cortical function, (Ramos & Arnsten, 2006), thus impacting cognitive functioning.

Dopamine is often considered the neurotransmitter that most influences motivation and gratification; it is also released when presented with something novel (Bisagno, Gonzalez, & Urbano, 2016). Brain lesions that affect dopamine cause cognitive deficits, but also significantly alter attention and drive (Nieoullon, 2002). Drugs that stimulate dopamine transmission tend to reinforce learning and behavior (Bisagno, Gonzalez, & Urbano, 2016).

GABA is an inhibitory neurotransmitter that has relevance for cognition and emotional processing (Gabriella & Giovanna, 2010). Glutamate is an excitatory neurotransmitter. Ratios of GABA and glutamate seem to change during aging in response to biological needs for memory and skill acquisition; a recent study showed that higher glutamate levels in children (but not adults) correlate with face identification, new skill acquisition, and neuroplasticity (Kadosh, Krause, King, Near, & Kadosh, 2015). Two types of glutamate receptors have been tied to cognition, AMPA (α-amino-3-hydroxyl-5-methyl-4-isoxazole-propionate) and NMDA (*N*-methyl-d-aspartate) receptors. AMPA receptors seem to regulate neuronal plasticity. NMDA receptors, normally blocked by magnesium, are activated when AMPA receptors are activated, which then triggers more AMPA receptors at the synapse (Urban & Gao, 2014). However, too much NMDA activity can overwhelm the brain, causing glutamate toxicity (Tun & Herzon, 2012).

More recent studies demonstrate that a compound called BDNF (Brain Derived Neurotrophic Factor) is the key molecule engaged in learning and memory. BDNF seems to be responsible for neurogenesis, neuron survival, and resilience, all necessary for learning and cognition (Gligoroska & Manchevska, 2012). BDNF is active throughout the brain, and levels vary, but decrease with age, vascular dementias, and affective, anxiety, and behavioral disorders (Levada & Cherenichenko, 2015). Infusion of BDNP in humans facilitates learning, while deficiency diminishes learning capacity (Gligoroska & Manchevska, 2012). Polymorphisms in BDNF potentiate cognitive decline, and represent risk factors for dementia and Alzheimer disease. Factors that influence BDNF include hormone levels (estrogen, corticosteroids, IGF-1) and neurotransmitter levels (glutamate, acetylcholine, GABA, serotonin, and NE) (Gligoroska & Manchevska, 2012).

I. Drugs
The four main classes of nootropic drugs are eugeroics, psychostimulants, ampakines, and racetams.

A. Eugerotics: or "good arousal" are drugs which promote wakefulness; these are less likely to be addictive or interfere with sleep than psychostimulants.

Modanafil (Provigil) is a schedule IV controlled drug approved for excessive daytime sleepiness (such as in narcolepsy, obstructive sleep apnea, or shift work disorder). It is also sometimes used off-label to treat depression, cocaine and nicotine addiction, schizophrenia, seasonal affective disorder, and to combat fatigue in cancer, in depressive patients, due to jet lag, or in military combat situations. In other countries, it is not classified as a controlled substance and used, perhaps, more widely as a nootropic drug. Modafinal is a weak inhibitor of the dopamine transporter (DAT) (Bisagno, Gonzalez, & Urbano, 2016); it increases dopamine reuptake, but does not increase dopamine release (Rxlist) and does so specifically in the prefrontal cortex (Bisagno, Gonzalez, & Urbano, 2016). Cocaine and methamphetamine also increase dopamine levels, but their action is much stronger, quicker, and less targeted. Modafinal also influences GABAergic, glutamergic, noradrenergic, histaminergic, and orexinergic systems (orexin regulates arousal, wakefulness, and appetite).

Modafinal increases perfusion into the cortex (Bisagno, Gonzalez, & Urbano, 2016), likely contributing to its nootropic effect. It improves pattern recognition memory, digit span recall, and mental digit manipulations (Urban, Gao, 2014) as well as information processing in the prefrontal cortex. Low doses seem to cause the prefrontal cortex to be more efficient at cognitive information processing, while decreasing anxiety signals from the amygdala (Urban & Gao, 2014).

In order to be considered a nootropic, not just eugeroic (wakefulness promoting) drug, it must have some neuroprotective effects. Modafinil protects against methamphetamine-induced brain toxicity (Bisagno, Gonzalez, & Urbano, 2016). As a modulator of dopamine (inhibitor of dopamine transporter, or DAT), it affects motivation, arousal, and reward-based behavior. Modafinal does reduce cocaine dependence and withdrawal phenomenon (Krishnan & Chary, 2015), likely due to DAT modulation. However, modafinil does not seem to increase the risk of schizophrenia, which is typically though to be influenced by high levels of dopamine. In fact, modafinal is associated with a decrease in negative symptoms of schizophrenia (apathy, lethargy, social withdrawal, and anhedonia) without increasing positive symptoms, such as hallucinations (Bisagno, Gonzalez, & Urbano, 2016).

The dose is 200 mg taken orally once a day in the morning, or 100mg taken every 12 hours. The max dose is 400 mg/day, with no consistent evidence that the increased dose provides additional benefit. Most common side effects are headache, nausea, nervousness, rhinitis, diarrhea, back pain, anxiety, insomnia, dizziness, and dyspepsia. Modafinal can also cause feelings of euphoria, with some potential for abuse/dependence. Of additional note, it may limit efficacy of the oral contraceptive pill and other medications by inducing clearance of CYP 3A4. Serious rashes, including Stevens-Johnson syndrome, may occur, even weeks after initiating therapy (Rxlist).

Modafinil seems to be more beneficial to cognitive performance in lower-performing individuals than higher performing individuals, and may even cause deficits in higher performing individuals (Urban & Gao, 2014). Thus, high achievers, either in school or work settings should approach this drug with some caution. Further, dopamine is tightly regulated in the adolescent brain. Modifications to dopamine levels could induce changes in neural plasticity or behavioral rigidity (Urban & Gao, 2014) at this critical time.

Additionally, we know that sleep enhances the immune system and cortisol inhibits it. Those experiencing sleep deprivation, or under significant stress, will have decreased immune function.

The use of eugerotics to enhance wakefulness and cognition, particularly if done so under stressful conditions, will further inhibit immune function. Although modafinal is considered a generally safe drug, it has been shown to increase CRP (a marker of inflammation) after a single dose, and has also been shown to reduce immunity, as exemplified by decreased resistance to the bacteria *Listeria monocytogenes* (Krishnam & Chary, 2015).

Armodafinil (Nuvigil), is an enantiomer of modafinil (R-modafinil) with a longer half-life, and is also approved for the treatment of excessive sleepiness. Dose is 150 mg to 250 mg taken orally once a day as a single dose in the morning, and it has the same potential side effects and warnings, including schedule IV designation due to potential for dependence. Nuvigil is brand name only; the older Provigil (modafinil) is also available as a generic.

Adrafinil is a pro-drug of modafinil that is converted to modafinil by the liver. Its manufacture was discontinued in 2011, but can be easily purchased online.
The dose is 600 to 1200mg per day. Indications and warnings are the same as for modafinal, with the additional strong warning about the risks of purchasing something that is truly a drug online.

B. Psychostimulants

Methylphenidate (MPH, Ritalin)
MPH is a schedule II drug approved for ADHD and narcolepsy. It is used off-label for depression, lethargy/fatigue, and obesity. MPH binds to both the dopamine transporter and the norepinephrine transporter in neuronal synapses and stimulates the release of more dopamine and norepinephrine in the prefrontal cortex. This specificity reduces both the risk of drug abuse and the drug's side effects. MPH may also bind to and activate the serotonin and muscarinic ACh receptors.

Low dose MHP can enhance cognition, likely due to increased dopamine. At optimal doses, MPH causes dopamine to bind to D1 receptors and NE to bind to α2 receptors, causing increased flow of information and enhanced neuronal communication (Urban & Gao, 2014). However, higher doses cause dopamine to bind to D2 receptors, and NE to bind to α1 receptors, which can facilitate distractibility (Urban, Gao, 2014) and alter response to stimuli (Bisagno, Gonzalez, & Urbano, 2016), significantly affecting cognition. There is no reliable method of determining the optimal dose for enhanced cognition (Urban & Gao, 2014).

Similar to modafinal, MPH shows neuroprotective effects against methamphetamine-induced toxicity. However, it has a much greater potential for abuse and dependence (Bisagno, Gonzalez, & Urbano, 2016), thus the schedule II designation.

MHP is taken 2-3 times daily, preferably 30 to 45 minutes before meals; average dosage is 20 to 30 mg daily. A long acting form is available and usually dosed at 20mg taken one a day. The most common side effects are nervousness and insomnia; loss of appetite (and weight loss in children) is also common, as are skin rashes. Sudden death, stroke, and myocardial infarction have been reported in children and adults taking standard dosages for ADHD. Underlying psychotic or manic symptoms are likely to be exacerbated on MPH, and the drug should be discontinued if this occurs. MPH should not be used in those with significant anxiety, tension, or agitation, or in within a 14-day window of use of MAOI drugs.

The alterations to dopamine and NE may have consequences, particularly in adolescents who may be interested in using MPH to aid in classwork and test taking. The alterations to neurotransmitters, at a time when the brain is particularly sensitive to dopamine and NE, may disrupt maturation of the prefrontal cortex, affecting behavior and thought processes. Further, treatment in early life with MPH may alter circadian rhythm, induce anxiety (in some cases, persisting into adulthood), and impair some types of memory such as object recognition. These effects can be seen even at doses thought to be therapeutic (Urban & Gao, 2014). Thus, treatment with MPH in adolescents who do not have ADHD may cause students *appear* to be more focused on classwork, though perhaps at the risk of decreased behavioral flexibility, object recognition, and healthy circadian rhythm. These changes may affect the development of interpersonal skills (Urban & Gao, 2014) and creative thinking.

Others

Adderall (dextroamphetamine / amphetamine salts) is also used to treat ADHD. Adderall has a higher abuse potential due to less targeted action and is more likely to cause weight loss due to decreased appetite. While this is certainly used as a cognitive enhancer, particularly among high school and college students, research on shows that those using the drug *think* they perform better, and yet objective measurements showed no improvement (Ilieva, Boland, & Farah, 2013).

Guanfacine is a selective α2A agonist used in hypertension and ADHD. Guanfacine is effective in patients with prefrontal cortex dysfunction such as ADHD, but it has not clearly shown benefit in neurotypical adults (Bisagno, Gonzalez, & Urbano, 2016). Thus it is not considered a neurohacking drug.

C. Ampakines

Ampakines are a class of drugs that bind to and enhance activity of the glutamatergic AMPA receptor, which has already been demonstrated to increase neuronal plasticity. These drugs are not currently FDA approved, but are under investigation as treatment for Alzheimer's disease, Parkinson's disease, ADHD, schizophrenia, depression, and autism; they have also been shown to improve memory and cognition in healthy adults. Ampakines are not stimulants, and thus are considered much safer for normal adults, or for military in combat situations, than MPH, amphetamines, or modafinil. Despite this, there are some safety concerns. Glutamate toxicity, which damages neuronal cells, can occur at high doses of these drugs. Increased neuronal plasticity, while positively affecting memory and cognition, might also increase emotional plasticity, leading to behavioral changes. Additionally, increased neuronal plasticity and heightened neuronal activity could trigger synaptic pruning, something seen in those on the autistic spectrum (Urban & Gao, 2014).

D. The "Racetams"

Corneliu E. Giurgea (creator of the term nootropic) created the first drug in this class, Piracetam, in 1964. Piracetam was originally created to address motion sickness; it was later discovered to effect memory, acquisition of new ideas, and to protect against hypoxia-induced amnesia. All drugs in this class are structurally close to the amino acid pyroglutaminc acid, with differing side chains (Malik, Sangwan, Saihgal, Dharam, & Piplani, 2007). Pyroglutaminc acid has an effect on ACh as well as GABA; altered levels have been implicated in Alzheimer's disease (Wang et al,

2014). Aniracetam is considered one of the most potent nootropics, but others, including piracetam, oxiracetam, and pramiracetam are also considered nootropics. The racetams are used in Alzheimer's disease, alcoholism, epilepsy, dementia, stroke, parkinsonism, schizophrenia, and dyslexia in other countries (Malik, Sangwan, Saihgal, Dharam, & Piplani, 2007); none of the aforementioned is approved as a drug in the United States. All revert amnesia included by scopolamine, electroconvulsive shock, and hypoxia, and are generally considered safe (Malik, Sangwan, Saihgal, Dharam, & Piplani, 2007). Levetiracetam (Keppra) is approved for the treatment of epilepsy; it has neuroprotective effects against scopolamine, but has much less cognitive enhancing properties than the other racetams.

II. Herbs

Caffeine, a methylxanthine, was one of the earliest psychoactive, or perhaps more specifically, eugerotic substances to be used. Caffeine is found in tea (*Camellia sinensis*), coffee (most commonly *Coffea arabica*), guarana (*Paullinia cupana)*, yerba mate (*Ilex paraguariensis)*, guayusa (*Ilex guayusa*), chocolate (*Theobroma cacao*), and cola (*Cola accuminata/nitida*).

Caffeine is a stimulant of the central nervous system and general metabolism and is used to maintain alertness and enhance concentration (Krishnam & Vengadaragava, 2015). Encapsulated caffeine is often added into nootropic products, or "stacks" for this purpose. However, caffeine seems to facilitate passive, but not active, learning, and hinder working memory-based tasks. High doses can induce anxiety, nervousness, palpitations, and jitters (Nehlig, 2010).

Bacopa Monnieri

Bacopa is an Ayurvedic herb with a long history of use. As a *medhya-rasayana* herb, it has been used to sharpen intellect and was historically used to facilitate the memorization of Vedic hymns. New studies demonstrate that Bacopa improves spatial learning and memory retention. Constituents include the triterpenoid saponins known as bacosides, with bacoside A being the most well studied. Bacopa also contains alkaloids (brahmine), D-mannitol, apigenin, herasaponin, monnierasides I-III, cucurbitacins, and plantainoside C (Aguiar & Borowski, 2013). Other botanical actions include anti-oxidant, hepatoprotective, anxiolytic, inflammation modulating, adaptogenic, analgesic, and antimicrobial (against H. pylori) properties.

Bacopa is a potent anti-oxidant (Aguiar & Borowski, 2013). The brain is particularly sensitive to oxidative damage because it is very metabolically active, contains high levels of iron (which is pro-oxidant), and because the blood brain barrier prevents entry of many anti-oxidant substances. Mouse studies have shown that Bacopa increases brain levels of glutathione, vitamin C, vitamin A, and vitamin E after exposure to toxins such as nicotine smoke. As an anti-oxidant, Bacopa appears to have greater potency than ascorbic acid. Rats administered colchicine, which induces cognitive decline via microtubule disruption, showed complete reversal of the drug-induced memory decline, as well as a restoration of levels of anti-oxidants such as glutathione reductase and glutathione S-transferase. Phenytoin is an anticonvulsant drug that is also known to decrease cognitive function. Rats administered Bacopa with phenytoin showed improved memory acquisition and retention, without an increase in seizures. Bacopa also reversed diazepam-induced amnesia (Aguiar & Borowski, 2013).

Additional mechanisms for its nootropic action include increased cerebral blood flow, increased cerebral ATP, inhibition of AChE (thus allowing more ACh to be available), potentiation of dopamine and serotonin, and inhibition of b-amyloid (plaque found in patients with Alzheimer's disease. It is important to note, though, that these effects were present when Bacopa was used chronically, not acutely (Aguiar & Borowski, 2013).

Clinical studies show that Bacopa is most effective in reducing the rate of forgetting, versus increasing new memory acquisition. In a study that compared modafinial, *Panax quinquefolius*, and Bacopa, Bacopa was the most effective intervention for supporting attention and information processing tasks. This efficacy was seen after chronic (3 month) dosing, but was not effective at increasing cognition in acute settings (Aguiar and Borowski, 2013).

Bacopa is a safe herb; the most common side effects are nausea and increased intestinal motility. One mouse study did show the herb, at high doses, to impair fertility in males (Aguiar & Borowski, 2013); it is not known whether this occurs in humans, but one might consider avoiding chronic dosing if fertility is the chief concern.

Other Ayurvedic *Medhya rasayana* herbs include *Centella asiactica* (gotu kola, *Mandakaparni*), *Glycyrrhiza glabra / uralensis* (licorice, *Yashtimadhu*), *Tinospora cordifolia* (*Goduchi*, amrit), *Acorus calamus* (calamus root, *Vaca*), and *Shankhpushpi* (*Convolvulus pluricaulis, Evolvulus alsinoides*).

Huperzia serrata

Huperzia serrata (club moss, *Lycopodium serratum, qian ceng ta*) is a Chinese medicine traditionally used for swelling, fever (Zangara, 2003), pain, contusion, and schizophrenia (Tun & Herzon, 2012). Much of the herb's activity is thought to be from the alkaloid Huperzine A. Huperzine A is a potent reversible inhibitor of acetylchoninesterase (AChE), which breaks down ACh. The importance of ACh to cognition has already been demonstrated; Huperzine A has greater potential to inhibit AChE than the Alzheimer's drug donepezil (Tun & Herzon, 2012).

Huperzine A is protective against organophosphate toxicity (Zangara, 2003). Pesticides, herbicides, and nerve agents such as sarin are sources of organophosphates; they damage by inhibiting AChE, which causes a buildup of ACh and symptoms such as salivation, lacrimation, urination, emesis, increased GI motility, and potentially, death. Huperzine A and other AChE inhibitors block the binding of the organophosphates, providing a protective effect. In a small animal study, those given Huperzine A before exposure survived, without any neurological deficits; animals given the typical antidote for organophosphates, pyridostigmine, suffered extensive neurological damage and 5/6 died (Tun & Herzon, 2012).

Huperzine A also protects against glutamate-enhanced excitotoxicity via inhibition of NMDA glutamate receptors, and acts as a potent anti-oxidant (Tun & Herzon, 2012). Huperzine A is able to pass through the blood brain barrier, thus can specifically affect neuronal cells, and promotes the growth of nerve dendrites (Malik, Sangwan, Saihgal, Dharam, & Piplani, 2007). Further, Huperzine A seems to enhance brain metabolism, diminish apoptosis, enhance neuronal glycemic control, and increase BDNF expression (Mao, Cao, Li, Yin, Wang, Zhang, Mao, Zhou, & Liu, 2014).

The isolated alkaloid Huperzine A is generally safe (Zangara, 2003), although higher doses could potentially cause cholinergic symptoms including salivation, nausea, diarrhea, vomiting, decreased gastrointestinal transit time, and muscle spasms. More typical side effects include dizziness and headaches. As a general precaution, it should be avoided in pregnancy and lactation. Interactions include anticholinergic drugs, D2 dopamine receptor blockers, calcium channel blockers, and beta blockers; Huperzine A is also a CYP3A4 inducer, thus may stimulate faster breakdown (and less efficacy) of drugs metabolized by 3A4 (Bentue-Ferrer, Tribut, Polard, & Allain, 2003). Use of the whole plant is typically avoided, as there have been case reports of liver and kidney toxicity.

Unfortunately, Huperzia yields very low amounts (0.011%) of Huperzine A (Tun & Herzon, 2012). *Huperzia serrata* plants growing in humid forests will contain significantly more Huperzine A than plants growing in more arid environments, and Huperzine A levels are highest if the plant is harvested mid-fall, and the lowest in the early spring (Ma, Tan, Zhu, Gang, 2005). While other sources of Huperzine A have been identified within the Huperziaceae species, the highest content was found in *Phlegmariurus carinatus* (keeled tassel fern), which is endangered. Perhaps most promisingly, the endophytic fungal strain ES026, isolated from Huperzia, is able to produce huperzine A (Shu, Zhao, Wang, Zhang, Cosoveanu, Ahn, & Wang, 2014), presenting perhaps a more sustainable source of this alkaloid.

Salvia officinalis, Saliva lavandulaefolia (garden sage, Spanish sage)
Salvia was utilized by the Greeks and Romans for memory (Kennedy & Scholey, 2006). Sage has a variety of other uses, including carminative, antimicrobial, anti-oxidant, astringent/antihidrotic, and anti-inflammatory.

Both types of sage contain a variety of volatile oils, as well as polyphenols. Of note, Spanish sage does not contain the toxic terpenes α-thujune and β-thujone, which allows encapsulated volatile oils to be a safe delivery system (Kennedy & Scholey, 2006).

Spanish sage volatile oil demonstrated dose-dependent inhibition of AChE, however, no single constituent has been identified as responsible for this action. It is theorized that synergy between constituents provides this action. In another study, the ethanolic extract of sage leaves also exhibited AChE effects. Both types of sage are also potent anti-oxidants, with effects comparable to *Gingko biloba* and *Panax ginseng*. While many nootropic herbs have anti-oxidant properties, this seems unlikely as the main mechanism of its nootropic effect. One of the constituents, rosmarinic acid, has neuroprotective properties. Rosmarinic acid is also found in rosemary, another herb often used to enhance memory and alertness. Phytoestrogenic activity is theorized to contribute to increased cerebral blood flow, decreased inflammation, enhanced synaptic activity, and neo-protective and neurotrophic effects on brain tissue system (Kennedy & Scholey, 2006).

Those taking Spanish sage oil showed significant improvements in immediate and delayed word recall; both types of sage also increased ratings of immediate word recall (Hamidpour, Hamidpour, Hamidpour, & Shahlari, 2014), "alertness", "contentedness" and "calmness"(Kennedy and Scholey, 2006). Inhalation of sage volatile oils demonstrate most, but not all of the effects of oral ingestion; the mood-enhancing properties (Hamidpour, Hamidpour, Hamidpour, & Shahlari, 2014) can help with drive and productivity.

Salvia officinalis / lavandulaefolia are considered relatively safe herbs; S. *lavandulaefolia* being the safer of the two due to absence of α-thujune and β-thujone, which should be avoided in pregnancy.

Large internal doses of the essential oil of *Salvia officinalis* should also be avoided. The interaction with anticholinergic drugs already discussed (in Huperzia) is a potential here, as well.

Salvia *miltiorrhiza* (danshen, Chinese sage, red sage) is a Chinese herb in the same sage family, traditionally used to promote blood flow and treat vascular disease. Unlike the other *Salvia sp.* discussed, which utilize the leaves, the root of *Salvia miltiorrhiza* is used. While less often considered a nootropic, it does demonstrate neuroprotective activity against inflammatory and oxidative neurotoxicity (Lin & Hsieh, 2010). Additionally, cryptotanshinone, a diterpene constituent, has been demonstrated to have AChE inhibiting activity. Rat studies suggest that *Salvia miltiorrhiza* improves task learning and attenuates scopolamine-induced cognitive impairment (Wong, Ho, Lin, Lau, Lau, Rudd, Chung, Fung, Shaw, & Wan, 2010).

Melissa officinalis (lemon balm)

Paracelsus described lemon balm as appropriate for "all complains supposed to proceed from a disordered state of the nervous system" (Kennedy & Scholey, 2006), which certainly relates to cognition. Melissa has anti-viral, antispasmodic, mild sedative, anti-oxidant, anti-inflammatory properties and tends to elevate the mood. Constituents include monoterpenoid aldehydes, flavonoids, and polyphenols such as rosmarinic acid, a potent anti-oxidant and neuroprotective.

The volatile oil of Melissa has AChE inhibiting properties; stronger when the fresh plant is utilized, although only about half as strong as the sages. Melissa binds to nicotinic and muscarinic ACh receptors in human brain tissue; the dried plant has a particular affinity for muscarinic receptors. Different strains of Melissa produce distinct amounts of each constituent; strains with low cholinergic binding activity have anxiolytic activity but no memory enhancing effect. Strains with high ACh muscarinic/nicotinic binding properties demonstrate the same mood effects, but with increased memory and performance. It is unclear if this mechanism can be attributed to the AChE inhibition alone (Kennedy & Scholey, 2006).

Since Melissa has mild sedative activity at higher doses, low doses should be more effective in tasks requiring speed and drive. A human study demonstrated this, with lower doses effective on memory and timed memory tasks, and higher doses inhibiting timed memory tasks. At all doses, participants reported increased calmness (Kennedy & Scholey, 2006).

Melissa is a very safe herb, often used in children. Caution should be used in hypothyroidism, as it can suppress thyroid action in those with thyroid conditions. When considering this as part of a cognitive enhancing formula, lower doses should be utilized, not for safety purposes, but to avoid a strongly relaxing effect.

Rosemarinus officinalis (rosemary)

Rosemary was also associated with cognition by the Greeks and Romans. Students wore sprigs or garlands of rosemary when taking exams (Kennedy & Scholey, 2006). Rosemary contains volatile oils (including 1,8 cineole), diterpenes, flavonoids, phenolic acids (such as rosmarinic acid), and tannins. It is considered a circulatory stimulant with affinity for the brain and a nootropic, as well as a spasmolytic, anti-inflammatory, carminative, nervine, cholertic/cholagogue, and antimicrobial.

Rosemary has mild AChE activity, but much less pronounced than that of sage or lemon balm (Kennedy & Scholey, 2006), so this is unlikely to be the mechanism for its nootropic action. More likely, neuroenhancement is mediated by volatile oils such as 1,8 cineole, or a combination of mechanisms.

Inhalation, as well as oral administration, of rosemary essential oil was found to result in serum 1,8-cineole levels. It is thought that the volatile oil is absorbed through nasal or lung mucosa and is transmitted through the blood brain barrier to either act directly, or indirectly though enzymatic activity, to stimulate neurons (Moss, Oliver, 2012). In a study done with rosemary aromatherapy used for 3 minutes, EEG showed decreased frontal alpha and beta power, which was interpreted as increased alertness. Another aromatherapy study found enhanced memory and performance, but reduction in speed; increased subjective reports of alertness and contentedness (Kennedy & Scholey, 2006).

Its action as a mood enhancer could be due to activity on noradrenergic and dopaminergic systems (Moss & Oliver, 2012), which themselves affect cognition. Interestingly, human studies have demonstrated a correlation between *positive* mood and performance, but no correlation between *stimulated* mood and performance (Moss & Oliver, 2012). Rosemary is very safe herb that grows well in Arizona's arid climate.

Vinca major / minor (greater/lesser periwinkle)
Vinca major/minor are common decorative plants traditionally used as styptic/astringents. An alkaloid found in both plants (leaves are typically used), vincamine, has action as a vasodilator that increases blood flow, oxygen, and glucose to the brain; it also increases neuronal ATP utilization (Malik, Sangwan, Saihgal, Dharam, & Piplani, 2007). Vincamine also blocks excitotoxicity and attenuates neuronal damage due to cerebral ischemia/reperfusion (Ogunrin, 2014) and scopolamine administration (Pepeu & Spignoli, 1989). A synthetic derivative of vincamine, vinpocetine, is available as a supplement and drug, and is often used in research studies, although appears to be less safe the whole plant.

Vinpocetine has cognition-enhancing effects and improves the recall and retention of information (Ogunrin, 2014). In a study that examined the effects of vinpocetine on cognitive damage in those with epilepsy and dementia, vinpocetine was most effective in those with the least amount of cognitive decline (Ogunrin, 2014), making this herb an ideal consideration for the neurohacker (who is assumed to have *no* cognitive decline).

Vinca should be avoided in pregnancy, in those trying to get pregnant (also the male partner), those with a brain tumor, or acute brain injury. It has a hypotensive effect, so use caution in those with low blood pressure or bradycardia. Vincamine should not be administered parentally due to several reports of torsade des pointes, a life-threatening arrhythmia. Avoid before surgery due to blood thinning effect. As an astringent, use general precautions in those with constipation or malabsorption.

Hericium erinaceus (lion's mane, Yamabushitake)
Lion's mane is a mushroom that grows on living and dead broadloaf trees; it has been used as food and medicine for centuries (Brandalise et al, 2017). The parts used are the fruiting body and mycelium; the mycelium is thought to be the most potent.

Lion's mane has a beneficial, strengthening effect on the immune system and has promising research on improvement of cognitive function in those with dementia (Brandalise et al, 2017). However, it has also shown beneficial effects on cognition in healthy subjects.

Two constituents, hericenones (in fruiting body) and erinacines (in mycelium) (Li et al, 2014), have been shown to significantly induce nerve growth factor (NGF) in neurons. NGF is a protein that has an essential role in neurogenesis and memory (Lei et al, 2013); it also stimulates the release and prolongs the availability of ACh (Auld, Mennicken, Day, & Quirion, 2001). Mice given lion's mane for 2 months showed changes in neural architecture, particularly in the hippocampus, which plays a key role in declarative memory (items than can be explained, such as facts). Lion's mane also increases novelty/exploratory behavior and ability to recall past events (Brandalise et al, 2017). Thus, it appears to facilitate nerve growth (Lei et al, 2013) and increased cognition. Studies have not shown it to be neuroprotective against oxidative stress, however. Interestingly, lion's mane also decreased depression and anxiety in human females after 4 weeks of use (Brandalise et al, 2017). Enhanced mood supports many of the aspects of cognition of interest to neurohackers, such as motivation and drive to complete tasks.

Lion's mane is a very safe herb; even very high doses showed no adverse effects in animal studies (Li et al, 2014).

III. Non-herbal interventions

Exercise, Yoga, Meditation
It has been well demonstrated that physical activity increases cognition; possible mechanisms include increased blood flow to the brain, increased release of the neurotransmitters NE, epinephrine, and serotonin, and increased vascularization of the cerebral cortex. Additionally, exercise increases BDNF by decreasing the stress-induced glucocorticoids that suppress BDNF expression. Exercise also stimulates neurogenesis in the hippocampus, facilitating learning (Gligoroska & Manchevska, 2012).

Physical activity improves executive function, cognitive speed, and episodic memory. Sedentary subjects who started a program of cardio demonstrated significantly increased levels of grey and white matter in their brains (Gligoroska & Manchevska, 2012).

In a study using **yoga**, *Medhya rasayana* herbs, and control, those taking the herbs had the most pronounced increase in memory using objective measurements, but those practicing yoga showed increased concentration, calmness, and memory, and the largest subjective increase in measurements associated with learning and retention (Sarokte & Rao, 2013). **Meditation / mindfulness** practices have been shown to increase cerebral blood flow (Newberg, Wintering, Khalsa, Roggenkamp, & Waldman, 2010) and neuroplasticity (Xiong & Doraiswamy, 2009), which certainly relate to cognition.

Sleep has a vital role in cognition. It facilitates consolidation of memories previously learned as well as acquisition of new memories; it also affects attention, reasoning, decision-making, and language. Sleep deprivation reduces reaction time, focused attention, and strategic planning (Diekelmann, 2014). Sleep alone does not enhance cognition, but a lack of sleep decreases cognitive function (Diekelmann, 2014). Sleep can thus be considered part of the groundwork necessary for optimal cognitive function.

Diet

Certain foods have long been associated with cognitive function; perhaps most prominently walnuts and almonds. In a 27-day trail, rats were administered almond paste or water. The almond group demonstrated increased memory and spatial memory acquisition. Almonds contain tryptophan, a serotonin precursor, as well as essential fatty acids, which are utilized in serotonin metabolism. Normalizing serotonin levels, especially in those with depression, increases cognition. Almonds also contain choline, a precursor to ACh; the role of ACh in cognition has already been well covered. Interestingly, although almonds are high in fat, the rats that consumed the almonds decreased their overall caloric intake and demonstrated decreased cholesterol levels at the end of the study (Haider & Haleem, 2012). Researchers found similar effects using walnuts (*Juglans regia*) on serotonin and learning/memory after a 28-day trial (Haider et al, 2011).

Fasting is another technique that affects cognition. Restricting caloric intake has long been known to increase lifespan, decrease the risk of cancer formation and kidney disease, and play a protective role against neuronal dysfunction in Alzheimer's, Parkinson's, and stroke (Anson et al, 2003). Fasting increases production of ketones, which are used by the brain for energy instead of glucose, and provides protective activity toward neurons and thus resistance to seizures in epileptics (Anson et al, 2003).

Intermittent fasting is a new technique that is easier for people to maintain and offers many of the same benefits. Mice put on an intermittent fasting program showed increased memory, acquisition skills, beneficial alterations to brain anatomy, and decreased oxidative stress when compared to mice on a regular diet (Li, Wang, & Zuo, 2013). Interestingly, intermittent fasting, but not caloric restriction ("dieting") had a protective role against neuronal excitotocicity in another mouse study (Anson et al, 2003). In both studies, the intermittent fasting was administered as fasting every other day.

Intermittent fasting has become a culture for neurohackers (likely less so among students). Many companies support fasting periods of 14 to 30 hours, with workers reporting increased productivity and cognition on fasting days. It also decreases distractions from work, since no meal breaks are necessary. Group "break fasts" solidify a working community. The online community https://wefa.st supports those interested in intermittent fasting in this context.

Since at least some of the benefits of fasting / intermittent fasting seems attributable to the ketone bodies generated, following a ketogenic diet may provide similar benefits. In the ketogenic diet, carbohydrates are severely restricted, with most calories coming from fats. The ketogenic diet minimizes glucose levels in the body without restricting calories or causing malnutrition (Hallböök, Maudsley, & Martin, 2012). There are variations in how the diet is implemented, but typically about 75% of calories comes from fat, 20% from protein, and only 5% from carbohydrates. The ketogenic diet has been shown to enhance cognitive function in healthy, as well as in pathophysiologic animal models (epilepsy, traumatic brain injury, dementia, ALS, seizures). Additionally, increased alertness and behavior has been consistently reported in children on the ketogenic diet (Hallböök, Maudsley, & Martin, 2012). Fat rich diets can cause decreased alertness, but only if this differs from habitual intake (Gibson & Green, 2002). Thus, consistency is key.

D. Context

Many people, particularly students and those in high pressure, competitive jobs, might consider nootropics useful. Whether use of these substances is ethical, and should be considered "cheating" is a topic of much contention within the neurological and medical ethics communities (Cadic, 2009, *Neuropharmacology* 2013).

Certainly, it is hard to define "cognition": stimulant nootropics increase drive and, in some cases, retention, but sometimes at the detriment of emotional and behavioral plasticity. This a particular concern for adolescents who use nootropic drugs, and in whom such use may permanently alter cognitive architecture. Is it beneficial to be able to memorize facts for a test when the context for these facts is missed?

Additionally, studies looking at cognitive function typically use animal models, but how well cognition in a mouse correlates to cognition in a human remains to be determined.

Stimulant drugs, when used by those already chronically stressed, will tend to decrease sleep and increase underlying anxiety. Sleep clearly has a role in cognition (Diekelmann, 2014); while sleep deprivation may allow for short-term gains in memory and productivity, it is unlikely to have beneficial long-term effects, and may decrease ability to process complex information as well as emotional stability. Lack of sleep also decreases immune function. Certainly those using eugerotic substances should take regular break days without the substances.

Despite the relative safety of nootropic drugs, there is still potential for side effects, and in some cases, addiction. Supplements, which are often comprised of combinations, or "stacks", of nootropic drugs and herbs, may not be ideal either. If someone already has stable levels of neurotransmitters, modulation of these can cause unwanted side effects.

Herbs are much safer, particularly when used as singles or customized compounds. Herbs tend to have a normalizing effect; there is no evidence that they force a neurotransmitter pathway at the expense of another. Interestingly, evidence suggests that nootropic drugs tend to have an anxiolytic effect; the herbs discussed in this paper also have this, perhaps more effectively. Perhaps, when mood is no longer an impingement to drive and productivity, one can process and remember more efficiently.

Bacopa and the alkaloids Huperzine A (*Huperzia serrata*) and vincamine (*Vinca major/minor*) have some of the best evidence for supporting increased cognition in those without neurodegererative disease. It is important to note that some of the herbs discussed, such as Bacopa and Lion's mane, may need to be used in a chronic manner for best results. Intermittent fasting or the ketigenic diet may offer the best evidence for longevity, cognition, and overall well-being. However, exercise, yoga, adequate sleep, and meditation also confer benefits.

References

Aguilar, S. & Borowski, T. (2013). Neuropharmacological Review of the Nootropic Herb *Bacopa Monnieri*. *Rejuvenation Research*. 16(4), 313-326.

Anson, R. M., Guo, Z., de Cabo, R., Iyun, T., Rios, M., Hagepanos, A., ... Mattson, M. P. (2003). Intermittent fasting dissociates beneficial effects of dietary restriction on glucose metabolism and neuronal resistance to injury from calorie intake. *Proceedings of the National Academy of Sciences of the United States of America*. *100*(10), 6216–6220. http://doi.org/10.1073/pnas.1035720100.

Auld, D.S., Mennicken, F., Day, J.C., & Quirion, R. (2001) Neurotrophins differentially enhance acetylcholine release, acetylcholine content and choline acetyltransferase activity in basal forebrain neurons. *J Neurochem.* Apr;77(1):253-62.

Bentue-Ferrer, D., Tribut, O., Polard, E., & Allain, H. (2003). Clinically significant drug interactions with cholinesterase inhibitors: a guide for neurologists. *CNS Drugs.* 17(13):947-63.

Bisagno, Veronica, Gonzalez, Betina, & Urbana, Francisco (2016). Cognitive Enhancers versus addictive psychostimulants: The good and the bad side of dopamine in prefrontal cortical circuits. *Pharmacological Research.* 109 (108-118)

Brandalise, F., Cesaroni, V., Gregori, A., Repetti, M., Romano, C., Orrù, G., ... Rossi, P. (2017). Dietary Supplementation of *Hericium erinaceus* Increases Mossy Fiber-CA3 Hippocampal Neurotransmission and Recognition Memory in Wild-Type Mice. *Evidence-Based Complementary and Alternative Medicine : eCAM.* 3864340. http://doi.org/10.1155/2017/3864340

Cadic, V. (2009). Smart dugs for cognitive enhancement: ethical and pragmatic considerations in the era of cosmetic neurology. *J Med Ethics.* 35:611-615. Doi:10.1136/jme.2009.030882.

Diekelmann, S. (2014). Sleep for cognitive enhancement. *Frontiers in Systems Neuroscience. 8*, 46. http://doi.org/10.3389/fnsys.2014.00046.

Gabriella, G. & Giovanna, C. (2010). γ-Aminobutyric acid type A (GABA(A)) receptor subtype inverse agonists as therapeutic agents in cognition. *Methods Enzymol.* 485:197-211. doi: 10.1016/B978-0-12-381296-4.00011-7.

Gibson, Leigh & Green, M.W. (2002). Nutritional influences on cognitive function: mechanisms of susceptibility. *Nutr Res Rev.* Jun;15(1):169-206. doi: 10.1079/NRR200131.

Gligoroska, Jasmina Pluncevic & Manchevska, Sania. (2012). The Effect of Physical Activity on Cognition – Physiological Mechanisms. *Mater Sociomed.* 24(3): 198–202. doi: 10.5455/msm.2012.24.198-202.

Gonzalez-Burgos, I., & Feria-Velasco, A. (2008). Serotonin/dopamine interaction in memory formation. *Prog Brain Res.*172:603-23. doi: 10.1016/S0079-6123(08)00928-X.

Gouliaev, Alex Haahr & Senning, Alexander. (1994). Piracetam and other structurally related nootropics. *Brain Research Reviews*. 19:(180-222)

Haider, S. & Haleen, D. J. (2012). Nootropic and hypophagic effects following long term intake of almonds (*Prunus amygdalus*) in rats. *Nutr Hosp.* 27(6): 2109-2115.

Haider, S. et al. (2011). Effects of walnuts (*Juglans regia*) on learning and memory function. *Plant Foods Hum Nutr.* 66(4): 335-340.

Hamidpour, M., Hamidpour, R., Hamidpour, S., & Shahlari, M. (2014). Chemistry, Pharmacology, and Medicinal Property of Sage (*Salvia*) to Prevent and Cure Illnesses such as Obesity, Diabetes, Depression, Dementia, Lupus, Autism, Heart Disease, and Cancer. *Journal of Traditional and Complementary Medicine.* 4(2), 82–88. http://doi.org/10.4103/2225-4110.130373.

Hallböök, T., Ji, S., Maudsley, S., & Martin, B. (2012). The effects of the ketogenic diet on behavior and cognition.

Epilepsy Research. 100(3), 304–309. http://doi.org/10.1016/j.eplepsyres.2011.04.017

Ilieva, I., Boland, J. & Farah, M.J. (2013). Objective and subjective cognitive enhancing effects of mixed amphetamine salts in healthy people. *Neuropharmacology.* Jan;64:496-505. doi: 10.1016/j.neuropharm.2012.07.021. Epub 2012 Aug 1.

Kadosh, Cohn, Krause, B, King, A, Near, J, & Kadosh, Cohen. (2015) Linking GABA and glutamate levels to cognitive skill acquisition during development. *Hum Brain Mapp.* Nov;36(11):4334-45. doi: 10.1002/hbm.22921. Epub 2015 Sep 9.

Kennedy, David O. & Scholey, Andrew B. (2006) The Psychopharmacology of European Herbs with Cognition-Enhancing properties. *Current Pharmaceutical Design.* 23, 4613-4623.

Krishnam, Raman & Chary, Krishnan Vengadaragava. (2015). A rare case modafinil dependence. *J Pharmacol Pharmacother.* Jan-Mar; 6(1): 49–50.
doi: 10.4103/0976-500X.149149.

Lai, P.L., Naidu, M., Sabaratnam, V., Wong, K.H., David, R.P., Kuppasamy, U.R., Abdullah, N., & Malek, S.N. (2013). Neurotrophic properties of the Lion's mane medicinal mushroom, *Hericium erinaceus* (Higher Basidiomycetes) from Malaysia. *Int J Med Mushrooms.* 5(6):539-54.

Levada, O.A. & Cherenichenko, N.V. (2015). Brain-dervied neurotrophic factor (BDNF): neurobiology and marker value in neuropsychiatry. *Lik Sprava.* Apr-Jun;(3-4):15-25.

Li, I.C., Chen, Y.L., Chen, W.P., Tsai, Y.T., Chen, C.C., & Chen, C.S. (2014) Evaluation of the toxicological safety of erinacine A-enriched *Hericium erinaceus* in a 28-day oral feeding study in Sprague-Dawley rats. *Food Chem Toxicol.* Aug;70:61-7. doi: 10.1016/j.fct.2014.04.040. Epub 2014 May 6.

Li, L., Wang, Z., & Zuo, Z. (2013). Chronic Intermittent Fasting Improves Cognitive Functions and Brain Structures in Mice. *PLoS ONE.* 8(6), e66069. http://doi.org/10.1371/journal.pone.0066069

Lin, Tsai-Hui & Hseih, Ching-Liang. (2010). Pharmacological effects of *Salvia miltiorrhiza* (*Danshen*) on cerebral infarction. *Chinese Medicine.* 5:22. DOI: 10.1186/1749-8546-5-22

Ma, X., Tan, C., Zhu, D., & Gang, D.R. (2005). Is there a better source of huperzine A than Huperzia serrata? Huperzine A content of Huperziaceae species in China. *J Agric Food Chem.* Mar 9;53(5):1393-8.

Malik, Ruchi, Sangwan, Abhijeet, Saihgal, Ruchika, Jindal, Dharam Paul, & Piplani, Poonam.(2007). Towards Better Brain Management: Nootropics. *Current Medicinal Chemistry.* 123-131.

Mao XY, Cao DF, Li X, et al. (2014). Huperzine A ameliorates cognitive deficits in streptozotocin-induced diabetic rats. *Int J Mol Sci.* 15(5):7667-7683. doi: 10.3390/ijms15057667

Moss, Mark & Oliver, Lorraine. (2012). Plasma 1,8-cineole correlates with cognitive performance following exposure to rosemary essential oil aroma. *Ther Advanced Psychopharmacol.* Jun; 2(3): 103-113.

Nahata, A., Patil, U.K., & Dixit, V.K. (2010) Effect of Evolvulus alsinoides Linn. on learning behavior and memory enhancement activity in rodents. *Phytother Res.* Apr;24(4):486-93. doi: 10.1002/ptr.2932.

Nehlig, A. Is caffeine a cognitive enhancer? (2010) *J Alzheimers Dis.* 20 Suppl 1:S85-94. doi: 10.3233/JAD-2010-091315.

Newberg, A.B., Wintering, N., Khalsa, D.S., Roggenkamp, H., & Waldman, M.R. (2010). Meditation effects on cognitive function and cerebral blood flow in subjects with memory loss: a preliminary study. *J Alzheimers Dis. 20(2):517-26. doi: 10.3233/JAD-2010-1391.*

Nieoullon A. (2002). Dopamine and the regulation of cognition and attention. *Prog Neurobiol.* May;67(1):53-83.

Pepeu, Giancarlo & Spignoli, Giacomo (1989). Nootropic Drugs and Brain Cholinergic Mechanisms. *Prog. Neuro-Psychopharmacol. & Biol. Psychiat.* (13) S77-S88.

Ogunrin, A. (2014). Effect of Vinpocetine (CognitolTM) on Cognitive Performances of a Nigerian Population. *Annals of Medical and Health Sciences Research.* 4(4), 654–661. http://doi.org/10.4103/2141-9248.139368.

Ramos, Brian & Arnsten, Amy. (2006). Adrenergic Pharmacology and Cognition: Focus on the Prefrontal Cortex. *Pharmacol Ther.* Mar; 113(3): 523–536. Published online 2006 Dec 28. doi: 10.1016/j.pharmthera.2006.11.006.

Schmidt, J.A., Wingen, M., Ramaekers, J.G., Evers, E.A., & Riedel, W.J. (2006) Serotonin and human cognitive performance. *Curr Pharm Des.* 12(20):2473-86.

Sarokte, Atul Shankar & Rao, Mangalagowri V. (2013). Effects of *Medhya Rasayana* and *Yogic* practices in improvement of short-term memory among school-going children. *Ayu.* Oct-Dec; 34(4): 383–389. doi: 10.4103/0974-8520.127720.

Shu, Shaohua , Zhao, Xinmei, Wang, Wenjuan, Zhang, Guowei, Cosoveanu, Andreea, Ahn, Youngjoon, & Wang, Ahn. (2014). Identification of a novel endophytic fungus from *Huperzia serrata* which produces huperzine A. *World J Microbiol Biotechnol.* Dec;30(12):3101-9. doi: 10.1007/s11274-014-1737-6. Epub 2014 Sep 12.

Tun, Maung Kyaw Moe & Herzon, Seth B. (2012). The pharmacology and therapeutic potential of (−)-huperzine A. *J Exp Pharmacol.* 4:113-123.

Urban, Kimberly & Gao, Wen-Jun. (2014). Performance enhancement at the cost of potential brain plasticity: neural ramifications of nootropic drugs in the healthy developing brain. *Frontiers in Systems Neuroscience.* (8) 1-10.

Wang, H., Lian, K., Han, B., Wang, Y., Kuo, S.-H., Geng, Y., ... Wang, M. (2014). Age-Related Alterations in the Metabolic Profile in the Hippocampus of the Senescence-Accelerated Mouse Prone 8: A Spontaneous Alzheimer's Disease Mouse Model. *Journal of Alzheimer's Disease : JAD*, 39(4), 841–848. http://doi.org/10.3233/JAD-131463.

Wong, K.K.,Ho, M.T., Lin, H.Q., Lau, K.F., Rudd, J.A., Chung. R.C., Fung, K.P., Shaw, P.C., & Wan, D.C. (2010). Cryptotanshinone, an acetylcholinesterase inhibitor from Salvia miltiorrhiza, ameliorates scopolamine-induced amnesia in Morris water maze task. *Planta Med.* Feb;76(3):228-34. doi: 10.1055/s-0029-1186084. Epub 2009 Sep 11.

Xiong, G.L. & Doraiswamy, P.M. (2009). Does meditation enhance cognition and brain plasticity? *Ann N Y Acad Sci.* Aug;1172:63-9.

Zangara, A. (2003). The psychopharmacology of huperzine A: an alkaloid with cognitive enhancing and neuroprotective properties of interest in the treatment of Alzheimer's disease. *Pharmacol Biochem Behav.* Jun;75(3):675-86.

The Problem of Proton Pump Inhibitors

Dr Jillian Stansbury

GERD AND THE CASE FOR ACID PROTECTORS OVER ACID BLOCKERS

- Proton-pump inhibitors (PPIs) and Histamine (H2) acid blocking drugs are the mainstay of acid reflux treatment, with sales topping 10 billion dollars per year, and an estimated 100 million people experiencing occasional symptoms, and 15 million suffering from heartburn on a daily basis. However, the innocuous public opinion regarding ant-acid use is undeserved. Regular use of antacids can promote dysbiosis of the small intestinal bacterial flora1 - SIBO, and exacerbate the tendency of NSAIDS to injure the intestinal mucosa.2

- Furthermore, the list of side effects and consequences from chronic reliance on acid blocking drugs grows each year, with papers published linking antacids to an increased risk of peritonitis in some patients, and *Clostridium difficile* infection, both associated with harmful shifts in intestinal flora.3,4 One study reported that children on acid blocking drugs are at an over 4 fold risk of developing *Clostridium difficile* infections, over other children.5

- PPIs are specifically shown to exacerbate intestinal erosions and inflammation seen with aspirin and steroid use.6 Additional issues becoming associated with the use of acid blocking drugs include an increased risk of pneumonia in stroke patients7, fracture in osteoporotic adults8, lower respiratory tract infections in susceptible individuals9, and chronic kidney disease10, as well as impaired semen quality11, and COPD exacerbation12.

- With such serious complications with the use of such drugs, it seems best to not start such medications in the first place, and instead work on improving GI health, motility, protect mucous membranes and barriers, and gastrointestinal flora. And because most of the millions of people who use such drugs on a regular basis suffer rather immediately when skipping the meal's dose, alternative practitioners have an extreme need for safe and rapidly effective alternatives.

- Most readers will be aware of the need to consider special diets, increase fiber, decrease difficult to digest foods such as meat or common allergens, and so on, all of which help support a beneficial intestinal ecosystem. The most commonly offensive foods for reflux disease are alcohol, chocolate, citrus, tomatoes, peppermint, coffee, and onions, however the big picture of the diet, transit time, fiber content, and other factors should all be considered in overall food choices.

• Weight loss often improves reflux for patients who are overweight, and smoking cessation will also offer improvement in those able to do so. All patients should be coached to avoid large meals, and eat instead frequent small meals. Most GERD patients will benefit from elevating the head of the bed, and avoiding laying down for a full 3 hours after eating. Some patients may require digestive enzymes,

• others biliary support and cholagogues, some may require antimicrobials, or even pharmaceutical antibiotics when *Helicobacter* or SIBO (small intestinal bacterial overgrowth) are present, and others still, may benefit from nervines and stress relief. Some of these ideas are exemplified in the formulary that follows. What all patients with GERD usually benefit from are demulcent herbs in a variety of forms, probiotics to help support beneficial flora, and agents that support optimal gastric emptying and intestinal motility.

DEMULCENTS FOR GERD AND
AN INTRODUCTION TO ALGINATES

• Allopathic medicine involves opposing symptoms – it opposes microbial infections with anti-biotics, inflammation with anti-inflammatories, and GERD with antacids. An alternate medical philosophy for GERD might aim to build gastric mucosal membrane protective barriers instead of oppose the acid. In addition to all the long term consequences associated with antacid use, listed above, blocking acid acutely can create a vicious cycle whereby pH sensors note insufficient acid and a mount an effort to produce more, compelling a person to use more antacids.

• Botanical agents to support mucous membranes include the demulcent herbs, listed in herbals for centuries to help treat heartburn. Herbs such as *Althea* and *Ulmus* are classic for this purpose, and are most effective as teas, compared to tinctures, and better yet, as medicinal foods such as the traditional Slippery Elm gruel. *Aloe* gel can improve reflux symptoms13, and may be included in teas and smoothies wherever possible. Recipe ideas are listed below.

• Simply making the stomach contents more viscous by consuming demulcent "snacks" prior to meals, may thicken fluids to such a degree, that reflux is inhibited.14 Licorice, *Glycyrrhiza glabra* is shown to improve the quality and quantity of mucous released from intestinal goblet cells15. While these herbs can help as part of a broad protocol, overtime, they are unlikely to provide substantial relief of severe reflux in the short term.

So what *can* help quickly, even immediately, for a patient we are trying to wean off of acid blocking drugs? Alginates

• are one tool that can be added to our tool kits. While alteratives, diet changes, motility enhancing therapies, probiotics, and enzymes can gradually help improve the integrity of the gastroesophogeal sphincter, and health of the entire gastrointestinal ecosystem, alginates may help give us some quick relief.

SEAWEED FOR GERD

- Alginates are named for algae, such as seaweed where they occur in the cell walls of brown algae including the kelps and bladderwracks. Like demulcents, alginates are polysaccharides with mucilaginous, mucous-like physical properties. These seaweeds are currently the world's largest sea "crop" as they are used in large quantity as raw materials to produce purified crude alginates, presently used as stabilizers and emulsifiers in the food industry, to make gums and gel that can be fashioned into artsy foods, or simple foods such as grain-free seaweed "noodles".

- Alginates may also be processed into fibers used to make bandages for wound care, and into beads impregnated with various drugs and nutrients to enhance their delivery, including herbal medicines.[16] Kelp, *Macrocystis pyrifera* is used in alginate production in California, and *Laminaria japonica, Laminaria hyperborean*, and *Ascophyllum nodosum* are used in other regions of the world.

- Alginates can be highly useful in allaying acute GERD symptoms[17,18,19,20]. Alginates can bind stomach acid and form a gel of neutral pH, which is less easily refluxed into the esophagus. The gel-forming physical nature of alginates can bind stomach acid at the gastroesophageal junction and create a barrier that helps resist reflux. Because stomach acid often floats on top of ingested food in the stomach, a situation referred to as an "acid pocket", the consumption of sodium or magnesium alginate after meals may bind the acid, and cap off the gastroesophageal sphincter by forming a gel.

- Alginates impregnated with calcium carbonate are also being developed to remedy reflux.[21] Gaviscon™ is a commercial prescription containing alginates and magnesium carbonate, however the product also contains aluminum hydroxide. In China, alginates impregnated with *Coptis chinensis* and *Evodia rutecarpa* are shown to protect the gastric mucosa from alcohol-induced injury.[22] Sodium alginate is available and included in some herbal products aimed at treating GERD.

ENHANCING MOTILITY TO TREAT GERD

- Impaired motility may contribute to GERD, as inability to pass stomach contents along predisposes to reflux. Gastric emptying is controlled by hormonal factors, but there is also a foundational electrical rhythm in the stomach, acting like a pacemaker in digestive smooth muscle.[23]

- Delayed gastric emptying and gastroparesis may contribute to dysbiosis and allow *Helicobacter pylori* to become established. Stomach pain and belching, have been found to positively correlate to delayed gastric emptying[24], as has Crohn's disease.[25]

- Chewing stimulates saliva flow, and digestive motility, and thereby may reduce GERD and gastroparesis. Studies suggest that chewing alone, may reduce reflux26, and medicinal chewing gum is now available for this purpose, such gum containing licorice and papain.27 Gum chewing speeds the clearance of refluxate from the esophagus, a benefit that endures for at least 3 hours after 1 hour of gum chewing.

- Because xylitol chewing gum has shown benefits to dental health, and to reduce childhood ear injections, it has already received some research and sugar-free products are on the market. Xylitol chewing gum is also shown to increase gastrointestinal motility recovery following major surgeries. As it could do no harm, patients with GERD might use the following formulas, and chew gum for one hour after all meals.

GLUTAMINE FOR THE GI

- Glutamine is the most abundant amino acid in the human body, with important roles acid in illness, stress, and injury. In the gut, glutamine is an essential nutrient to support the rapid cell turnover rate of intestinal mucosal cells, and the small bowel takes up more glutamine than any other tissue28. Glutamine can easily be added to teas, the days drinking water, and medicinal foods in protocols for GERD.

MUCOADHESIVITY IDEAS FOR GERD

- In some cases, loss of mucosal integrity may contribute to esophageal reflux. The barrier integrity, and general moist spongy nature of the digestive mucosa may lose structure due to old age, dysbiosis, infection, and other limitations in mucosal regeneration.

- Nourishing, connective tissue supportive herbs, such as *Centella* is classic for healing ulcers, trauma, and skin rashes, and may make a nutritive base for teas intended for long term use for GERD patients. *Calendula* may help improve circulation to the mucosa and be another, safe and gentle herb for long term use.

- When reflux induces esophagitis, sore throats, erosive lesions, or Barrett's esophagitis, there is a need for pain relief, as well as a concern over increased risk of malignant transformation. Herbs that improve the ability of a formula to adhere to mucosal surfaces may boost efficacy.

- Alginates, described above have useful mucoadhesivity, as well as pectin29, hyaluronic acid30,31 and Locust Bean/Guar gum from *Parkia biglobosa*32, Polysaccharides from *Tamarindus indica* seeds yield a mucoadhesive polymer33,34 and Licorice Solid Extract has anti-inflammatory and ulcer healing effects to mucous membranes.

INCREASED RISK OF GASTROESOPHOGEAL CANCER IN GERD PATIENTS

- The gradual replacement of esophageal epithelium with cells more typical of the lower digestive track, known as Barret's esophagus, increases the risk for esophageal cancer. Insufficient saliva and mucosal secretions contribute to Barrett's esophagitis, and may be improved by prolonged mastication35, such as chewing gum mentioned above.

- *Curcuma*, noted for numerous anti-cancer affects, helps protect an irritated esophagus from undergoing Barret's transformation.36 *Panax ginseng* may ameliorate inflammatory changes that occur with chronic GERD37, and is especially indicated when GERD occurs with chronic stress and emotional symptoms. Berries and their flavonoids are known to protect vascular and other tissues in many research models of inflammatory stress and can be included in the diet and formulas to reduce the risk of gastric cancer associated with GERD and *Helicobacter* infections.

HELICOBACTER AND GERD

- *Helicobacter* infections are one factor contributing to the development of GERD and peptic ulcer. Herbs with activity against Helicobacter are indicated in therapies for GERD. However, the digestive ecosystem may allow, if not invite, this microbe to proliferate such that antimicrobial therapies are incomplete in and of themselves.

HELICOBACTER AND GERD

- Many herbs including *Matricaria38*, and *Hydrastis* have been found to deter *H. pylori* and may be superior to pharmaceutical antibiotics by simultaneously offering anti-inflammatory and digestion enhancing effects, as well as antimicrobial effects.

HELICOBACTER AND GERD

- *Matricaria* has significant gastroprotective effects39, protecting against alcohol-induced ulceration, and optimizing glutathione regulation and detoxification40,41 increasing sulfur bioavailable, and supporting anti-oxidant pathways.42 A short list of herbs shown to deter Helicobacter are offered in the sidebar.

HELICOBACTER INFECTIONS

- *Helicobacter pylori* has been shown to be highly associated with peptic ulcer diseases as well as proven to be a potent carcinogen associated with gastric carcinoma43, particularly gastric B cell lymphoma. A long list of herbs has been shown to have activity against *Helicobacter* 44,45,46,47 including...

- *Achillea millefolium, Azadirachta indica, Carum carvi, Coptis, Curcuma longa, Elettaria cardamomum, Foeniculum vulgare, Gentiana lutea, Hydrastis canadense, Juniper communis, Lavandula angustifolia, Mahonia aquifolium, Matricaria chamomilla, Melissa officinalis, Mentha piperita, Myristica fragrans, Origanum majorana, Passiflora incarnata, Pimpinella anisum, Rheum palmatum, Rosmarinus officinalis, Sanguinaria canadense,* and *Zingiber officinale*

INHIBITNG GASTRIC ACID HAS MANY HARMFUL SIDE AFFECTS

- Proton-pump inhibitors (PPIs) and Histamine (H2) acid blocking drugs such as Tagamet are the mainstay of acid reflux treatment but may provoke dysbiosis of the small intestinal bacterial flora - SIBO, as well as exacerbate nonsteroidal anti-inflammatory drug-induced small intestinal injury. Acid blocking drugs may increase the risk of peritonitis in some patients, due to dysbiosis, and allow pathogenic bacteria, such as *Clostridium difficile*, to thrive., In fact, children put on acid blocking drugs are at an over 4 fold risk of developing *Clostridium diffficile* infections. PPIs may also exacerbate the damaging effects of aspirin and steroids on the intestinal mucosa. Acid blocking drugs may increase the risk or pneumonia in stroke patients, impair semen quality, exacerbate COPD, increase the risk of chronic kidney disease, increase the risk of fracture in osteoporotic adults, and increase the risk of lower respiratory tract infections in susceptible individuals. It may be wise to treat GERD without such drugs in the first place, given how difficult *Clostridium* infections are to eradicate and how serious the complications.

POST-PRANDIAL GUM CHEWING TO REDUCE GERD

- Chewing stimulates saliva flow, digestive motility and can reduce GERD and gastroparesis. Studies suggest that chewing alone, may reduce reflux, and companies now offer medicinal chewing gum for this purpose, such gum containing licorice and papain.

POST-PRANDIAL GUM CHEWING TO REDUCE GERD

- Gum chewing improves the clearance of refluxate from the esophagus , a benefit that endures for at least 3 hours after 1 hour of gum chewing. The chewing of xylitol gum has many benefits to dental health and may also help reduce childhood ear infections, and xylitol chewing gum is also shown to increase gastrointestinal motility recovery following major surgeries.

SEAWEED ALGINATES FOR GERD

- Alginates are found in the cell walls of brown algae including the kelps and bladderwracks, and are polysaccharide chains of manuronic and guluronic acid. These seaweeds are currently the world's largest sea "crop" as they are used in large quantity as raw materials to produce purified crude alginates, presently used as stabilizers and emulsifiers in the food industry, as well as processed into fibers used to make bandages for wound care, and into beads impregnated with various drugs and nutrients to enhance their delivery, including herbal medicines. Kelp, *Macrocystis pyrifera* is used in alginate production in California, and *Laminaria japonica, Laminaria hyperborean,* and *Ascophyllum nodosum* are used in other regions of the world.

SEAWEED ALGINATES FOR GERD

- The gel-forming physical nature of alginates can bind stomach acid at the gastroesophageal junction and create a barrier that helps resist reflux.
- Several clinical trials have shown alginates to help relieve symptoms in GERD patients.,, Because stomach acid often floats on top of ingested food in the stomach, referred to as an "acid pocket", immediately consuming sodium or magnesium alginate at the close of all meals may bind the acid, cap off the gastroesophageal sphincter, and reduce reflux without antacids.
- Alginates impregnated with calcium carbonate are also being developed to remedy reflux.

Sweet and Sour Alginate "Cordial" for GERD

- Mg or Na Alginate 1 TBL (Available with a bit of searching)
- Pectin   ½ tsp
- Tamarind paste   ¼ tsp
- Licorice solid Extract   ¼ tsp
- Hyaluronic Acid   ¼ tsp
- Hot Water or Tea   1 Cup

Combine all ingredients available in the hot water or tea, stirring vigorously. Drink immediately. May take with digestive enzymes to offer further digestive support. Use after meals

---

Carminitive Tea Formula for GERD and Helicobacter Infection

- *Foeniculum vulgare*   4 oz whole seeds or powder
- *Achillea millefolium*   2 oz, finely ground flowers
- *Matricaria chamomilla* 2 oz flowers
- *Rosmarinus officinalis* 2 oz fine cut leaves
- *Zingiber officinale* 2 oz finely cut dried root
- *Glycycrrhiza glabra*   2 oz shredded root

Place 2 -3 tsp of the herb blend per cup of hot water in a sauce pan. Bring to a gentle simmer and remove immediately from the heat, and let stand covered for 10 minutes. Strain and drink freely, at least 3 cups per day.

Anti-Microbial Tincture Formula for GERD and Helicobacter Infections

- *Achillea millefolium*   8 ml
- *Curcuma longa*   8 ml
- *Hydrastis canadense*   4 ml
- *Rosmarinus officinalis*   4 ml
- *Gentiana lutea*   4 ml
- *Zingiber officinale* 4 ml
- Fennel Essential oil 20 drops

Take 1-2 tsp 5-6 times a day reducing as symptoms improve.

Licorice –Aloe Paste for GERD and Esophagitis

- Aloe gel – 1 ounce
- Tamarind paste – 1 Tbl
- Licorice solid extract – 1-2 tsp
- Glutamine Powder
- Place all in a small bowel and blend vigorously with a fork. Take 1 tsp 3 times a day, off the spoon, or diluted with one of the teas shown in this chapter. Additional doses may be used as needed for acute symptom relief. Use the entire recipe over the course of the day, and make fresh each day.

Licorice Syrup for Barrett's Esophagitis

- *Curcuma longa*   1/3 oz
- *Panax ginseng*   1/3 oz
- *Fucus*   1/3 oz
- *Glycyrrhiza* solid extract   1 oz

The licorice solid extract can help the other herbs cling, at least momentarily, to the esophagus. The formula can also be stirred into berry powder such as *Crataegus* or *Vaccinium* powders.

BLOOD MOVER BASICS

Dr Jillian Stansbury

General Poor Circulation

- *Allium*
- *Angelica*
- *Crataegus*
- *Gingko*
- *Hibiscus*
- *Lepidium*
- *Rhodiola*
- *Zingiber*
- *Achillea*

- "Blood movers" can be used to improve all aspects of circulation; stasis, blood clots, vascular congestion, vascular insufficiency and hypertension.
- Herbs that affect nitric oxide, platelet activation, blood lipids and inflammatory markers, and endothelial reactivity may be some of the mechanisms behind traditional blood movers.

Poor Circulation with Diabetes

- *Allium*
- *Ceanothus*
- *Curcuma*
- *Opuntia*
- *Syzygium*
- *Trigonella*
- *Zingiber*
- *Cinnamomum*

- Poor circulation may result from high cholesterol and high glucose, and diabetes.
- These herbs are particularly indicated for Metabolic Syndrome and the Deadly Quartet.

Circulatory Congestion and Fluid Stasis

- *Gingko* –Improves peripheral circulation
- *Angelica* – Improves peripheral circulation
- *Calendula* – enhances microcirculation to the basement membrane enhancing wound healing
- *Centella* – Enhances connective tissue regeneration
- *Crataegus* – Supports general circulation and has a stabilizing effect on inflamed vasculature
- *Echinacea* – Promotes the healing of ulcers due to supporting hyaluronic acid and inhibits secondary infections
- *Hydrastis* – Can be used topically as a skin wash for secondary infections and to astringe purulent secretions.
- *Mahonia* - Can be used topically as a skin wash for secondary infections and to astringe purulent secretions.
- *Phytolacca* – May be included in formulas to promote lymphatic circulation and immune response
- *Symphytum* – May be used topically and internally to promote wound healing and connective and epithelia cell repair.
- Stasis ulcers are common in diabetics and others with circulatory insufficiency.
- Blood movers, connective tissue restoratives, antimicrobial, and wound healing agents are all helpful.
- Treating the underlying diabetic condition if present would also be important

---

HERBS HISTORICALLY RECOMMENDED FOR ANGINA

Gingko biloba
Crataegus oxyacantha
Strophanthus hispidus
Adonis vernalis
Arnica montana
Viscum flavens
Ammi visnaga
Leonurus species
Lobelia
Nervines
Platelet anti-aggregators
Beta Blocking Herbs

- Angina is a profound symptoms of vascular congestion and heart disease.

PLATELET ANTI-AGGREGATORS/PAF INHIBITORS

- Apiacea family members -
- *Allium sativa* (Garlic) - May prevent the conversion of arachidonic acid to thromboxane.
- *Allium cepa* (Onions) - May block thromboxane synthesis. Sulfur compounds are responsible for the platelet anti-aggregating activity.
- *Angelica sinensis* (Dong quai) - Ferulic acid inhibits platelet aggregation.
- *Astragalus membranceous*
- Bromelain has been noted to reduce platelet aggregation

- *Capsicum frutescens* (Cayenne Pepper) – the capsaicin resin inhibits platelet aggregation.
- Coumarins, in general display platelet aggregating activity Osthole, for example.
- *Gingko biloba* - Ginkgolide competes with PAF for binding sites and minimizes the effects.
- Glycine max (Soy beans)
- *Glycyrrhiza glabra* – Glycyrrhizin, a triterpenoid saponin found in Licorice root has been shown to inhibit thrombin.
- *Vaccinium myrtyllis* (Bilberry) - anthocyanosides promotes prostacyclin which dilates blood vessels and inhibits platelet aggregation.

PLATELET ANTI-AGGREGATORS/PAF INHIBITORS

- Vitis vinifera – Grape juice, skins, and seeds contain polyphenolic compounds known improve microcirculation by having an anti-oxidant and protective effect on the vasculature.
- Eugenia (Cloves) - eugenol is credited as being a PAF inhibitor
- Cucuma longa (Turmeric) - inhibits platelet aggregation by inhibiting the formation of thromboxanes, and promoting the formation of prostacyclin.
- Zingiber officinale (Ginger) - inhibits thromboxane synthetase, while promoting the formation of prostacyclin.
- Commiphora mukul (Gugul) - steroidal compounds may inhibit platelet aggregation.
- Procyanidolic Oligmers (Pycnogenols, leukocyanindins) - these flavinoid have been shown to inhibit platelet aggregation.
- Galphimia glauca - inhibits PAF response.

- Picrorrhiza kurroa - shown to inhibit PAF induced bronchoconstriction in animal studies.
- Vit E – decrease can potentiate pharmaceutical anticoagulants
- Psoralea corylifolia -
- Fragaria- Lipids occurring in the leaves, fruits (achenes) and pollen of strawberry plants have been found to inhibit PAF.
- Linum usitatissimum- Flax seed oil is high in alpha linolenic acid known be have anti-atherogenic properties. Lignins act as PAF receptor agonists.
- Panax ginseng- the non-saponin or lipophilic fraction inhibits thrombin induced platelet aggregation. It is presently proposed that Panax acts via cGMP and thromboxane A2 to inhibit thrombin.
- Petrosellinum -

COUMARIN CONTAINING PLANTS

- *Apiacea* plants produce coumarin compounds to help defend against microbes , and coumarins have numerous vascular and hormonal effects in humans.
- The primary coumarin coumpounds having extensive research include psoralen, umbelliferone, aescultetin, Osthole, bergapten, xanthotoxin and imperatorin.

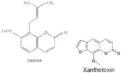

COUMARIN CONTAINING PLANTS

- In a concentrated and isolated form, coumarin is toxic due to internal hemorrhage, and liver and kidney toxicity, and pure coumarins have been banned as a food additive for over 50 years in the US.
- Coumarin is also considered to be a lung carcinogen, though this is in part due to its history as a flavorant in tobacco products.
- However, in the organic matrix of other plant molecules, coumarin compounds appear to be safe and gentle, as with celery, carrots, fennel seeds and other Apiacea family plants

COUMARIN CONTAINING PLANTS

- Coumarins offer many vascular benefits including hypotensive action and hypolipidemic affects.
- Oral absorption of coumarins is moderate due to extensive liver conversion into umbelliferone, however enough can be absorbed from plant to be physiologically active.

HERBS FOR CEREBROVASCULAR CIRCULATION

- Herbs for vascular dementia include *Salvia miltiorrhiza, Huperzia serrata, Ligusticum chuanxiong, Ginkgo biloba*, and *Panax ginseng*.
- Controlling cholesterol and inflammation in the blood is vital to controlling plaque build-up in the carotid arteries and some severe cases will require surgical approaches to help clear the carotid arteries.

Don't Confuse Coumarin with Coumadin

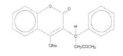

- These is an erroneous but persisting myth in some herbal practices that coumarin has a blood thinning effect such that it could be used instead of pharmaceutical coumadin medication.
- Some coumarins, such as those found in several *Angelica* species have been noted to act as platelet anti-aggregators, but not act as coumadin-like anticoagulants.

Don't Confuse Coumarin with Coumadin

- *Dicoumarols* however, the agents which pharmaceutical Warfarin anticoagulants are based, have potent anticoagulant action.
- *Dicoumarol* is structurally similar to Vitamin K and acts as an antagonist, competing with Vitamin K and reducing the effects of this blood clotting vitamin to promote the clotting factors VII, IX, and X.

DiCoumarol

SPONTANEOUS DICOUMEROL FORMATION

- *Dicoumarols* may form naturally from the fermentation of *coumarin* in plant leaves, such as decayed Sweet Clover and Sweet Vernal Grass.
- Therefore, anticoagulant action from dried plant material such as *Melilotus officianalis* or *Trifolium pratense* is theoretically possible but not emphasized in historic or modern literature on *coumarins* except in the case of accidental poisoning of livestock.

SPONTANEOUS DICOUMEROL FORMATION

- Livestock who graze on large amounts of *Trifolium*, Red Clover or other legumes or umbels as forage are noted to develop gas and bloating, as do humans consuming a high legume diet, but blood clotting difficulties are not observed.
- However, livestock who graze on large amounts of spoiled Yellow clover, *Melilotus officianlis,* or Sweet Vernal Grass, *Anthoxanthum odoratum* ARE reported to suffer hematologic and bleeding disorders which can be fatal when a large amount is ingested, due to the conversion of coumarin to dicoumarol, a potent anticoagulant.

SPONTANEOUS DICOUMEROL FORMATION

- Although coumarin itself is not found to be anticoagulant like the dicoumerol category of drugs or like heparin, many plants high in coumarin-like compounds are noted to affect platelets, blood cells and the vasculature such *aesculin* in *Aesculus, Umbelliferone* in the Umbell/Apiace Family, and the *coumarin* in *Melilotus officinalis*.

Aesculin

NATURAL COUMARINS THAT SUPPORT CIRCULATION

- Coumarins do not inhibit necessary and appropriate blood clotting, but rather act on capillary, venule, and vein permeability, increasing fluid uptake and return from the tissues to general circulation.

HIGH COUMARIN PLANTS

- Coumarins may inhibit aberrant clotting by having anti-inflammatory and platelet anti-aggregating effects.
- Such coumarin constituents appear to act in tandem with "Permeability factors" such as rutin and quercitin and improve venous return.
- High rutin plants include *Ruta graveolans* or Rue, *Fagopyrum esculentum,* Buckwheat, and Citrus peels as well as the *Apiacea* plants.

WORMS, GERMS, AND KINASE ENZYMES
TO DISSOLVE CLOTS AND PROTECT AGAINST ISCHEMIC INJURY

- Acute stroke requires agents that can permeate the blood brain barrier, immediate infusion of thrombolytic and most patients will remain on long term anti-coagulant therapy thereafter.
- While immediate thrombolytic drug therapy can help restore perfusion before major neuronal death of neurons occurs and may improve stroke recovery, such drugs can also cause intracranial bleeds, which can be fatal.

- Longterm use of such Vitamin K antagonists can also cause gastrointestinal and traumatic bleeds, and are tricky to combine with many other drugs, herbs, or even foods, as blocking the drugs may lead to new clots, and synergizing drug effects may lead to internal bleeding.

WORMS, GERMS, AND KINASE ENZYMES

- Thrombolytic drugs are used to dissolve fibrin in blood clots following MIs and thromboembolic strokes, as well as to treat deep vein thrombosis, and pulmonary embolism.
- Such pharmaceuticals can help clear blood vessel occlusion, but there is a high incidence of reocclusion and prolonged circulatory insufficiency, necessitating long term coumarin, with its many concerns such bleeding risk.
- Herbal and naturally sourced anticoagulants may be highly valuable to reduce the tendency to further clots or emboli, and may complement, or in some cases replace pharmaceutical anticoagulants.

WORMS, GERMS, AND KINASE ENZYMES

- Microorganisms have been recognized as source of thrombolytic agents, such as streptokinase from *Streptococcus hemolyticus* and staphylokinase from *Staphylococcus aureus*, and traditional foods fermented with these bacteria have been safely consumed for generations in Asia.
- Tissue plasminogen activators, streptokinase and urokinase activate plasminogen into active plasmin, which promotes degradation of fibrin in the blood clots, but are expensive and side affects are common, especially allergic reactivity.

WORMS, GERMS, AND KINASE ENZYMES

- While streptokinase doesn't have excellent penetration through the blood brain barrier, it and related microbe-derived kinase enzymes, are being explored as a maintenance therapy for those with an increased risk for clots, thrombi, emboli, and stroke, cardiac ischemia and infarct risk.
- Streptokinase should be administered as rapidly as possible, within 3 hours ideally, following a stoke

NATURAL THROMBOLYTIC AGENTS

- Similar enzymes are produced by earthworm and leeches.
- Earthworm, *Lumbricus* genera, have anticoagulant properties due to a serine protease enzyme with thrombolytic and fibrinolytic activity.
- The earthworm enzymes may be able to help dissolve clots due to direct fibrinolytic effect on fibrin, and is well absorbed in the intestines.
- Earthworm kinases show great potential in the management of ischemic vascular disease, preventing platelet activation, protecting neuronal tissue, and helping to dissolve thrombi.

NATTOKINASE

- Nattokinase from *Bacillus natto* or *Pseudomonas aeruginosa* is a potent thrombolytic agent.
- Nattō is a fermented soy product, used as a traditional food in Asia, and the enzyme nattokinase in the food may improve blood pressure, and may directly lyse thrombi in vivo, as well as enhance fibrinolytic activity in plasma and increase plasmin.
- Nattokinase interacts with heparin and interferes with heparin's binding and activation of various clotting cascades, supports antithrombin, and limits fibroblast growth factors.

NATTOKINASE

- Nattokinase can inhibit platelet aggregation by blocking thromboxane.
- Nattokinase may be included in protocols for reducing cardiovascular disease and improving risk factors, due to decreasing plasma levels of fibrinogen, and clotting factors VII and VIII, and improving blood pressure via inhibition of angiotensin II.

NATTOKINASE

- Although human studies are limited, single doses of nattokinase may reduce clotting factors and increase antithrombin in healthy subjects.
- It should be emphasized that substituting nattokinase for a pharmaceutical anticoagulant is not a simple matter, and should not be attempted without experience, vigilant monitoring, and expert guidance, especially in those with artificial values or other high clot risk situations.

NATTOKINASE

- Nattokinase appears most appropriate to reduce blood coagulation for those with varicosities, heart diseas and cardiovascular risk factors, to improve blood circulation and reduce clotting risk.

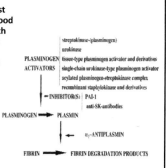

NITRIC OXIDE PROMOTORS

- **Angelica** has been shown to promote vasodilation via nitric oxide promotion.
- **Trifolium has** been shown to activate nitric oxide synthase in endothelial cells through genomic influences that involve the beta type of estrogen receptors. *Trifolium* Isoflavones appear to act synergistically with 17beta-estradiol to increase endothelial nitric oxide synthase activity and expression.
- **Apium graveolans**
- **Cnidium**
- **Osthole**

CALCIUM CHANNEL BLOCKERS

- *Allium sativum*
- *Ammi visnaga.*
- *Daucus carota*
- *Angelica species*
- *Apium*
- *Cnidium*
- *Zingiber officianlis*
- *Cinamomon*
- Osthole, a coumarin in the Apicacea family has Ca(2+)-channel blocking properties.

THROMBOXANE INHIBITORS

- Thromboxane is powerful vasoconstrictor, that once activated, the effects persist for several days.
- Thromboxane is increased by smoking, essential fatty acid deficiency, and high fats, and is deterred by these, and other herbs.
- These herbs are commonly thought of as "blood movers", and this is one more mechanism by which they offer cardiovascular benefits.
- **Angelica** Osthole reduces platelet aggregation induced by ADP, arachidonic acid, PAF, collagen and thrombin via direct thromboxane inhibition.
- *Allium sativum ,*
- *Curcuma longa*
- *Foeniculum vulgare*
- *Zingiber*
- *Piper methysticum-* Kavain- a pyrone from the roots of Kava inhibits arachidonic acid, cyclooxygenase, and thromboxane synthase

BLOOD MOVER
MATERIA MEDICA

PUERARIA LOBATA

- *Pueraria lobata*, Gegen or Kudzu is a rich source of polyphenolic compounds, including isoflavones, isoflavonoid glycosides, coumarins, and puerarols, all contributing to hypotensive and vascular protectant effects.
- Many mechanisms of action have been identified, including blockade of beta adrenergic receptors, and inhibiting angiotensin converting enzyme both of benefit to hypertension, and thereby suppressing the progression of atherosclerosis.

Salvia miltiorrhiza

- *Salvia miltiorrhiza*, Danshen or Red Sage, is longstanding traditional Chinese medicinefor the protecting the vasculature.
- *Salvia miltiorrhiza* has hypotensive, and endothelial protective properties, and numerous anti-oxidant, anti-inflammatory, and anti-proliferative properties, and is widely used in China medicine for treating coronary artery disease, hypertension, diabetes, atherosclerosis, and chronic heart failure.

- Tanshinone is credited as one active constituent against stroke and coronary artery disease. The salvianolic acids increase cerebral blood flow after ischemia and inhibit thrombosis, via modulating effects on thromboxane B2 formation and platelet aggregation.

ANGELICA SINENSIS

- Angelica sinensis is considered to be a "blood mover" in traditional Chinese medicine and modern research has identified numerous cardiovascular benefits.

- Angelica may reduce congestion in the tissues through enhanced blood and lymph circulation , and vasodilating effects via both nitric oxide and calcium channel inhibition are demonstrated.

ANGELICA SINENSIS

- *Angelica sinensis*, Dong Quai, has many anti-inflammatory mechanisms in the vasculature, and reduces inappropriate platelet activation and aggregation, and has anti-allergy, and anti-histamine effects.

Angelica for Cardiovascular Formulas

- *Angelica sinensis,* Dong Quai, is vasodilating, especially to the pelvic vasculature.
- *Angelica* inhibits platelet aggregation and has antihistamine, anticholine, and antiserotonin effects, all helping to reduce vascular inflammation and allergic reactivity.

Angelica for Cardiovascular Formulas

- *Angelica* also has immune enhancing, and anti-tumoractivity.
- *Ferulic acid* is credited with many of the cardiovascular benefits, having hypolipidemic and platelet anti-aggregating effects, helping to reduce blood cholesterol and triglylcerides, and improve blood viscosity.

Angelica for Cardiovascular Formulas

- *Ferulic acid* acts as an antioxidant in plant cell and may also protect animal tissues from oxidative damage.
- Coumarins from *Angelica* species have been noted to possess platelet anti-aggregating effects either equal to or greatly surpassing that of aspirin.

Angelica for Cardiovascular Formulas

- The coumarin compounds also display an inability to calm arachidonic acid and thromboxane induced inflammatory and platelet aggregating activity.
- Mild hyperlipidemic effects have also been demonstrated by Apiaceae coumarins such as umbelliferone

Coumarin   4-hydroxycoumarin

Dicoumarol   Warfarin

ANGELICA SINENSIS

- Angelica has protective and antiproliferative effects on vascular smooth muscle, and Angelica coumarins, ferulic acid, and lugistilide all inhibit platelet aggregation.
- Numerous anti-allergy and anti-histamine effects are identified which also contribute to the ability of *Angelica* to reduce vascular inflammation.

Ginkgo and Circulatory Enhancement

- *Ginkgo* has been well documented to improve cerebral blood flow and provide an antioxidant action to nerves and vasculature.
- *Ginkgolide*-B has been shown to act as a PAF (platelet activity factor) antagonist.

Ginkgo and Circulatory Enhancement

- *Ginkgo* is useful in cases of arterial insufficiency, intermittent claudication, ischemic heart disease, and other cases of tissue hypoxia, and is being explored as a means of reducing tumor, cancer, and degenerative disease processes.

GINKGO HAS MANY VASCULAR BENEFITS

- *Ginkgo* will also relax the vasculature and enhance perfusion, which is one proposed mechanism which heart muscle improves activity, memory and senility.
- In cases of cerebral insufficiency, one clinical study showed cerebral blood flow to be increased severity percent following the ingestion of Ginkgo.

GINKGO FOR CIRCULATORY INSUFFICIENCY

- Since *Ginkgo* enhances peripheral circulation, it may benefit peripheral vascular disease.
- Several studies have shown *Ginkgo* to promote blood flow in both healthy and compromised blood vessels.
- *Gingko* has been investigated in numerous human trials and has shown to be useful in cases of arterial insufficiency, intermittent claudication, ischemic heart disease, and other cases of tissue hypoxia.

GINKGO FOR CLAUDICATION

- *Gingko* supplementation has been shown to reduce symptoms of tissue hypoxia in human trials.
- One clinical trial noted comfortable walking distance to be lengthened in those suffering from arterial insufficiency.
- Thromboxane synthesis and thrombus formation have been inhibited in animal studies.
- Animal studies have also shown vasospasms to be reduced with the administration of *Ginkgo*.

GINKGO AND ANTI-COAGUANTS

- Ginkgo is readily available in a variety of forms and formulations and are safe to use in tandem with pharmaceutical heart medicines, perhaps even anticoagulants as one very large clinical investigation found no increased risk of bleeding or other adverse effects in those use *Gingko* in tandem with warfarin.

CRATAEGUS

- *Crataegus*, the Hawthorn berry, is one of the most widely used western herbs in a variety of cardiovascular formulas. The flavonoids are credited with hypolipidemic effects.
- *Crataegus* may help protect the tunica intima from atherosclerotic changes, promote oxidation enzymes in the liver helping to metabolize lipids and, and upregulated the influx of cholesterol from the plasma into the liver for processing.

ROSA CANINA - ROSE HIPS

- Rose hips and Hawthorn berries are both in the rose family, and rose hips too, have cardioprotective effects.
- Rosehips can be added to teas, and takes as a solid extract, and rose hips have been shown to promote brown fat, supporting of lipolysis and favorable fat metabolism.

COMMIPHORA MUKUL

- *Commiphora* mukul, Guggul, supports thyroid function, and via this and other mechanisms, can help reduce hyperlipidemia.
- *Commiphora* compounds known as guggulsterones inhibit the development and maturation of fat storing cells, called adipocytes.
- Guggulsterones exert direct inhibitory effect on adipocytes, inducing decreased synthesis of new cells, decreased fat accumulation in existing cells, and increased destruction (apoptosis) of fat cells.

Allium cepa and *Allium sativum*
Onions and Garlic

- *Allium cepa*, Onions, and *Allium sativum,* Garlic, support healthy blood glucose, cholesterol, and blood pressure, with much of the action credited to sulfur compounds, alliin and allicin

Allium sativa

- *Allium sativa* improves cholesterol, triglyceride, and lipid ratios, has a vasodilating action, and have cardioprotective effects via a variety of molecular mechanism including cyclooxygenase inhibitIon , improved elasticity of the aorta, nitric oxide promotion, and inhibition of platelet aggregation.

Allium sativa

- *Allium* may also reduce vascular inflammation in diabetes, reducing blood glucose, improving insulin sensitivity, and reducing oxidative stress in animals fed a high fructose diet.
- Human clinical trials have shown that the consumption of 400 mg of garlic powder can help reduce body weight and person body fat in patients with nonalcoholic fatty liver disease.

LIGUSTICUM AND GASTRODIA

- Ligustrazine, from *Ligusticum chuanxiong* helps protect against reperfusion injury.
- *Gastrodia elata* is a traditional Chinese medicine for treating stroke, epilepsy, dizziness and dementia, and the constituent gastrodin has been shown to prevent reperfusion injury.

SAMPLE BLOOD MOVING FORMULARY

All Purpose Cardio-Vascular Support Tea

- *Salvia miltiorrhiza*
- *Pueraria lobata*
- *Angelica sinensis*
- *Mahonia aquifolium*
- *Arctium lappa*
- *Cinnamomun*
- *Zingiber officinalis*
- *Hibiscus* flowers
- *Rosa canina* chopped hips
- *Glycyrrhiza glabra*
- Combine several ounces of each ingredient and store in an airtight container. Simmer 2 TBL in 6 cups of water for 10 minutes, let stand covered, for 10 minutes more, strain, and drink throughout the day.

Blood Cell Reactivity, Hives

- *Angelica*   ½ oz
- *Ephedra*   ½ oz
- *Petasites* ½ oz
- *Tanacetum*   ½ oz

Take as much as a tsp every half hour for acute hives and atopic reactivity reducing as symptoms subside.

- Platelets harbor histamine, serotonin and other inflammatory substances and may be involved in initiating hives, eczema, and atopic phenomena.
- Modern research has demonstrated that many herbs used folklorically for hives, asthma and allergies reduce inappropriate platelet activation.

Vascular Protection Formula Based on Classic Traditional Chinese Medicine Duo

- *Angelica sinensis* root   ½ pound
- *Astragalus* roots   ½ pound

Blend the two herbs and decoct 1 tsp per cup of hot water. Drink 3 or more cups per day.

- *Angelica sinensis* and *Astragalus* roots have been used at least since the 1200s in combination to treat vascular inflammation such as diabetic nephropathy, pulmonary fibrosis, liver fibrosis and heart disease.

Formula for General Vascular "Heat" and Inflammation

- *Tanacetum*   ½ oz
- *Petasites*   ½ oz
- *Crataegus*   ½ oz
- *Gingko*   ½ oz

Take 1-2 droppers of tincture 3 or more times daily.

- Because platelets harbor histamine and white cells harbor cytokines and inflammatory mediators, using herbs that act directly on blood cells may help treat blood vessel inflammation, clotting disorders, and atherosclerosis.
- Those with atopic tendencies, hives, or allergies occurring in tandem with cardiovascular complaints would especially benefit from herbs such as *Petasites* and *Tanacetum*, both known to reduce the release of inflammatory products from blood cells and have general anti-inflammatory effects.

General Formula for "Cold" Vascular Stasis

- *Angelica* 25 ml
- *Salvia miltiorrhiza*   25 ml
- *Zingiber* 10 ml

Take 5 ml 3 or more times a day.

- Those with cold hands and feet, vascular congestion, and a tendency to clots, might be said to have "coldness" in the blood in the various energetic traditions of the world.
- The use of warming and "blood moving" herbs is appropriate in such situations.
- Warming herbs might include *Zingiber* or *Capsicum*, and blood moving herbs might include *Achillea, Ginkgo, Angelica,* or *Salvia miltiorrhiza.*

High Lipids or Inflammatory Markers Concomitant with Excessive Clotting

- *Allium*   1 oz
- *Angelica*   ½ oz
- *Salvia miltiorrhiza* ½ oz

Take 1 tsp 3 or more times a day, along with 500-1000 mg of Bromelain between meals 3 or 4 times daily.

- Those with a history of blood clots and/or elevated platelets or C Reactive protein, may benefit from herbs that are known "platelet anti-aggregators."
- Bromelain would be an excellent supplement to complement this formula to reduce the tendency to excessive or inappropriate platelet activation and clotting.
- Patients on Coumadin should use under attempt use under a doctor's supervision, as lab work will be required to monitor progress.

High Lipids with Liver Congestion and/or Intestinal Dysbiosis

- *Aesculus*   15 ml
- *Silybum marianum* 15 ml
- *Allium*   10 ml
- *Curcuma*   10 ml
- *Iris*   10 ml

Take one to three droppers, three times per day. Complement with two lipotropic capsules with each meal.

- **High lipids can sometimes be the result of weak liver function where fats are not emulsified, processed, or metabolized readily.**
- **Herbs that support liver function and intestinal health can be helpful here.**
- **Consider a formula such as this, especially when patients have symptoms of toxemia, digestive issues, acne or other skin issues.**
- **This tincture would be complemented by the use of a commercial "Lipotropic" encapsulation formula.**

Tincture Formula for Angina

- *Gingko*   15 ml
- *Angelica*   15 ml
- *Crataegus*   15 ml
- *Viscum*   10 ml
- *Arnica*   5 ml

Take 1 -2 tsp 3 to 6 times daily.

- **This formula is a basic circulatory and platelet anti-aggregating blend, while the one that follows is a more powerful vasorelaxant.**
- ***Arnica* is not often ingested orally, but one of the folkloric recommendations is chest pain that is aching and sore, as if bruised in character.**

Angina with Acute Squeezing Pain

- *Angelica*
- *Lobelia*
- *Valerian*

Take 1 -2 tsp every 5 minutes for acute chest pain, reducing as symptoms improve. Take 1-2 tsp 3 times a day for maintenance dosing.

- ***Lobelia* is a natural beta blocker for coronary vasospasm and angina. *Angelica* also relaxes many muscle types in the body via effects on calcium channels plus is a platelet anti-aggregator and general anti-inflammatory blood mover.**
- **This formula may be more effective in alleviate acute angina than the above formula which is more nourishing and tonifying that this formula.**
- **In the upper dosing ranges for acute angina, *Lobelia* may promote salivation and nausea and can only be dosed as tolerated.**
- **Taking the dose in mint or chamomile tea may alleviate this problem, but there would not always be time to prepare tea in acute situations.**

Sini Tang/decoction to Improve Cardiac Ejection after Myocardial Infarction

- *Aconitum carmichaelii*
- *Zingiber officinale*
- *Glycyrrhiza uralensis,*
- *Cinnamomum cassia*

- **This traditional formula is used in China for MI patients, to improve cardiovascular function.**

Post MI Recovery Tincture

- *Terminalia arjuna*   15 ml
- *Cactus grandiflorous*   15 ml
- *Crataegus oxyacantha* 25 ml
- *Piper nigrum*
       5 ml

Take by the dropper full, 3 or 4 times per day.

- **The herbs in this formula are noted to improve cardiac enzyme levels, and improve lipid and anti-oxidant levels.**

Rhodiola Simple for Ischemic Heart Disease

- *Rhodiola* capsules

Take 2-3 capsules, 2 to 3 times day

- ***Rhodiola* is a traditional medicine for improving energy, stamina, mood, and athletic performance, and the plant has been used in formulas for angina pectoris, coronary artery disease, and heart failure.**
- **Numerous clinical studies suggest that the plant improves EKG reading and improves the symptoms of ischemic heart disease.**

Classic Chinese Duo for Protecting the Heart

- *Ligusticum chuanxiong*
- *Angelica sinensis*

Combine equal parts of tincture and take 1-2 droppers at a time, 3 or 4 times daily.

- *Angelica sinensis* and *Ligusticum chuanxiong* are a traditional duo used to support circulation and protect the vasculature.
- Numerous mechanisms of action have been proposed, but the pair are featured here due to an ability to inhibit the proliferation of vascular smooth muscle from oxidative and hypertensive stress, and promote vasodilation via nitric oxide and intracellular Ca^{2+}.

Umbell Tea for Tachyarrhythmias

- *Angelica archangelica*
- *Apium seeds*
- *Rosa canina hips*
- *Salvia miltorrhiza*

Combine the dry herbs and decoct 1 heaping tsp per cup of hot water, strain and drink freely.

- Osthole can reduce the frequency of action potential in neurons via inhibition of calcium channels.
- In animal studies, osthole has been shown to relax the thoracic aorta by virtue of its Ca (2+)-channel blocking properties and by elevating cGMP levels in vascular smooth muscle.
- This is presently presumed to be the mechanism whereby some Apiacae plants such as *Cnidium*, *Angelica*, and *Apium* are able to reduce blood pressure.
- Osthole was noted to reduce hyperexcitability of the atrial electrical fibers when subjected to electrical stimulation.
- The protection against excessive electrical activity has been credited to calcium channel inhibition. This research suggests that Apiaciae plants might be useful for tachyarrhthmias as well as hypertension.

Poor Circulation with Damp Symptoms and Doughy Skin

- *Allium*   15 ml
- *Angelica*   15 ml
- *Ceanothus*   15 ml
- *Iris*   8 ml
- *Cinnamomum* 7 ml

Take 5 ml a minimum of 3 times daily.

- Longstanding poor circulation can allow metabolic waste products to remain in the lymphatic and interstitial spaces and cause congestion, a tendency to infection – sometimes referred to as "dampness".
- Diabetics with impaired circulation often develop thick doughy skin following many years of such vascular stasis. The following herbs may improve circulation and reduce tissue congestion.

Poor Circulation in Healthy Very Elderly

- *Panax*   20 ml
- *Angelica*   10 ml
- *Gingko*   10 ml
- *Lepidium* 10 ml
- *Zingiber*   10 ml

Take 1-2 droppers of tincture 3 or more times daily.

- *Panax* is an herb with broad application for the elderly and those with weakness, deficiency and poor circulation.
- Research is mounting showing that *Lepidium* may also improve heart function and may be used in tinctures and the powder in smoothies.
- The general blood movers *Gingko* and *Angelica* may complement these heart tonics. T
- his formula may benefit elderly patients who are generally healthy and without frank heart disease, but whose limbs fall asleep readily and are becoming weak, dizzy, and exercise intolerant.

Tincture for Poor Circulation to the Kidneys, with Renal Insufficiency

- *Salvia miltiorrhiza* 30 ml
- *Crataegus*   15 ml
- *Lepidium*   10 ml
- *Thuja occidentalis* 5 ml

Take one to two dropper fulls of tinctures 3 times a day or as often as hourly for conditions of renal failure.

- This formula combines agents that support general circulation with a small amount of *Thuja* to act as a counter irritant.
- *Thuja* is slightly irritating to the urinary tissues and may promote glomerular filtration but should only be used in small doses as it can irritate and inflame the kidneys.

Tea for Poor Circulation to the Kidneys, with Renal Insufficiency

- *Gingko*   4 oz
- *Urtica* species 4 oz
- *Petroselinum*   4 oz
- *Equisetum*   4 oz

Combine the herbs to yield a pound of tea and store in a large glass jar in a dark cupboard. Steep 1 Tbl of the blend per cup of hot water for 10 minutes. Strain and drink 3 or more cups a day.

- This tea would complement the above tincture formula. These herbs all support diuresis but are nourishing, non-irritating, and can be used in a long term way.
- This formula is unflavored, so mint, *Stevia* or other herbs may be added as preferred by the patient.

Poor Circulation Leading to Stasis Ulcer

- *Gingko*   20 ml
- *Echinacea*   20 ml
- *Phytolacca*   20 ml

Take 1dropper every 2 or 3 hours, reducing as the ulcer heals.

- Tibial ulcers due venous stasis occur in the elderly, diabetics and anyone else with poor circulation.
- Elevating the legs is essential to promote healing.
- *Echinacea* can reduce the breakdown in hyaluronic acid helping skin lesions heal and inhibiting opportunistic infections.
- *Phytolacca* can improve lymphatic stasis and *Gingko* improves peripheral circulation.
- Reduce the *Phytolacca* should any oral irritation occur.

Topical Compress for Stasis Ulcers

- *Calendula* flower powder
- *Achillea* powder
- *Symphytum* root powder
- *Centella* powder
- *Equisetum* powder
- Tea Tree Oil
- Lavendar Oil

Combine 1 oz of each of the dry powders in a ziplock bag or glass jar and blend well. At the time of use remove 1 tbl of the powder blend and place in a small bowl. Pour 1 cup of hot water over the herbs and stir. Allow to sit for 15 minutes. Soak a soft clean cloth or sterile gauze pad in the mixture, add 1 or 2 drops each of lavender and tee tree oils to the pad and apply to the ulcer. Repeat as many times per day as possible with the legs elevated.

- Stasis ulcers are due to poor circulation so topical applications alone are rarely effective.
- However, topical compresses skin washes can deter opportunistic infections and be complementary to oral circulatory enhancing agents.
- Chronic stasis ulcers can also be foul smelling so the use of essential oils is pleasant for both the doctor and the patient.

Poor Circulation in Legs with Claudication

- *Achillea*   20 ml
- *Angelica*   15 ml
- *Gingko*   15 ml
- *Zingiber*   10 ml

Take 5 ml 3 or more times a day.

- The herbs in this formula can act as peripheral vasodilators getting more blood to the limbs, as well as reduce abnormal clotting tendencies to improve blood viscosity.
- *Achillea* can act as an alterative as well as a peripheral vasodilatory helping improve the absorption of the formula and support general digestion.
- Magnesium, Vitamin C and Inositol hexaniacinate are complementary nutrients to this formula.

Herbal Tincture Formula for Intermittent Claudication

- *Ginkgo biloba*
- *Crataegus species*
- *Angelica sinensis*
- *Achilliea millefolium*
- *Cinnmomun*

Combine equal parts and take 3 or more times per day.

- Intermittent Claudication represents fairly advanced circulatory insufficiency and those affected will likely require life long circulatory support.
- A tincture such as this may be complemented by Ginkgo capsules, and nattokinase or similar product to prevent clot risk.

General Circulatory Weakness and Underlying Deficiency State

- *Panax ginseng* ½ oz
- *Lepidium*   ½ oz
- *Crataegus*   ½ oz
- *Capsicum*   ½ oz

Take 5 ml 3-4 times a day.

- General weakness and deficiency states may be constitutional or may develop secondary to stress, adrenal fatigue illness and other causes.
- General deficiency may manifest as low energy and stamina, a weak voice, and coldness.
- When deficiency extends specifically to the heart exercise tolerance, general fatigue, shortness of breath and dizziness may also accompany.
- The pulse may be weak or thin, the complexion pale or even greyish or bluish, and the body especially the hands and feet cold.
- This formula features the "Chi Tonic" *Panax ginseng* and combines it with circulatory tonics *Lepidium* and *Crataegus* and the warming agent *Capsicum*.

Formula for Poor Circulation in the Head with Impaired Cognition

- *Gingko*
- *Rosmarinus*
- *Salvia*
- *Centella*
- *Curcuma*

Combine equal parts of the herbal tinctures, and take 1-2 droppers, 3 or 4 times a day, decreasing as symptoms improve.

- This formula is to enhance cerebral circulation when hypoxic symptoms such as tinnitus and frequent faintness and dizziness are present.
- *Ginkgo* is a noted cerebral circulatory stimulant, and clinical trials suggest that *Gingko biloba* can improve cognition in cases of vascular dementia.
- *Rosmarinus* and *Salvia officinalis* have circulatory enhancing effects as well as cholinergic effects making them appropriate for memory loss and confusion related to poor circulation to the head.
- *Centella* and *Curcuma* are both noted to reduce fibrosis and scarring in the brain related to hypoxia, injuries, toxin exposure and inflammation.
- Most of the herbs in this formula could also be prepared as a tea rather than a tincture.

Tincture for Poor Circulation to the Head with Dizziness or Tinnitus

- *Gingko*   20 ml
- *Rhodiola* 10 ml
- *Rosmarnius*10 ml
- *Salvia officinalis* 10 ml
- *Vinca* 10 ml

Take 1-2 droppers 3 or more times a day long term.

- Carotid artery insufficiency, low blood pressure, or elderly patients with poor circulation may all experience dizziness, especially with standing.
- The herbs in this formula all improve circulation to the head. This formula may be simplified and just several of the herbs selected as preferred.
- Ringing in the ears, tinnitus, may also occur with poor circulation to the ears, and *Ginkgo* is a traditional remedy for the complaint.

Poor Circulation to the Brain with TIAs Transient Ischemic Attacks

- *Gingko*   10 ml
- *Curcuma*   10 ml
- *Centella*   10 ml
- *Rosmarinus*   10 ml
- *Salvia miltiorrhiza*   10 ml
- *Salvia officinalis*   10 ml

Take 1-2 droppers 3 or more times a day long term.

- TIAs are small warning strokes that should be taken very seriously.
- TIAs are treated in the same manner as significant ischemic strokes.

Tea Formula to Protect Against Stroke in Patients with Heart Disease, Atrial Fibrillation

- *Gingko*
- *Salix*
- *Apium*
- *Salvia miltiorrhiza*

Combine equal parts of tincture, and take 1 dropper 3 or 4 times a day.

- *Gingko* is approved in China for the treatment of stroke. *Ginkgo* reduces capillary fragility, terpenoids may inhibit platelet activation, and improve viscosity, and reduce the risk of stroke.
- Salicylates are cyclooxygenase inhibitors that inhibit platelet activation.
- Aspirin is widely used to reduce the risk of clots, thrombi, and stroke, but salicylate containing herbs may also work in similar ways.
- Celery seeds, *Apium graveolans*, are high in butylphthalide noted to protect again ischemic brain injury.
- *Salvia miltiorrhiza* is shown to reduce the impact of ischemia/reperfusion injury in the brain, and support regeneration of neural stem cells following stroke.

Tea for History of Blood Clots

- *Trifolium*
- *Zingiber*
- *Cinamomum*
- *Ceanothus*
- *Quercus*

Combine the dry herbs and blend. Gently simmer 1 tsp per cup of hot water for just 1 minute. Cover the pan and let stand for 10 to 15 minutes off of the heat source. Strain and house in a covered jar or thermos.

- Those with a history of a blood clot, are at an increased risk for a recurrence.
- Lifelong circulatory support with blood moving herbs, may be helpful.
- Quitting smoking is essential.
- Complementary approaches include Ginkgo capusles and nattokinase, regular excersice, and regular use of garlic, onions, ginger, turmeric, and other blood moving herbs.

OPTIMIZING GASTRIC MOTILITY

DR JILLIAN STANSBURY

GASTRIC MOTILITY

- MOTILITY DURING THE DIGESTIVE PERIOD INVOLVES BOTH NEURAL AND HORMONAL INPUT.
- MOTILITY INVOLVES GALLBLADDER CONTRACTIONS, STIMULATION OF PANCREATIC SECRETION, AND SPHINCTER OF ODDI RELAXATION.
- UP TO 30–40% OF GALLBLADDER EMPTYING AND 25% OF PANCREATIC SECRETION OCCURS DURING THE CEPHALIC PHASE VIA VAGAL INPUT
- ANOTHER 10–20% OF THE RESPONSE OCCURS DURING THE GASTRIC PHASE VIA VASOVAGAL PATHWAYS.
- HOWEVER, THE GALLBLADDER EMPTIES MOST OF ITS REMAINING CONTENTS AND THE PANCREAS UP TO 50% OF ITS TOTAL SECRETION DURING THE INTESTINAL PHASE.

REGULATION OF GASTRIC MOTILITY

- GASTRIC MOTILITY INVOLVES THE RELEASE OF CHOLECYSTOKININ (CCK) AND SECRETIN FROM THE DUODENUM AND PROXIMAL JEJUNUM.
- DUODENAL CCK CONTRACTS THE GALLBLADDER, RELAXES THE S.O., AND CAUSES PANCREATIC EXOCRINE DIGESTIVE ENZYME SECRETION VIA DIRECT ACTIONS ON CCK RECEPTORS AND INDIRECTLY THROUGH CHOLINERGIC NEURONS.
- ATROPINE BLOCKS CCK INDUCED GALLBLADDER CONTRACTION AND PANCREATIC SECRETION INDUCED BY A PROTEIN-FATTY MEAL

HORMONES INVOLVED IN GASTRIC MOTILITY

- MOTILIN, SOMATOSTATIN, AND OCTREOTIDE HORMONALLY INFLUENCE S.O. FUNCTION.
- MOTILIN, SECRETED BY THE DUODENUM AND JEJUNUM, INDUCES CONTRACTION OF GB SMOOTH MUSCLE AND STIMULATES BILE SECRETION.
- SOMATOSTATIN, PRESENT IN ENDOCRINE CELLS THROUGHOUT THE GASTROINTESTINAL TRACT, EXERTS INHIBITORY EFFECTS ON BOTH GALLBLADDER CONTRACTION AND RELAXATION OF THE S.O.

SEROTONIN'S ROLE IN METABOLISM AND GASTRIC MOTILITY

- SEROTONIN, A CENTRAL NEUROMODULATOR WITH ANCIENT TIES TO FEEDING AND METABOLISM, IS A MAJOR DRIVER OF BODY FAT LOSS.
- SEROTONIN CONTROLS FOOD INTAKE AND FEEDING BEHAVIOUR, MOOD, ADIPOSITY, LOCOMOTION AND ENERGY EXPENDITURE.
- THE NEUROENDOCRINE RELEASE OF SEROTONIN RESPONDS TO NUTRIENT SENSORS, INCLUDING TACHYKININ RECEPTORS IN THE INTESTINE THAT ALSO DRIVE FAT LOSS VIA THE ADIPOCYTE TRIGLYCERIDE LIPASES.

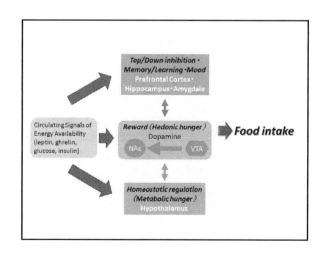

GUT BRAIN AXIS AND GLUCOSE HOMEOSTASIS

- THE GUT–BRAIN AXIS IMPACTS METABOLIC FUNCTION AND IS A POTENTIAL THERAPEUTIC TARGET FOR DEFECTIVE GLUCOSE HOMEOSTASIS.

- GLUCOREGULATORY PEPTIDES ARE RELEASED BY BOTH THE GUT AND BRAIN, AND MAY BE DERANGED FOLLOWING ACUTE PANCREATITIS AND OTHER AILMENTS.

- GLUCOREGULATORY PEPTIDES INCLUDE: GLUCAGON-LIKE PEPTIDE, GLICENTIN, OXYNTOMODULIN, PEPTIDE YY, GHRELIN, CHOLECYSTOKININ, VASOACTIVE INTESTINAL PEPTIDE (VIP), AND SECRETIN, AND ALL ARE BEING TARGETED AS POSSIBLE TARGETS TO TREAT DIABETES, WEIGHT LOSS, INTESTINAL MOTILITY, CHRONIC PANCREATITIS, AND OTHER DISORDERS.

- THESE GLUCOREGULATORY PEPTIDES AFFECT PANCREATIC ISLET CELLS AND ARE SECRETED BY ENTEROENDOCRINE CELLS AND BY THE BRAIN, AND THE INTERACTIONS BETWEEN THESE COMPOUNDS ARE REFERRED TO AS THE GUT-BRAIN AXIS, KNOWN TO ACT BIDIRECTIONALLY TO REGULATE ENERGY AND METABOLIC FUNCTIONS. PEPTIDES OF THE GUT–BRAIN AXIS EXERT THEIR ACTIONS THROUGH G PROTEIN-COUPLED RECEPTORS SUPERFAMILY.

GASTRIC EMPTYING AND FOOD INTAKE

- ANOREXIA NERVOSA IS ASSOCIATED WITH SLOWER GASTRIC EMPTYING AND HEIGHTENED VISCERAL PERCEPTION COMPARED TO OBESE AND NORMAL WEIGHT INDIVIDUALS.

- IN CONTRAST, OBESE INDIVIDUALS HAVE A DELAYED ONSET OF FULLNESS OR SATIATION. THEREFORE, GASTRIC EMPTYING AND MOTILITY MAY CONTRIBUTE TO BOTH OF THESE DISORDERS.

KEY HORMONES OF HUNGER AND SATIETY

- LEPTIN - THE SATIETY HORMONE
- ADIPONECTIN - THE APPETITE-STIMULATING HORMONE
- GHRELIN – THE HUNGER HORMONE

GHRELIN – THE HUNGER HORMONE

- GHRELIN, DISCOVERED IN 1999, AND RECOGNIZED TO STIMULATE OF GROWTH HORMONE SECRETION, AS WELL AS TO PLAY ROLES IN ENERGY HOMEOSTASIS, APPETITE STIMULATION AND ENERGY EXPENDITURE REGULATION.

- GHRELIN INDUCES POSITIVE ENERGY BALANCE, AND LOW LEVELS MAY PLAY A ROLE IN THE CANCER CACHEXIA SYNDROME. OPTIMIZING GHRELIN MAY SUPPORT WEIGHT GAIN AND NUTRITION.

HELICOBACTER'S EFFECT ON GHRELIN

- HELICOBACTER PYLORI INFECTION AND GASTRIC MUCOSAL ATROPHY AFFECT GHRELIN LEVELS, AND TREATING THIS INFECTION AS WELL AS RESTORING MUCOSAL INTEGRITY MAY NORMALIZE GHRELIN LEVELS.

GHRELIN PATHWAYS

- GHRELIN IS A PEPTIDE HORMONE WITH NUMEROUS CENTRAL AND PERIPHERAL EFFECTS.

- THE CENTRAL EFFECTS INCLUDE PROMOTION OF GH SECRETION, FOOD INTAKE, AND ENERGY HOMEOSTASIS AND ARE PARTLY MEDIATED BY KISS1- KISSR SIGNALING PATHWAY.

GHRELIN'S EFFECT ON INSULIN

- GHRELIN AND ITS RECEPTOR ARE ALSO EXPRESSED IN THE PANCREATIC ISLETS AND ARE ONE OF THE KEY METABOLIC FACTORS CONTROLLING INSULIN SECRETION FROM THE ISLETS OF LANGERHANS.

- GHRELIN MAY INHIBIT BOTH PANCREATIC ISLETS AND HYPOTHALAMUS HORMONES.

GHRELIN AND HORMONES OF DIGESTION

GHRELIN

- THE EXACT ROLE OF GHRELIN IN REGULATION OF INSULIN SECRETION IS NOT DEFINITELY UNDERSTOOD.

- GHRELIN WAS FOUND TO INHIBIT INSULIN SECRETION IN SOME EXPERIMENTS BUT TO STIMULATE IT IN OTHERS.

- GHRELIN IS SECRETED MAINLY FROM THE STOMACH.

- GHRELIN IS AN ENDOGENOUS LIGAND OF THE GROWTH HORMONE RECEPTOR, ALSO NOW REFERRED TO THE GHRELIN RECEPTOR.

- LIKE DOPAMINE, GHRELIN SUPPRESSES THE PULSATILE LUTEINIZING HORMONE (LH) SECRETION.

- GHRELIN REGULATES FOOD INTAKE, GASTROINTESTINAL MOTILITY, AND ENERGY HOMEOSTASIS.

- GHRELIN HAS OREXIGENIC EFFECT AND IS THEREFORE REFERRED TO AS "THE HUNGER HORMONE".

- GHRELIN PASSES THROUGH THE BLOOD–BRAIN BARRIER AND ACTS ON BRAIN NUCLEI INVOLVED IN FOOD INTAKE.

- GHRELIN IS ALSO PRODUCED CENTRALLY IN THE ARCUATE NUCLEUS OF THE HYPOTHALAMUS WHICH HAS A KEY ROLE IN REGULATION OF FOOD INTAKE.

- KISSPEPTINS (KSS) ARE PEPTIDES EXPRESSED IN THE HYPOTHALAMUS IS SENSITIVE TO NUTRITIONAL STATE, AND MAY CONTRIBUTE TO THE SUPPRESSION OF REPRODUCTIVE FUNCTION IN SUCH CONDITIONS AS NEGATIVE ENERGY BALANCE PERIODS, SUCH AS IN ANOREXIA.

- KISSPEPTINS HAS BEEN DETECTED IN THE CENTRAL NERVOUS SYSTEM AS WELL AS PERIPHERAL TISSUES SUCH AS PLACENTA, TESTES, AND PANCREAS.

- KISSPEPTIN AND ITS G PROTEIN-COUPLED RECEPTOR PLAY ESSENTIAL ROLES OF CONTROLLING GHRELIN EXPRESSION IN THE HYPOTHALAMUS.

- PANCREATIC BETA CELLS EXPRESS KISS-1 AND PLAY A ROLE IN HUNGER, METABOLISM, AND EXOCRINE FUNCTIONS.

FACTORS INFLUENCING GASTRIC EMPTYING TIME

Factors	Influence on Gastric Emptying
Volume	The larger the starting volume, the greater the initial rate of emptying, after this initial period, the larger the original volume, the slower the rate of emptying.
Type of meal	Reduction in rate of emptying to an extent directly dependent upon concentration of carbohydrate,lipid and protein type food
Osmotic pressure	Reduction in rate of emptying to an extent dependent upon concentration for salts and nonelectrolytes
Physical state of gastric contents	Solutions or suspensions of small particles empty more rapidly
Body position	Rate of emptying is reduced in a patient lying on left side.
Viscosity	Rate of emptying is greater for viscous solutions.

GASTROPARESIS

- GASTROPARESIS IS A CONDITION OF DELAYED GASTRIC EMPTYING, AND CAUSES PAIN, GAS, AND BLOATING, BUT NO ACTUAL OBSTRUCTION, AND PREDISPOSES TO DYSBIOSIS, AND SIBO.
- GASTROPARESIS MAY OCCUR IN METABOLIC DISORDERS SUCH AS DIABETES, PARTICULARLY THOSE WITH ADVANCED AUTONOMIC NEUROPATHY.
- HISTOLOGIC STUDY IN SEVERE GASTROPARESIS SHOWS ENTERIC NEURONAL, SMOOTH MUSCLE, INTERSTITIAL CELL, AND INFLAMMATORY ABNORMALITIES.

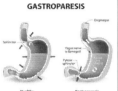

GASTROPARESIS

Healthy   Gastroparesis

GHRELIN AGONIST AND MOTILITY DRUGS

- MOTILITY ENHANCING AGENTS INCLUDE GHRELIN AGONISTS, AND GASTRIC ELECTRICAL STIMULATORS.
- PROKINETIC DRUGS INCLUDE SEROTONIN 5-HT4 AGONISTS, MOTILIN AGONISTS, DOPAMINE D2 ANTAGONISTS, MUSCARINIC ANTAGONIST AND ACETYLCHOLINESTERASE INHIBITORS.

motility stimulants

- = prokinetic drug
- domperidone (Motilium) - D_2 antagonist, also antiemetic
  - ↑ oesophageal sphincter pressure...GERD
  - ! hyperprolactinemia
- metoclopramide (Paspertin) - DA antagonist and Ach agonist
  - increases gastric emptying - GERD
  - ! extrapyramidal side effects
- cisapride (Prepulsid) - 5-HT$_4$ rec. agonist....Ach release
  - ↑ gut motility, no antiemetic action
  - withdrawn due to QT prolongation

GASTRIC MOTILITY IMPAIRMENT IN PARKINSON'S DISEASE

THE MOTILITY ISSUES OF PARKINSON'S DISEASE CAN AFFECT THE NERVES OF THE ENTIRE GASTROINTESTINAL TRACT AND CAUSE CONSTIPATION, SMALL INTESTINAL BACTERIAL OVERGROWTH, AND GASTROPARESIS.

CAPRYLIC ACID HAS AN OREXIGENIC EFFECT

- CAPRYLIC ACID IS A MEDIUM-CHAIN SATURATED FATTY ACIDS (MCFAS) WITH PHYSICAL AND METABOLIC PROPERTIES.
- CAPRYLIC ACID IS SHOWN TO BIND GHRELIN, THE ONLY PEPTIDE HORMONE WITH AN OREXIGENIC EFFECT.
- CARNITINE MAY PROMOTE GASTRIC SECRETION.

BASIC DIGESTION AND INTESTINAL MOTILITY

THE FAILURE TO ADEQUATELY BREAK DOWN, ABSORB, AND ASSIMILATE INGESTED FOOD MAY BE DUE TO:

- AGING
- BILIARY INSUFFICIENCY
- HYPOCLORHYDRIA
- HCL FROM THE STOMACH, OR
- PANCREATIC ENZYME INSUFFICIENCY
- GENETIC DEFECTS SUCH AS CELIAC'S DISEASE, OR LACTASE DEFICIENCY
- SHORT BOWEL SYNDROME.

GERIATRIC DIGESTIVE ISSUES

- THE ELDERLY ARE PARTICULARLY LIKELY TO HAVE HYPOCHLORHYDRIA AND PANCREATIC INSUFFICIENCY.
- COMMON NUTRITIONAL DEFICIENCIES INCLUDE CALCIUM, ZINC, MAGNESIUM, VITAMIN B(12), FOLIC ACID, AS WELL AS TRACE MINERALS AND GENERAL MALNUTRITION.
- HYPOCLORHYDRIA ALSO MAKES THE ELDERLY SUSCEPTIBLE TO SMALL BOWEL BACTERIAL OVERGROWTH, SIBO

MALABSORPTION SYMPTOMS

THE SYMPTOMS OF MALABSORPTION ARE:

- WEIGHT LOSS
- POOR WOUND HEALING
- DIGESTIVE GAS AND BLOATING

SYMPTOMS OF SPECIFIC NUTRIENT DEFICIENCIES:

- B VITAMIN - GLOSSITIS, PARESTHESIAS
- MINERALS AND ELECTROLYTES - MUSCLE CRAMPS AND SPASMS
- PROTEIN - LACK OF LUSTER AND INTEGRITY OF HAIR AND FINGERNAILS
- VITAMIN C – BRUISING AND BLEEDING GUMS
- CALCIUM - TETANY, MUSCLE CRAMPS, BONE PAIN.
- IRON – ANEMIA, FATIGUE, HEART PALPITATIONS

HERBS FOR MALABSORPTION

- TREAT MALABSORPTION AS SPECIFICALLY AS POSSIBLE.
- TREAT BILIARY INSUFFICIENCY WITH *TARAXICUM, SILYBUM, CURCUMA,* AND *CHELIDONIUM.*
- TREAT PANCREATIC INSUFFICIENCY WITH DIGESTIVE ENZYMES

SYMPTOMS OF PANCREATIC INSUFFICIENCY

- PANCREATIC INSUFFICIENCY MAY BE SUSPECTED BY OILY OR FATTY STOOLS (STEATORRHEA) THAT FLOAT IN THE TOILET OR ARE PARTICULARLY STICKY AND MALODOROUS, AND DIFFICULT TO FLUSH AWAY
- LARGE MALODOROUS STOOLS ALSO OCCUR WITH CELIAC DISEASE.
- FAIRLY IMMEDIATE BELCHING, HEARTBURN AND STOMACH PAIN IS MOST TYPICAL OF HYPOCHLORHYDRIA HIGH UP IN THE DIGESTIVE SYSTEM.

FOOD ALLERGENS AND MALABSORPTION

- INTESTINAL CRAMPING AND FLATULENCE ARE MOST TYPICAL OF MILK INTOLERANCE OR OTHER FOOD ALLERGEN AGGRAVATING THE INTESTINES.
- IF THE SYMPTOMS AND DIAGNOSTIC TESTS DO NOT HINT AT A SPECIFIC UNDERLYING CAUSE, A SIMPLE TRIAL ELIMINATION DIET MAY BE APPROPRIATE.

A TRIAL AND ERROR APPROACH IS REASONABLE

SINCE PATIENTS USUALLY RESPOND READILY TO HCL SUPPLEMENTS IF THEY ARE HYPOCHLORHYDRIC, TO PANCREATIC ENZYMES IF THERE IS ENZYME INSUFFICIENCY, AND TO BILIARY SUPPORT IF THERE IS INSUFFICIENT BILE, SUCH THERAPIES MAY SIMPLY BE ATTEMPTED FOR A WEEK OR TWO EVALUATING THE RESULTS.

DIGESTIVE BITTERS AND ALTERATIVE HERBS

- BITTERS AND ALTERATIVES SUCH AS *ARTEMISIA, JUGLANS, CURCUMA, TARAXICUM, RUMEX, ARCTIUM* STIMULATE HCL, BILE, AND PANCREATIC ENZYMES ARE APPROPRIATE IN MOST CASES OF MALABSORPTION.
- LIVER HERBS AND THE B VITAMIN RELATIVES, CHOLINE AND INOSITOL IMPROVE BILE QUANTITY AND QUALITY, AND MAY HELP THOSE WITH FAT INTOLERANCE AND THE ELDERLY WITH GENERAL DIGESTIVE INSUFFICIENCY.

INTESTINAL DEMULCENTS

WHEN PATIENTS ARE SUSPECTED TO HAVE INTESTINAL MUCOSA INFLAMMATION DUE TO INGESTION OF FOOD ALLERGENS, THE ADDITION OF DEMULCENTS AND ANTI-INFLAMMATORIES ARE INDICATED, ALONG WITH SPECIFIC DIETARY CHANGES.

LIQUIDS OVER PILLS FOR GI ISSUES

- WHEN PATIENTS HAVE BECOME MALNOURISHED, NUTRITIONAL SUPPLEMENTS MAY HELP REBUILD AND RESTORE THE BODY, HOWEVER TAKING CARE TO NOT USE TOO MANY PILLS AS THEY ARE UNLIKELY TO BE WELL UTILIZED OR ASSIMILATED.
- LIQUIDS NUTRIENTS SUCH AS TEAS AND TINCTURES OR THE ADDITIONAL OF LIQUID NUTRIENTS TO SMOOTHIES OR JUICES WILL BE THE EASIEST TO ABSORB.

MINERAL HERBS AND HOT HERBS

- HIGH MINERAL HERBS SUCH AS *EQUISETUM, MEDICAGO, CENTELLA, SYMPHYTUM* ARE APPROPRIATE TO HELP REBUILD AND RESTORE CONNECTIVE TISSUE, SKIN, HAIR, AND NAILS.
- ADDITIONS OF SMALL AMOUNTS OF HOT SPICY HERBS SUCH AS *ZINGIBER, CAPSICUM,* AND *PIPER NIGUM,* DUE TO LOCAL VASODILATION IN THE INTESTINES MAY IMPROVE THE ABSORPTION OF NUTRIENTS ESPECIALLY IN THE ELDERLY AND THOSE WITH A COLD DEFICIENT CONSTITUTION.

BLACK PEPPER TO INCREASE ABSORPTION

PIPER NIGRUM (BLACK PEPPER) HAS BEEN SHOWN TO MAKE INTESTINAL MUCOSAL TIGHT JUNCTIONS LESS PERMEABLE, AND YET *PIPER NIGRUM* HAS BEEN FOUND TO INCREASE THE ABSORPTION OF MANY BENEFICIAL NUTRIENTS BY 100 FOLD.

PIPER NIGRUM ENHANCES ASSIMILATION

PIPER NIGRUM MAY ENHANCE THE ABSORPTION OF NUTRIENTS THROUGH VASODILATORY EFFECTS ON THE SUBMUCOSAL VASCULATURE, AND BY A YET TO BE EXPLAINED MECHANISM THAT INCREASES THE LENGTH AND GIRTH OF INTESTINAL MICROVILLI AND THEREBY INCREASES THE ABSORPTIVE SURFACE AREA. PREPARATION OF THESE HERBS IN VINEGAR IS A USEFUL VEHICLE FOR PROMOTING DIGESTION FUNCTION.

DIGESTIVE VINEGAR

- 1 QUART APPLE CIDER VINEGAR
- FRESH GINGER ROOT CHOPPED
- FRESH HABENEROS PEPPERS
- GARLIC CLOVES
- ONION
- TURMERIC ROOT, CHOPPED
- 1 LEMONS, ZEST, AND JUICE
- *MEDICAGO* (ALFALFA) DRIED ½ CUP
- *MAHONIA* ROOT (OREGON GRAPE) ½ CUP
- *ARCTIUM* (BURDOCK ROOT) ½ CUP
- *ARTEMESIA* (WORMWOOD) ½ CUP

PLACE ALL IN A BLENDER AND LIQUEFY AS FINELY AS POSSIBLE. TRANSFER TO A LARGE CANNING JAR AND SHAKE DAILY FOR 6 WEEKS. STRAIN THE HERBS AND STORE THE VINEGAR IN INDIVIDUAL BOTTLES.

THIS VERSION OF THE CLASSIC "FIRE CIDER" ADDS BITTER HERBS TO STIMULATE DIGESTION. THE RECIPE CAN BE AMENDED FOR TASTE AND PURPOSE, MAKING HOTTER OR MILDER, AND USING MORE OR LESS BITTER HERBS. FRUITS SUCH AS MANGOS, PINEAPPLES, AND PAPAYAS, INCLUDING PAPAYA SEEDS, CAN ALSO BE BLENDED INTO THE VINEGAR, BOTH TO MAKE THE BLEND SWEETER, AS WELL TO PROMOTE HYDROCHLORIC ACID, AND HELP TREAT UNDERLYING DIGESTIVE INSUFFICIENCY AND DYSBIOSIS.

TINCTURE FOR MALABSORPTION DUE TO HYPOCHLORHYDRIA

- *ARTEMESIA* 15 ML
- *JUGLANS* 15 ML
- *RUMEX* 15 ML
- *MATRICARIA* 15 ML
- *ZINGIBER* 4 ML

THIS FORMULA IS BEST TAKEN ON AN EMPTY STOMACH 15 -20 MINUTES BEFORE MEALS. ANOTHER OPTION IS TO PREPARE AN APERATIV USING 1-2 TSP OF THE TINCTURE, THE JUICE OF A LEMON SLICE, AND A BIT OF WATER OR CHAMOMILE TEA TO SIP BEFORE MEALS.

BITTER HERBS STIMULATE BILE, HCL AND DIGESTIVE ENZYMES, BUT ALL ON THEIR OWN MIGHT BE NAUSEATING AND TOO STIMULATING.

THE BITTER HERBS ARE COMBINED WITH THE DIGESTIVE TONIC AND CARMINATIVE *MATRICARIA* AND *ZINGIBER* IN THIS FORMULA.

MALABSORPTION IN THE ELDERLY

- *GINKGO* 15 ML
- *GENTIAN* 15 ML
- *ARTEMESIA* 15 ML
- *PANAX* 15 ML
- *ZINGIBER* 4 ML

THIS FORMULA IS BEST TAKEN ON AN EMPTY STOMACH 15 -20 MINUTES BEFORE MEALS. ANOTHER OPTION IS TO PREPARE AN APERATIF USING 1-2 TSP OF THE TINCTURE, THE JUICE OF A LEMON SLICE, AND A BIT OF WATER OR CHAMOMILE TEA TO SIP BEFORE MEALS.

SOME PATIENTS, ESPECIALLY THE ELDERLY MAY HAVE BOTH HYPOCHLORHYDRIA AND POOR CIRCULATION IN THE DIGESTIVE ORGANS CONTRIBUTING TO MALABSORPTION.

NOTE HOW THIS FORMULA USES HALF BITTER AGENTS AND HALF CIRCULATORY ENHANCING HERBS.

POOR DIGESTION FOLLOWING A LONG ILLNESS

- *CURCUMA* 15 ML
- *PANAX* 15 ML
- *TARAXICUM`* 15 ML
- *ZINGIBER* 4 ML

- THIS FORMULA IS BEST TAKEN ON AN EMPTY STOMACH 15 -20 MINUTES BEFORE MEALS. ANOTHER OPTION IS TO PREPARE AN APERITIF USING 1-2 TSP OF THE TINCTURE, THE JUICE OF A LEMON SLICE, AND A BIT OF WATER TO SIP BEFORE MEALS.

- WHEN PATIENTS HAVE UNDERGONE SURGERY, BEEN HOSPITALIZED, ARE ON MANY MEDICINES, OR HAVE BEEN BED-RIDDEN DUE TO ANY ILLNESS, THE DIGESTIVE SYSTEM CAN BE WEAKENED AND MAY BENEFIT FROM A "JUMP START".

- THE USE OF CHI TONICS, BITTERS, ALTERATIVES, AND STIMULANTS IN THIS FORMULA, MAY QUICKLY IMPROVE APPETITE, BOWEL FUNCTION, AND DIGESTION.

BITTER TEA FOR HYPOCHLORHYDRIA

- *ACHILLEA*- FLOWERS
- *RUMEX* – ROOT, FINELY CHOPPED
- *MATRICARIA* - FLOWERS
- *CINNAMOMUM* - SMALL CHIPS

STEEP 1 -2 TSP PER CUP HOT WATER, STRAIN AND DRINK 1-2 CUPS 3 TIMES DAILY BEFORE EACH MEAL. MAY ADD A TSP OR TWO OF FRESH SQUEEZED LEMON JUICE TO EACH CUP.

BITTER TEA MAY BE CHALLENGING FOR SOME PATIENTS TO CONSUME, WHILE OTHERS MAY PREFER IT OVER TINCTURES, BEING LESS EXPENSIVE AND ALCOHOL-FREE.

THE USE OF CINNAMON BOTH IMPROVES THE FLAVOR AND ACTS AS CARMINATIVE STIMULANT

HERBAL VINEGAR FOR MALABSORPTION

- 2 TBL *ARTEMESIA* LEAVES
- 2 TBL NETTLE LEAVES
- 1 CAYENNE PEPPER, SMALL, SEEDED AND COARSELY CHOPPED
- 2 TBL FRESH GINGER ROOT, COARSELY CHOPPED

PLACE ALL IN A BLENDER AND COVER WITH APPLE CIDER VINEGAR AND PUREE. TRANSFER TO A GLASS JAR AND SHAKE DAILY FOR SEVERAL WEEK AND THEN STRAIN THROUGH A FINE STRAINER. USE FINISHED VINEGAR ON STEAMED VEGETABLES AND TO PREPARE SALAD DRESSINGS. THE VINEGAR MAY ALSO BE PREPARED INTO AN APERATIV TO SIP IN WATER OR TEA.

PATIENTS WITH MALDIGESTION CAN BE TAUGHT HOW TO MAKE THEIR OWN HERBAL VINEGAR AT HOME INEXPENSIVELY, OR YOU CAN PREPARE SOMETHING LIKE THIS FOR THEM.

VINEGAR ALONE IS GREAT FOR DIGESTION, AND ESPECIALLY ONE WITH APPROPRIATELY CHOSEN BITTER AND STIMULANT HERBS, AS IN THIS EXAMPLE.

ADJUVENT THERAPIES FOR MALABSORPTION AND MALDIGESTION

- OX BILE
- HCL
- PANCREATIC LIPASE, AMYLASE, AND PROTEASES
- BROMELAIN
- CHOLINE, INOSITOL

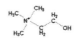

Choline

BOTANICAL THERAPIES FOR MALABSORPTION, BILIARY INSUFFICIENCY, HYPOCHLORHYDRIA

- *ARCTIUM LAPPA*
- *ARTEMESIA ABSINTHINUM*
- *BERBERIS SPECIES (MAHONIA)*
- *CHELIDONIUM MAJUS*
- *CINNAMOMUM*
- *GENTIANA LUTEA*
- *IRIS VERSICOLOR*

- *JUGLANS NIGRA*
- *MAHONIA*
- *PODOPHYLLUM PELTATUM*
- *RUMEX*
- *STILLINGIA*
- *TARAXICUM OFFICINALE*
- *ZINGIBER*

PANCREATIC INSUFFICIENCY

EXOCRINE PANCREATIC INSUFFICIENCY CAN RESULT IN MALABSORPTION, AND POSSIBLY IMPAIRED MOTILITY.

PANCREATIC INSUFFICIENCY CAN BE DUE TO CHRONIC PANCREATITIS, CYSTIC FIBROSIS, AND EXTENSIVE NECROTIZING ACUTE PANCREATITIS, AND HEAVY ALCOHOL CONSUMPTION.

PANCREATIC INSUFFICIENCY

- THE USE OF PANCREATIC ENZYMES MAY BE REQUIRED FOR LIFE.
- LIPASE LEVELS JUST 5–10% BELOW OF NORMAL CAN RESULT STEATORRHEA, WEIGHT LOSS, AND A POTENTIAL DECREASE IN QUALITY OF LIFE.
- DECREASED BICARBONATE OUTPUT ASSOCIATED WITH CYSTIC FIBROSIS OR CHRONIC PANCREATITIS CAUSES LOW INTESTINAL PH, IMPAIRS MICELLE FORMATION OF FATS AND FURTHER DAMPENING HYDROLYSIS OF INTRALUMINAL FAT.

PANCREATIC INSUFFICIENCY

- PANCREATIC INSUFFICIENCY RESULTS IN CLAY-COLORED, LOOSE, GREASY, FOUL-SMELLING LARGE STOOLS, ABDOMINAL DISCOMFORT, BLOATING, AND WEIGHT LOSS.
- ALTHOUGH FLOATING STOOLS ARE OFTEN THOUGHT OF BEING INDICATIVE OF STEATORRHEA, EVEN MORE TYPICAL, STOOLS THAT CLING TO THE TOILET BOWL, AND WON'T FLUSH AWAY, IS EVEN A MORE SPECIFIC SIGN

PANCREATIC INSUFFICIENCY

IN CELIAC DISEASE, ALTHOUGH EXOCRINE PANCREATIC FUNCTION IS INTRINSICALLY NORMAL, REDUCED LEVELS OF CHOLECYSTOKININ RELEASE AS A RESULT OF THE DUODENAL VILLOUS ATROPHY, ACCOUNTS FOR IMPAIRED GALL BLADDER CONTRACTION AND REDUCED EXOCRINE PANCREATIC SECRETION.

Pancreatic Insufficiency: Possible Causes
- Chronic pancreatitis (most common)
- Alcoholism
- Smoking
- Surgery
- Pancreatic obstruction
- Cystic fibrosis
- Autoimmune related
- Crohn's disease
- Celiac disease

Medscape

PANCREATIC INSUFFICIENCY

DIABETICS MAY ALSO DEVELOP PANCREATIC INSUFFICIENCY AS THE PART OF THE AUTOIMMUNE DISEASE.

PANCREATIC INSUFFICIENCY

ALL INFANTS, ESPECIALLY PRETERM INFANTS HAVE LOW PANCREATIC EXOCRINE FUNCTION, COMPENSATED FOR BY AMYLASE AND LIPASE PRESENT IN BREASTMILK, HOWEVER MANY INFANTS HAVE SOME DEGREE OF PANCREATIC INSUFFICIENCY, WHICH WOULD BE WORSE IN NON-BREAST-FED INFANTS AND PLAY A ROLE IN EARLY NUTRIENT DEFICITS.

DOSE OF LIPASE

- 25,000 –80,000 LIPASE UNITS PER MAIN MEAL IN ADULTS.
- PANCREATIC ENZYME REPLACEMENT THERAPY - ENTERIC-COATED PANCREATIC ENZYMES ARE MOST EFFECTIVE AT A PH > 6, SO THE ENTERIC COATED PILLS MIGHT BE TAKEN WITH LEMON JUICE, OR VINEGAR, OR WITH HCL SUPPLEMENTS.

IF THERE IS A POOR RESPONSE, CONSIDER CONCOMITANT COMORBIDITIES SUCH AS LACTOSE INTOLERANCE, ENTERIC BACTERIAL INFECTION, PARASITES (ESPECIALLY GIARDIA), SMALL INTESTINAL BACTERIAL OVERGROWTH, BILIARY DISEASE (CHOLESTASIS), COLITIS, CELIAC DISEASE, SHORT BOWEL SYNDROME, AND CROHN'S DISEASE.

SPHINCTER OF ODDI

- THE SPHINCTER OF ODDI IS A SMOOTH MUSCLE VALVE REGULATING THE FLOW OF BILIARY AND PANCREATIC SECRETIONS INTO THE DUODENUM
- THE SPHINCTER OF ODDI PREVENTS OF DUODENAL REFLUX AND REGULATES GALLBLADDER FILLING BY DIVERTING BILE INTO THE GALLBLADDER WITH SPHINCTER CLOSURE.

SPHINCTER OF ODDI DYSFUNCTION AND BILIARY DYSKENESIA

- SCINTIGRAPHY CAN HELP REVEAL BILIARY AND SPHINCTER OF ODDI DYSKINESIA, AND IS ONE CAUSE OF IMPAIRED GASTRIC MOTILITY.
- BILIARY DYSKINESIA IS A SEPARATE ENTITY.
- BOTH CAN CAUSE ABDOMINAL PAIN AND BE ASSOCIATED WITH ELEVATED LIVER ENZYMES.

SPHINCTER OF ODDI DYSFUNCTION

SO DYSFUNCTION IS A BROAD TERM REFERRING TO NUMEROUS BILIARY, PANCREATIC, AND HEPATIC DISORDERS RESULTING FROM SPASMS, STRICTURES, AND RELAXATION OF THIS VALVE AT INAPPROPRIATE TIMES.

SOD SPHINCTER OF ODDI DYSFUNCTION

- VARIOUS FACTORS THAT INCREASE THE RISK OF SPHINCTER OF ODDI DYSFUNCTION, INCLUDING CHOLECYSTECTOMY, OPIATES, AND ALCOHOL.
- SPHINCTER OF ODDI DYSFUNCTION MAY CONTRIBUTE TO PANCREATITIS AND BILIARY SYMPTOMS WITH HEPATIC ENZYME ELEVATION.
- PHARMACOLOGIC TREATMENTS OF SOD MAY INCLUDE CALCIUM-CHANNEL BLOCKERS, GLYCERYL TRINITRATE, AND TRICYCLIC ANTIDEPRESSANTS.

CLINICAL PRESENTATIONS OF SOD

- SPHINCTER OF ODDI DYSFUNCTION CAN INVOLVE THE BILIARY SPHINCTER, THE PANCREATIC SPHINCTER, OR BOTH.
- BILIARY SOD TYPICALLY PRESENTS WITH RECURRENT BILIARY PAIN, CHARACTERIZED AS DISABLING EPIGASTRIC OR RIGHT UPPER QUADRANT PAIN LASTING 30 MIN TO SEVERAL HOURS WITH OR WITHOUT HEPATIC ENZYME ELEVATION.

- IT MAY RADIATE TO THE BACK, SHOULDER, OR SCAPULA AND MAY BE ACCOMPANIED BY NAUSEA AND VOMITING, MIMICKING A GALLBLADDER ATTACK.
- PAIN IS NOT CONSISTENTLY POSTPRANDIAL AND IS NOT RELIEVED BY POSTURAL CHANGES, ANTACIDS, OR BOWEL MOVEMENTS.

PANCREATITIS AND MOTILITY

PANCREATIC SOD MAY CAUSE RECURRENT EPISODES OF ACUTE PANCREATITIS.

PATIENTS WILL HAVE MID-ABDOMINAL, PANCREATIC PAIN, RADIATING TO THE BACK, ASSOCIATED WITH ELEVATIONS IN SERUM AMYLASE AND LIPASE.

SYMPTOMS INVOLVING THE PANCREATIC SPHINCTER ARE FREQUENTLY EXACERBATED BY FOOD INTAKE.

NO OTHER CAUSES FOR PANCREATITIS ARE USUALLY FOUND IN THESE PATIENTS, AND THEY MAY BE CLASSIFIED AS HAVING IDIOPATHIC ACUTE RECURRENT PANCREATITIS.

CHOLECYSTIKININ – CKK
VASOACTIVE INTESTINAL POLYPEPTIDE - VIP

- THE MOST IMPORTANT HORMONE INVOLVED IN SO FUNCTION IS CCK.
- CCK IS RELEASED FROM ENTEROENDOCRINE CELLS IN RESPONSE TO A MEAL AND EXERTS DIRECT HORMONAL EFFECTS AS WELL AS INDIRECT EFFECTS.
- CCK BY INTERACTING WITH NEURAL PATHWAYS, LEADING TO GALLBLADDER CONTRACTION AND PANCREATIC ENZYME SECRETION.
- CCK DECREASES SO BASAL PRESSURES AND INHIBITS PHASIC CONTRACTIONS, THEREBY PROMOTING ANTEROGRADE FLOW.

VIP AND NO

VASOACTIVE INTESTINAL POLYPEPTIDE AND NITRIC OXIDE, PRESENT IN THE INTRINSIC NEURONS OF THE SO, ARE INVOLVED IN THE RELAXATION RESPONSE TO CCK AS WELL AS THE RELAXATION OBSERVED IN THE CEPHALIC PHASE OF THE MEAL.

CREATING HERBAL FORMULAS FOR SIBO
SMALL BACTERIAL INTESTINAL OVERGROWTH

- SMALL INTESTINAL BACTERIAL OVERGROWTH (SIBO) INVOLVES EXCESSIVE AND UNBALANCED BACTERIA IN THE SMALL INTESTINE, CAUSING BLOATING, PAIN, GAS, AND DIARRHEA.
- THE OPTIMAL SMALL INTESTINAL BACTERIA BECOMES REPLACED WITH COLONIC SPECIES, AND POSSIBLY MORE PATHOGENIC SPECIES. SIBO CAN CAUSE SYSTEMIC COMPLICATIONS SUCH AS OSTEOPOROSIS AND MACROCYTIC ANEMIA AS ABSORPTION OF MINERALS AND NUTRIENTS IS IMPAIRED.

DX AND TX OF SIBO

- GUT INFLAMMATION MAY INTERFERE WITH GENE EXPRESSION INVOLVED WITH MUCUS SECRETION, LINKING SIBO TO CYSTIC FIBROSIS, IRRITABLE BOWEL SYNDROME, AND CHRONIC ABDOMINAL PAIN.
- GLUCOSE AND LACTULOSE BREATH TESTS, SMALL INTESTINAL ASPIRATION AND CULTURES HELP DIAGNOSE SIBO.
- SOME CLINICIANS SIMPLY ATTEMPT A 2 WEEK COURSE OF A BROAD SPECTRUM ANTI-BIOTICS, AND IF UNRESPONSIVE, REPETITIVE CYCLES OF ANTIBIOTICS.

CAUSES AND THERAPIES FOR SIBO

- PROMOTILITY DRUGS, DIETARY MODIFICATIONS, ARE WARRANTED.
- ACID SUPPRESSING DRUGS USED FOR REFLUX DISEASE ARE ASSOCIATED WITH SIBO DYSBIOSIS AND SHOULD BE ELIMINATED.
- PPIS EXACERBATE NONSTEROIDAL ANTI-INFLAMMATORY DRUG-INDUCED SMALL INTESTINAL INJURY.
- GASTROPARESIS AND HYPOTHYROIDSM ALSO PREDISPOSE TO SIBO DUE TO IMPAIRED GI MOTILITY.

FIBER FOR INTESTINAL HEALTH

- THE NECESSITY OF A HIGH FIBER DIET, CAN NOT BE OVER EMPHASIZED.
- IN GENERAL, THE GREATER THE FIBER CONTENT, THE FASTER GASTRIC EMPTYING.
- GUAR GUM, APPLE PECTIN, AND PSYLLIUM CAN SIGNIFICANTLY MODIFY INTESTINAL MICROBIOTA AND EXERT PREBIOTIC EFFECTS, ENCOURAGING POPULATION OF THE GUT BY BENEFICIAL INTESTINAL PROBIOTIC SPECIES.

FIBER FOR INTESTINAL HEALTH

- FIBER SUPPLEMENTATION MAY HELP TREAT CONSTIPATION, IRRITABLE BOWEL SYNDROME (IBS), SMALL INTESTINE BACTERIAL OVERGROWTH (SIBO), AND OTHER COMPLAINTS.
- FIBER SUPPLEMENTATION MAY BOOST THE EFFICACY OF ANTIBIOTICS IN TREATING SIBO.
- CONSUMPTION OF FRESH FRUITS AND VEGETABLES WILL PROVIDE

DIET TO SUPPORT MOTILITY

AVOID
- AVOID BREAD, GLUTEN, PASTA, CRACKERS, PRETZLES, AND ALL FLOUR PRODUCTS
- AVOID ALCOHOL
- AVOID SUGAR, FRUITS JUICE, JAM, SUGARY SNACKS, DRIED FRUITS, APPLES, PEARS, CHERRIES, PLUMS, WATERMELON
- AVOID CARBOHYDRATE-RICH VEGETABLES: POTATOES, CORN, PEAS,

ENJOY
- FERMENTED FOOD: SAUERKRAUT, KIMCHEE, MISO, APPLE CIDER VINEGAR
- SEAWEEDS: IN BROTHS, SALADS, CONDIMENTS
- LOW FODMAP VEGGIES: CABBAGE, GREEN BEANS, ARUGALA, SPINACH, ZUCHHINI, SQUASH, TURNIPS, CARROTS, BELL PEPPER
- LOW FODMAP FRUITS: BERRIES, MELON, PINEAPPLES, CITRUS, GRAPES
- LOW FODMAP STAPLES: LENTILS, QUINOA, NUTS, CHEESE, QUALITY MEATS

IMPAIRMENT OF INTESTINAL MOTILITY BY ADHESIONS

- ABDOMINAL ADHESIONS CAN CONTRIBUTE TO INTESTINAL FUNCTION AND MOTILITY. ADHESIONS MAY RESULT FROM ABDOMINO-PELVIC SURGERY, RADIATION THERAPY, AND INFLAMMATORY PROCESSES.
- POST-SURGICAL: NEARLY 90% OF ABDOMINAL ADHESIONS FORM AS A RESULT OF PRIOR ABDOMINAL SURGERY, PRIMARILY LAPAROTOMY
- POST-INFLAMMATORY OR INFECTIOUS: ENDOMETRIOSIS AND PELVIC INFLAMMATORY DISEASE ARE THE MOST COMMON ETIOLOGIES OF NON-SURGICAL ADHESIONS IN WOMEN. OTHER ETIOLOGIES AFFECTING EITHER SEX INCLUDE DIVERTICULAR DISEASE (PARTICULARLY OF SMALL BOWEL), CROHN'S DISEASE, AND ABDOMINAL TUBERCULOSIS (IN ENDEMIC AREAS).
- POST-RADIATION: ABDOMINOPELVIC RADIATION USED FOR TREATMENT OF A VARIETY OF MALIGNANCIES
- ANN MED SURG (LOND). 2017 MAR; 15: 9–13. ABDOMINAL ADHESIONS: A PRACTICAL REVIEW OF AN OFTEN OVERLOOKED ENTITY N. TABIBIAN,A E. SWEHLI,A A. BOYD,A A. UMBREEN,A AND J.H. TABIBIANB

SYMPTOMS OF INTESTINAL ADHESIONS

- CHRONIC (PERSISTENT OR INTERMITTENT) BLOATING.
- ABDOMINAL CRAMPING AND BORBORYGMI.
- ALTERED BOWEL HABITS, INCLUDING CONSTIPATION OR FREQUENT LOOSE STOOLS (E.G. FROM DEVELOPMENT OF SMALL INTESTINAL BACTERIAL OVERGROWTH).
- NAUSEA WITH OR WITHOUT EARLY SATIETY.
- BOWEL OBSTRUCTION, WHICH MAY BE TRANSIENT, PARTIAL, OR COMPLETE (AND MAY CAUSE THE AFOREMENTIONED SYMPTOMS).
- FEMALE INFERTILITY AND DYSPAREUNIA.
- RECTAL BLEEDING AND DYSCHEZIA (I.E. PAINFUL DEFECATION) DURING MENSES, WHICH TYPICALLY INDICATE COLORECTAL INVOLVEMENT OF ENDOMETRIOSIS.
- IN ADDITION, MANY PATIENTS, PARTICULARLY IF THEIR SYMPTOMS ARE UNPREDICTABLE, GO UNDIAGNOSED, AND/OR WITHOUT EFFECTIVE TREATMENT, CAN DEVELOP ADJUSTMENT DISORDER AND DEMORALIZATION, WHICH MAY ERRONEOUSLY POINT TOWARD FUNCTIONAL BOWEL DISORDERS SUCH IS IRRITABLE BOWEL SYNDROME.

RIKKUNSHITO FOR GASTROPARESIS

RIKKUNSHITO IS A TRADITIONAL JAPANESE FORMULA USED TO TREAT UPPER GASTROINTESTINAL DISORDERS SUCH AS FUNCTIONAL DYSPEPSIA, GASTROESOPHAGEAL REFLUX, AND GASTRIC MOTOR FUNCTION VIA ENHANCING GHRELIN

- *GLYCYRRHIZA*
- *ZINGIBER*
- *ATRACTYLODIS LANCEAE*
- *ZIZYPHIS* FRUITS
- *CITRUS AURANTII* PEEL

PING WEI SAN (CALM THE STOMACH POWDER)

THIS FORMULA IS SPECIFICALLY INDICATED FOR DIGESTIVE SYMPTOMS HAVING A FULL HEAVY SENSATION, MUCOUS CONGESTION, AND "DAMPNESS", AND MAY IMPROVE APPETITE, SENSE OF TASTE, GERD, VOMITING, NAUSEA.

ATRACTYLODES	4 OZ
MAGNOLIA	3 OZ
CITRUS PEEL	2 OZ
GLYCYRRHIZA	2 OZ
ZIZYPHUS	2 OZ
ZINGIBER	1 OZ

COMBINE ALL AND DECOCT 1 QUARTER CUP IN 8 CUPS OF WATER, SIMMERING GENTLY DOWN TO 6 CUPS. STRAIN AND DRINK OVER THE COURSE OF THE DAY.

ZHIZHU FOR GASTROPARESIS

ZHIZHU PILL IS A TRADITIONAL CHINESE FORMULA USED FOR DYSPEPTIC SYMPTOMS. THIS DECOCTION ADAPTS THE TRADITIONAL FORMULA ADDING SEVERAL OTHER HERBS TRADITIONAL FOR GASTROPARESIS.

- *PINELLIA*
- *GLYCYRRHIZA*
- *PORIA*
- *GINSENG*
- *CODONOPSIS*
- *CITRUS PEEL*
- *ATRACTYLODES*
- *ZINGIBER*

COMBINE EQUAL PARTS OF EACH HERB AND BLEND. SIMMER 1 TSP/CUP OF HOT WATER FOR 10 MINUTES. LET STAND IN A COVERED PAN, AND DRINK 3 OR MORE CUPS PER DAY.

TINCTURE FOR FUNCTIONAL DYSPEPSIA AND GASTROPARESIS

HARPAGOPHYTUM	15 ML
COMMIPHORA MUKUL	15 ML
IRIS VERSICOLOR	10 ML
FOENICULUM	10 ML
ZINGIBER	10 ML

- ANETHOLE, A VOLATILE OIL IN FENNEL AND ANISE SEEDS, HAS BEEN SHOWN TO IMPROVE DYSPEPTIC SYMPTOMS AS WELL AS IMPROVE GASTRIC EMPTYING.
- THE ANTI-EMETIC EFFECTS OF GINGER, *ZINGIBER* MAY BE HELPFUL, BUT MINT MAY BE BE BEST AVOIDED DUE TO ACTING AS GASTRIC RELAXANT.
- *IRIS* IS A FOLKLORIC SECRETORY STIMULANT AND MAY ENHANCE DIGESTION AND MOTILITY.
- *HARPAGOPHYTUM PROCUMBENS*, DEVILS'S CLAW, MAY SUPPRESS APPETITE AND SUPPORT WEIGHT LOSS VIA THE GHRELINERGIC SYSTEM.
- THE GUGGULSTERONES IN *COMMIPHORA MUKUL* REDUCE FOOD INTAKE AND SUPPORTS WEIGHT LOSS IN PART VIA REDUCING PLASMA GHRELIN AND INCREASING PLASMA LEPTIN, SEROTONIN, AND DOPAMINE. THESE ACTIONS MAY ALSO ENHANCE GASTRIC MOTOR FUNCTIONS VIA EFFECTS ON GROWTH HORMONE RECEPTORS.

OOLONG TEA FOR GASTROPARESIS

CHIN-SHIN OOLONG TEA, IS SOMETIMES CALLED TEA GHRELIN BECAUSE IT HAS BEEN SHOWN TO BIND GROWTH HORMONE RECEPTORS LIKE GHRELIN.

OOLONG TEA

- STEEP 1 TBL PER CUP OF HOT WATER, AND DRINK THROUGH OUT THE DAY, ESPECIALLY AFTER EACH MEAL.

OOLONG IS A SEMI-FERMENTED GREEN TEA, ESPECIALLY FROM MOUNTAINOUS REGIONS OF TAIWAN.

SLOW MOTILITY WITH CONSTIPATION

IBERIS AMARA OR *RAPHANUS NIGRA*	20 ML
ANGELICA ARCHANGELICA	20 ML
CHELIDONIUM	20 ML
MATRICARIA CHAMOMILE	10 ML
FOENICULUM SEEDS	10 ML
SILYMARIN SEED POWDER	10 ML
MELISSA OFFCINALIS	10 ML
MENTHA PIPERTA	10 ML
GLYCYRRHIZA	5 ML
ZINGIBER	5 ML

THIS FORMULA WILL FILL A 4 OUNCE BOTTLE AND CAN BE TAKEN BY THE TEASPOON FULL 3 OR MORE TIMES PER DAY.

BASED ON A COMMERCIAL FORMULA SHOWN EFFECTIVE FOR FUNCTIONAL DYSPEPSIA AND GASTRIC SYMPTOMS, AND TO STIMULATE GHRELIN ACTIVITY, THIS FORMULA MAY BE PREPARED AS A TINCTURE OR A TEA TO TREAT IMPAIRED GASTRIC MOTILITY, AND IS FORMULATED HERE AS A COMPLEX TINCTURE.

AS *IBERIS*, OR CANDY TUFT, A BRASSICA FAMILY HERB MAY NOT BE READILY AVAILABLE, *RHAPHANUS*, SPANISH BLACK RADISH MAY BE A POSSIBLE SUBSTITUTE.

ACHILLEA MILLEFOLIUM
YARROW

- *ACHILLEA MILLEFOLIUM* INDICATED FOR IBS AND LIVER CONGESTION, SKIN LESIONS, ATONY TISSUE IN COLDER CONSTITUTIONS, DUE TO A WARMING AND EVEN DIAPHORETIC EFFECT.
- *ACHILLEA* IS STRONGLY ANTIMICROBIAL, AND DUE TO FAIRLY RELIABLE HEMOSTATIC EFFECTS, IS SPECIFIC FOR BLEEDING HEMORRHOIDS, BLOOD IN THE STOOL, AND PASSIVE HEMORRHAGE ASSOCIATED WITH ATONY OF THE TISSUES.

AESCULUS HIPPOCASTANUM

- *AESCULUS HIPPOCASTANUM* IS SPECIFIC FOR ENGORGEMENT IN THE LOWER BOWEL WITH HEMORRHOIDS, BACKACHE, AND SENSE OF FULLNESS AND PRESSURE IN THE ABDOMEN.
- *AESCULUS* MAY IMPROVE POOR DIGESTION WHEN ASSOCIATED WITH VENOUS STASIS AND PORTAL CONGESTION.
- *AESCULUS* IS SPECIFIC FOR FULL SENSATION]WITH TENDERNESS IN THE RIGHT UPPER QUADRANT, A SENSE OF WEIGHT IN THE STOMACH WITH GNAWING AND ACHING PAIN, AND HEMORRHOIDS WITH STICKING, OR SHARP SHOOTING PAIN, SWELLING OF THE RECTAL MUCOUS MEMBRANES WITH PAIN AND SORENESS IN THE ANUS. DUE TO ITS SPECIFICITY FOR PORTAL AND VENOUS CONGESTION.

ALLIUM SATIVUM

ALLIUM SATIVUM – MAY CORRECT INTESTINAL DYSBIOSIS, WITH ANTI-MICROBIAL EFFECTS FOR INFECTIOUS GASTROENTERITIS AND AMEOBIC DYSENTERY, AND IS A SAFE PREVENTATIVE AGENT WHEN TRAVELING OUT OF THE US.

ALLIUM IS WARMING, STIMULATING HERB BEST FOR COLD DAMP CONSTITUTIONS, CATARRHAL STATES, CONSTIPATION OR SLOW PERISTALSIS.

ALOE VERA

- *ALOE VERA* - ALOE RIND IS INDICATED FOR CHRONIC CONSTIPATION AND THE GEL AND JUICE MAY BE USED TO SOOTHE INTESTINAL PAIN, HEAL ULCERS, AND REDUCE INFLAMMATION OF DIGESTIVE MUCOUS MEMBRANES.
- BECAUSE *ALOE* JUICE CONTAINS IMMUNE POLYSACCHARIDES, CONSIDER *ALOE* ALSO FOR BOWEL CANCERS AND DYSPLASTIC CHANGES.

ARCTIUM LAPPA

- *ARCTIUM LAPPA* –IS AN IMPORTANT ALTERATIVE HERB AND CHOLAGOGUE THAT CAN BE INCLUDED IN FORMULAS FOR INTESTINAL DYSBIOSIS, MALABSORPTION, AND DYSPEPSIA.
- *ARCTIUM* IS SPECIFICALLY INDICATED FOR SYSTEMIC SYMPTOMS THAT SPECIFICALLY INDICATE ITS USE INCLUDE HYPERLIPIDEMIA, ACNE AND SKIN DISORDERS, HYPERESTROGENISM, AND GENERAL MALAISE RELATED TO TOXICITY.

ARTEMESIA SPECIES

- *ARTEMESIA ANNUA* – SPECIFIC FOR PARASITES, MALABSORPTION AND AMEOBIC DYSTENTARY, BUT MAY ALSO HAVE STIMULATING EFFECTS ON ALL GI SECRETIONS FOR INSUFFICIENCY AND ATONY OF THE LIVER AND BILIARY SYSTEMS
- *ARTEMESIA VULGARIS* – A BITTER HERB SPECIFIC FOR INSUFFICIENT DIGESTIVE SECRETIONS, AND PARASITES. DUE TO POTENTIALLY TOXIC VOLATILE OILS, ONLY SMALL SHORT TERM DOSES SHOULD BE USED AND THE ESSENTIAL OIL SHOULD NEVER BE CONSUMED ORALLY.

ANGELICA SINENSIS

ANGELICA SINENSIS- *ANGELICA'S* AREA OF ACTION IS MAINLY ON BLOOD CELLS AND CYTOKINES GIVING IT "BLOOD MOVING" PROPERTIES, ANTI-ALLERGY EFFECTS, AND AN ABILITY TO ENHANCE PERFUSION TO VARIOUS ORGANS.

ANGELICA MAY BE INCLUDED IN GASTROINTESTINAL FORMULAS WHEN FOR VASCULAR CONGESTION, PELVIC STAGNATION, MENSTRUAL CRAMPS, ALLERGIES ARE PRESENT AND CONTRIBUTORY.

ATROPA BELLADONNA

- *ATROPA BELLADONNA* – BELLADONNA IS A POTENTIALLY TOXIC HERB USED IN SMALL DOSES FOR SPASTIC COLON AND MUCOUS COLITIS AS IT WILL QUICKLY REDUCE EXCESSIVE INTESTINAL SECRETIONS PERISTALSIS.

- BELLADONNA OILS AND OINTMENTS CAN BE PAIN RELIEVING WHEN APPLIED TOPICALLY TO HEMORRHOIDS AND RECTAL FISSURES.

BETA VULGARIS

- *BETA VULGARIS* – BEETS AND BETAIN ARE SUPPORTIVE TO LIVER DETOXIFICATION PATHWAYS, AND CAN BE INCLUDED LIBERALLY IN THE DIET OR IN VARIOUS BEVERAGES.

- KVASS, A TRADITIONAL FERMENTED BEVERAGE PREPARED FROM BEETS, IS ALSO USEFUL AND MAY BE MADE AT HOME, OR MAY BE COMMERCIALLY AVAILABLE.

BUPLEURUM CHINENSE, FALCATUM

- *BUPLEURUM CHINENSE, FALCATUM* – IS WIDELY USED TO TREAT FEVER, HEPATITIS, JAUNDICE, NEPHRITIS, DIZZINESS.

- BUPLEURUM BAKED WITH VINEGAR IS USED TO TREAT LIVER DISEASE AND IS SPECIFIC FOR ORGANOMEGALY AND ABDOMINAL PAIN.

- *BUPLEURUM* IS OFTEN COMBINED WITH PEONY TO TREAT LIVER CONGESTION AND DISEASE IN TCM.

CEANOTHUS AMERICANUS

- *CEANOTHUS AMERICANUS* – SPECIFIC FOR LIVER CONGESTION, PELVIC AND PORTAL CONGESTION, SPLENOMEGALY, VASCULAR CONGESTION AND HYPERTENSION.

- CEANOTHUS HAS AN AFFINITY FOR THE LYMPHATIC SYSTEM, ALLEVIATING VASCULAR CONGESTION VIA ENHANCING ENTRY OF INTERSTITIAL FLUID INTO THE VASCULATURE AND ENHANCING VENOUS RETURN.

CHELIDONIUM MAJUS

- *CHELIDONIUM MAJUS* – A VALUABLE CHOLAGOGUE USED FOR PAIN OR FULLNESS IN THE RIGHT UPPER QUADRANT, PAIN THAT RADIATES TO RIGHT SHOULDER, JAUNDICE, BILIARY DISEASE, AND GALLSTONES.

- *CHELIDONIUM* TREATS NAUSEA AND PAIN DUE TO BILIARY INSUFFICIENCY.

- CHELIDONIUM IS SPECIFIC FOR A COATED FLABBY TONGUE WITH INDENTATIONS OF TEETH ON LATERAL MARGINS, AND CONSTIPATION WITH DRY HARD STOOLS.

- *CHELIDONIUM* IS ALSO SPECIFIC WHEN THE STOOL IS ABNORMAL, SUCH AS BRIGHT YELLOW, CLAY COLORED, OR LIGHT COLORED STOOLS THAT FLOAT, ALL INDICATIVE OF BILIARY INSUFFICIENCY.

- ALTHOUGH CHELIDONIUM IS ONE OF THE BEST REMEDIES FOR BILIARY AND HEPATIC CONGESTION, IT IS BEST AVOIDED IN ACUTE INFLAMMATIONS OF THE LIVER.

CHELONE

- *CHELONE* – IS AN ALTERATIVE AND CHOLAGOGUE USED FOR LIVER CONGESTION WITH JAUNDICE, DYSPEPSIA, AND TO HELP RECOVER FROM INFECTIOUS ILLNESS WHERE THE APPETITE AND DIGESTION HAVE BEEN AFFECTED.
- CHELONE IS SPECIFICALLY INDICATED FOR GI DEBILITY ACCOMPANIED BY JAUNDICE, FOR DYSPEPSIA FOLLOWING FEBRILE DISEASES AND EXHAUSTIVE ILLNESSES.

CHENOPODIUM

- *CHENOPODIUM* – A CLASSIC REMEDY FOR INTESTINAL WORMS, THE EXTREMELY BITTER VOLATILE OIL WAS GIVEN ON SUGAR CUBES, IN SYRUP, OR IN CASTOR OIL SEVERAL TIMES A DAY FOR 5 DAYS TO A WEEK.

CHIONANTHUS

- *CHIONANTHUS* – FRINGE TREE IS TRADITIONAL FOR JAUNDICE AND HEPATITIS, SPECIFICALLY INDICATED FOR LIVER PAIN AND FULLNESS, AND FROTHY OR CLAY COLORED STOOLS.
- *CHIONANTHUS* WAS HIGHLY REGARDED BY THE ECLECTIC PHYSICIANS FOR PORTAL CONGESTION AND HEPATIC ENLARGEMENT, AND ALSO RECOMMENDED FOR INFANTILE JAUNDICE.

COLLINSONIA CANADENSIS

- *COLLINSONIA CANADENSIS* – IS SPECIFIC FOR RECTAL TIGHTNESS, HEMORRHOIDS, AND A CONGESTED FEELING IN THE PERINEUM.
- THE ROOT AND WHOLE PLANT MAY IMPROVE VASCULAR CONGESTION IN THE PELVIS.
- *COLLINSONIA* IS A TRADITIONAL REMEDY FOR ALL MANNER OF RECTAL COMPLAINTS INCLUDING FISSURES, PROCTITIS, STRAINING WITH BOWEL MOVEMENTS, AND FISTULAS.

DIOSCORREA VILLOSA

DIOSCORREA VILLOSA – SPECIFIC FOR COLICKY PAINS IN ABDOMINAL ORGANS INCLUDING MENSTRUAL CRAMPS, POOR DIGESTION AND FLATULENCE, RUQ PAINS THAT RADIATE TO THE SHOULDER OR RIGHT NIPPLE, AND TWISTING AND BORING PAINS ABOUT THE UMBILICUS.

EUGENIA AROMATICA

- *EUGENIA AROMATICA* – ACTS AS A DIGESTIVE STIMULANT, PROMOTING DIGESTIVE SECRETIONS, STIMULATING APPETITE, AND STRENGTHENING PERISTALSIS.
- UNLIKE IRRITANT LAXATIVES, *EUGENIA* IS ALSO CARMINATIVE AND ANTIMICROBIAL, CAN RELIEVE NAUSEA AND VOMITING IN CASES OF INFECTIONS, AS WELL AS RELIEVE FLATULENCE, CRAMPING, AND DISTENSION.

FOENICULUM VULGARE

FOENICULUM VULGARE – GAS AND BLOATING, PEPTIC DISTENSION CAUSING FULLNESS AND DISCOMFORT, BURPING AND CRAMPING AND GURGLING IN THE INTESTINES, COLIC IN BABIES.

GENTIANA LUTEA

- *GENTIANA LUTEA* –IS BEST FOR ATONIC SITUATIONS IN THE DIGESTIVE TRACT, GIVEN BEFORE MEALS TO STIMULATE THE APPETITE IN CASES OF ANOREXIA.
- *GENTIANA* CAN HELP RECOVER ENFEEBLED DIGESTION FOLLOWING PROLONGED ILLNESSES.
- *GENTIANA* IS SPECIFICALLY INDICATED WHEN FATIGUE AND MENTAL LETHARGY ACCOMPANY THE PHYSICAL SYMPTOMS.

HYDRASTIS CANADENSIS

- *HYDRASTIS* – DIGESTIVE DISTURBANCE ASSOCIATED WITH MUCH THICK ROPY MUCOUS, MUCOUS IN DIARRHEA, ATONIC DYSPEPSIA, JAUNDICE, LIVER TENDERNESS, TRAVELER'S DIARRHEA, PULSATIONS IN THE STOMACH AND "ALL GONE" FEELING..
- MORNING NAUSEA AND VOMITING IN CHRONIC ALCOHOLICS, ANOREXIA AND GASTRIC CATARRH IN ALCOHOLISM.
- *HYDRASTIS* IS AN ANTI-MICROBIAL AND DRYING AGENT USEFUL IN CASES OF GASTRITIS, DIGESTIVE ULCERS, AND BOWEL CANCER.
- HYDRASTIS TONES AND TIGHTENS DAMP, BOGGY AND ATONIC DIGESTIVE TISSUES, USEFUL FOR INTESTINAL INFECTIONS, RECTAL PROLAPSE, ANAL FISSURES WITH STICKING PAIN IN THE RECTUM.

IRIS VERSICOLOR

- *IRIS VERSICOLOR* –STIMULATES CONGESTED LYMPHATIC TISSUES AND BODY GLANDS – LYMPH NODES, SPLEEN, LIVER, AND THYROID.
- *IRIS* INCREASES DIGESTIVE SECRETIONS USEFUL FOR DIGESTIVE INSUFFICIENCY, FAT INTOLERANCE WITH STEATORRHEA.
- *IRIS* IS SPECIFIC FOR ROUGH, GREASY SKIN, PIGMENTARY CHANGES AND A TENDENCY TO SEBACEOUS PAPULES OR PUSTULES.
- *IRIS* IS A WARMING STIMULATING HERB. USE SMALL DOSES ONLY TO GENTLY STIMULATE THE GLANDS.

MAHONIA AQUIFOLIUM

- *MAHONIA AQUIFOLIUM* - IS A BROAD ACTING ALTERATIVE ANTIMICROBIAL APPROPRIATE FOR EVERYTHING FROM INFECTIOUS HEPATITIS, TO DYSBIOSIS, TO TRAVELER'S DIARRHEA AND FOOD POISONING.
- *MAHONIA* IS SPECIFIC FOR LIVER CONGESTION WITH TENDERNESS AND SLOW DIGESTION, COATED TONGUE, AND SKIN ERUPTIONS DUE TO POOR LIVER AND DIGESTIVE HEALTH, CHRONIC CATARRH, WEAKNESS AND EMACIATION FROM CHRONIC DISEASE, DIGESTIVE DERANGEMENTS, AND MALNUTRITION.

MATRICARIA RECUTITA, CHAMOMILLA

- *MATRICARIA RECUTITA, CHAMOMILLA* – IMPROVES DIGESTIVE SYMPTOMS DUE TO EMOTIONAL UPSETS, AND DYSPEPSIA WITH GAS, BLOATING, STOMACH PAIN AND PRESSURE, NAUSEA, AND BURPING.
- *MATRICARIA* IS AN EXCELLENT BASE HERB IN FORMULAS FOR IRRITABLE BOWEL SYNDROME, DIARRHEA, INTESTINAL ULCERATIONS, COLITIS, AND INTESTINAL CRAMPING, FLATULENT COLIC, GERD AND BURPING WITH BITTER OR FOUL TASTE, WORSE COFFEE.

MENTHA PIPERITA

- *MENTHA PIPERITA* –ONE OF OUR BEST HERBS FOR QUEASY STOMACHS AND CAN BE VERY VALUABLE IN FORMULAS FOR NAUSEA AND BLOATING, COLIC IN INFANTS, DIGESTIVE UPSET WITH A LARGE AMOUNT OF PAINFUL GAS, BURPING, RUMBLING, AND FLATULENCE.
- *MENTHA* CAN BE INCLUDED IN TINCTURES AND TEAS AND USED TOPICALLY AS AN ESSENTIAL OIL FOR COLIC AND DISTENSIVE OR SPASTIC PAIN IN THE STOMACH AND INTESTINES.

MYRICA CERIFERA

- *MYRICA CERIFERA* – SPECIFIC FOR LIVER DISEASE AND HEPATIC CONGESTION, BILIARY INSUFFICIENCY WITH NAUSEA, AND FOR A BITTER TASTE IN THE MOUTH AND HALITOSIS.
- *MYRICA* IS ALSO INDICATED FOR LOSS OF APPETITE, STOMACH DISCOMFORT AFTER EATING, FOR DIGESTIVE SYMPTOMS THAT ARE BETTER WITH ACIDS OR FOR A CRAVING FOR ACIDS.
- MYRICA IMPROVES LIVER INFLAMMATION, JAUNDICE, RUQ PAIN, CONSTANT SENSE OF FULLNESS, AND CLAY COLOR STOOL.

PICRASMA EXCELSA

- *PICRASMA EXCELSA* – QUASSIA BARK IS A BITTER STOMACH TONIC SAID TO COMBINE WELL WITH VINEGAR OR LEMON JUICE.
- *PICRASMA* IS OFTEN SEEN IN OLD FORMULAS FOR DIGESTIVE COMPLAINTS OF CHRONIC ALCOHOLICS.

PODOPHYLLUM PELTATUM

- *PODOPHYLLUM* –IS POTENTIALLY CAUSTIC HERB, USED IN SMALL AMOUNTS ONLY.
- *PODOPHYLLUM* IS SPECIFICALLY FOR CHRONIC DIGESTIVE COLIC, JAUNDICE AND LIVER DISEASE, "BILIOUS VOMITING" ENLARGEMENT OF THE LIVER, PORTAL CONGESTION AND TENDENCY TO HEMORRHOIDS, UPPER ABDOMINAL PAIN, HEARTBURN, GAGGING, RETCHING.

QUERCUS ALBA

- *QUERCUS ALBA* – A DIGESTIVE ASTRINGENT FOR SWOLLEN ATONIC DIGESTIVE PASSAGES WITH EXCESSIVE MUCOUS DISCHARGES.
- *QUERCUS* IS HIGH IN TANNINS AND COMBINES WELL WITH MINT OR CINNAMON FOR DIARRHEA, AS WELL AS FLUID STASIS SECONDARY TO LIVER DISEASE AND ALCOHOLISM.
- *QUERCUS* IS SPECIFIC FOR PORTAL CONGESTION, HEMORRHOIDS, CHRONIC LIVER CONGESTION, INTESTINAL ATROPHY WITH MUCOUS DIARRHEA, BLOOD IN THE STOOL.

RAPHANUS NIGRA

- *RAPHANUS NIGRA* - HAS THE UNIQUE ABILITY TO RELAX BILIARY MUSCULATURE.
- RAPHANUS IMPROVE BILE FLOW IN CASES OF BILIARY COLIC, DYSPEPSIA AND CHRONIC CONSTIPATION.
- RAPHANUS IS SPECIFIC FOR LIVER AND SPLENIC PAIN, PAINFUL INCARCERATED FLATULENCE, DISTENDED, TYMPANIC HARD ABDOMEN, PERIUMBILICAL CRAMPING AND PAIN, LOOSE FROTHY PROFUSE STOOL PASSED WITH MUCH PAIN AND FLATULENCE, PUTRID ERUCTATIONS, RETCHING AND VOMITING, LOSS OF APPETITE.

RHAMNUS PURSHIANA

- *RHAMNUS PURSHIANA* – AN IRRITANT LAXATIVE MOST USED FOR LOSS OF PERISTALSIS, CONSTIPATION, ATROPHY OF INTESTINAL MUSCLES. A CARMINATIVE AGENT IS REQUIRED IN FORMULAS USING *RHAMNUS* TO PREVENT THE PLANT FROM CAUSING INTESTINAL CRAMPS AND EXPLOSIVE BOWEL MOVEMENTS.

RHEUM PALMATUM

- *RHEUM* –INDICATED FOR INSUFFICIENT SECRETIONS AND SLOW OR IMPAIRED GASTRIC AND DIGESTIVE MOTILITY.
- RHEUM IS SPECIFIC FOR A SOUR SMELL TO BODY, DIARRHEA, FOR THE SENSATION OF HUNGER BUT EASILY BECOMING OVERFULL, FOR COLICKY PAIN ABOUT THE UMBILICUS, AND FOR SOUR SMELLING STOOL PASSED WITH CRAMPING AND STRAINING.
- *RHEUM* WAS AN IMPORTANT INGREDIENT IN FORMULAS FOR DYSPEPSIA, OFTEN REFERRED TO AS "NEUTRALIZING CORDIALS" AND COMBINED WITH CINNAMON, MINT, AND POTASSIUM BICARBONATE.

RICINUS CASTORUS

- *RICINUS CASTORUS* – CASTOR OIL IS MOST OFTEN USED TOPICALLY OVER INFLAMED AND CONGESTED ORGANS, BUT MAY BE TAKEN INTERNALLY AS A LAXATIVE.
- A SINGLE DOSE MAY IMPROVE CHRONIC COLICKY BOWEL MOVEMENTS WITH GRAY, STICKY, OR OTHER POOR QUALITY STOOL.
- COMBINE CASTOR OIL WITH PEPPERMINT ESSENTIAL OIL AND LICORICE TEA TO IMPROVE THE FLAVOR AND THIN THE THICK STICKY VISCOUS QUALITY.

RUMEX SPECIES

- *RUMEX CRISPUS* – DOCK IS INDICATED FOR HYPOCHLORHYDRIA, MALABSORPTION, CONSTIPATION, DIGESTIVE INSUFFICIENCY. *RUMEX* IS SPECIFIC FOR SKIN ERUPTIONS SECONDARY TO DIGESTIVE INSUFFICIENCY, BILIARY INSUFFICIENCY, AND POOR ELIMINATION WITH TOXICITY.
- *RUMEX* IS ALSO SPECIFIC FOR A SORE COATED TONGUE, HEARTBURN, HICCUPS, CHRONIC GASTRITIS, NAUSEA AND ANOREXIA, FLATULENCE AND ABDOMINAL PAIN, MORNING DIARRHEA, PRURITIS RELATED TO LIVER AND DIGESTIVE DISTURBANCES

XANTHOXYLUM CLAVA-HERCULIS

- *XANTHOXYLUM CLAVA-HERCULIS* – BARK IS A WARMING, STIMULATING REMEDY THAT BRINGS HEAT AND BLOOD TO THE STOMACH, INCREASING FUNCTION.
- *XANTHOXYLUM* INCREASES CIRCULATION AND SECRETIONS IN CASES OF DIGESTIVE DEBILITY AND INSUFFICIENCY, AND IS BEST IN THOSE WITH COLD CONSTITUTIONS, WEAKNESS, LETHARGY, AND POOR CIRCULATION.
- *XANTHOXYLUM* HAS A CARMINATIVE AND ANTISPASMODIC ACTION, AND IS A MILD APATITE STIMULANT IN CASES OF DYSPEPSIA.

ZINGIBER OFFICINALE

- *ZINGIBER OFFICINALE* – A WARMING, STIMULATING CARMINATIVE IN CASES OF DYSPEPSIA AND FLATULENT COLIC.
- *ZINGIBER* USEFUL ANTI-INFLAMMATORY IN CASES OF ALCOHOL OR IRRITANT INDUCED GASTRITIS, AND FOR DIARRHEA DUE TO ATONY OF THE BOWELS.
- *ZINGIBER* ALSO HAS BROAD ACTIVITY AGAINST NUMEROUS MICROBES AND IS WELL TOLERATED IN TEAS, TINCTURES, AND ENCAPSULATIONS.

MEDICINES OF THE SOUL: THE RITUAL USE OF HERBS
©David Winston, RH (AHG) 2004 updated 2016

Ritual and ceremony are practices that developed early in human history. Creating ritual to help deal with the challenges of life (birth, death, maturation, war, hunting, agriculture, etc.) seems to be a necessity in every culture. Examples such as the cave paintings in Lascaux, France, the 11,000-12,000 year old gravesite known as Shanidar in Iraq, and the abundance of stone goddess figures dug up throughout the fertile crescent, Europe, and Asia (the earliest such figures have been dated to around 25,000 BC) are all testaments to the importance of ritual to early humans.

It is unlikely early people took the time to paint elaborate scenes of hunting and horned men simply to beautify their surroundings. The gravesite at Shanider contained the pollen of many plants known today for medicinal use and for their aromatic qualities, suggesting a ritual burial. It is quite likely that the addition of these plants served a purpose beyond aesthetics. Many indigenous cultures still perceive reality through a worldview that refuses to separate medicine, spirituality, ritual, language, history, myths, or culture. Even in Western dominant cultures, religion and ritual are still an every day part of many people's lives. Plants have always played a vital role in ritual and ceremony. In many Native American cultures herbs such as Sweet Grass (Hierochloë odorata), Cedar (Juniperus spp. or Thuja spp.), and Medicine Sage (Artemisia ludoviciana) are commonly burned to purify people and places. In Native American traditions herbs are also used as ritual paints, baths, amulets, and teas for emotional and spiritual cleansing, to bring good luck, success or wealth, to attract the opposite sex, to enhance hunting, and to create harmony and prevent discord. In Christian traditions, especially in Eastern Orthodox, Coptic and Catholic churches, the gum resins of Frankincense and Benzoin are still burned to perfume churches and make the congregation holy. In many Asian cultures, herb-based incense (sandalwood, aloeswood, benzoin, pine resin, etc.) is burned as an offering to the ancestors, to bring good luck and to keep possibly malevolent spirits appeased. The use of hallucinogenic plants and fungi for altering consciousness is another common ritual practice. These substances were inhaled, chewed, drunk as teas, smoked, and even used as enemas or applied topically (flying ointments). The purpose was not so much the need to escape a boring or painful life as is often seen today with recreational drug use, but an intentional desire to experience the worlds beyond our normal perceptions. In most indigenous cultures these substances were rarely used habitually or casually. The users needed to be trained or guided by an experienced medicine person. Often extensive periods of fasting, dietary restrictions, abstinence from sex, or elaborate ceremonies proceeded or were part of the taking of these "medicines".   The almost universal use of plants to affect the psyche and spirit of individuals and communities strongly suggests not a common superstition, but an underlying truth. That truth being that plants have the ability to not only affect us physically as medicines, but they can alter consciousness, enhance our connection to spirit, relieve fear, grief, envy, anger, and clear negativity as well.

In the following sections of herbs you will find many overlap one category. Even though a plant may be listed as an incense, it is not uncommon to find that a plant had other uses and could easily have been placed in another category as well.

A Selection of Plants Used in Ritual

Incense – a significant number of plants are burned either as incense (sticks/cones, etc.), or as a dried herb. Usually these herbs are aromatic and have strong, mostly pleasant aromas. In Eastern traditions, burning incense not only perfumes a home or temple but also placates ancestral spirits, promoting good will, health, and preventing bad luck and disease (Staub, et al, 2011). In Native American cultures the burning of herbs for purification is common. This practice, known as smudging or smoking, bathes people in fragrant smoke to clear negativity, grow the spirit, and make people and places holy.

Copal (*Protium sessiliflorium, Bursera spp.*) - also known as Pom, is sacred to the Maya peoples of Mexico and Central America. There are several types of Copal, the resin from Protium sessiliflorium is known as Copal Blanco, or White Copal. The resin from the tree is burned and produces a voluminous and fragrant cloud of smoke. Bathing in this relieves spiritual diseases such as susto (fear), envida (envy), and the evil eye. Treatment usually continues for 9 days with prayers and herbal baths as a part of the treatment (Arvigo & Epstein, 2004). Among ancient Mesoamerican cultures various types of Copal were burned as ritual foods for the gods. Corn fed the people and Copal nourished the gods, promoting a good harvest and adequate rain (Stross, 1993).

Flat Cedar (*Thuja occidentalis*) – is a fragrant member of the Cupressaeceae family, native to the Northern U.S. and Canada. The fresh leaves are used as a medicine (antiviral, antifungal, antibacterial, diuretic), and the dried leaves are burned by many northern native peoples (Anishinaabeg, Menominee, Potawatomi, Penobscot) to purify the heart and mind, to clear ill will and negative feelings. Flat Cedar used as a smudge or as a tea poured on hot rocks exorcised the harmful effects caused by evil spirits and it enhanced concentration and consciousness. The late Anishinaabeg herbalist, Keewaydinoquay made an infused oil from the buds, which was placed on a baby's "life spot" (the hollow of the throat) for failure to thrive and lack of life force. Other members of this aromatic plant family (Cupressus funebris, Juniperus squamata, J. formosana and Chamaecyparis obtusa) are commonly used by the Bai people in Southwest China to commune with ancestors, to enhance wellbeing and celebrate important evens such as weddings (Staub, et al, 2011). Many Juniperus spp, often referred to as Cedar are used in Native American traditions to clear physical and emotional illness and to remove residues of fear, doubt, envy, anger or jealousy. In Italy, branches of Juniperus communis along with Helichrysum italicum and Spartium junceum are burned to prevent the evil eye (Pieroni, 2002).

Frankincense (*Boswellia spp.*) – or Olibanum, is a gum resin extracted from several Boswellia spp. which grow in Somalia and the Arabian Peninsula. Along with Myrrh, these gum resins were two of the most important commodities in ancient Egypt and in ancient Middle Eastern cultures. Frankincense was used as a medicine (vulnerary), in cosmetics, perfumes, as incense, and for funerary practices. Frankincense was "one of the four ingredients of the incense used in the tabernacle (Exodus 30:34)" and it was burned at Roman funeral pyres to propitiate the gods and overcome the horrid smell of a burning body (Dayagi-Mendals, 1989). Today Frankincense is commonly used as part of a blend of resins (66% Frankincense, 27% benzoin, and 7% storax) that is burned in Eastern Orthodox, Catholic and Coptic Christian churches. Inhaling the smoke of Frankincense and the herb Buchu before sleeping induces vivid, colorful dreams.

Medicine Sage (*Artemisia ludoviciana*) – Various species of Artemisia are known as Sage to the native peoples throughout the Western U.S. Medicine Sage or Peji hota is used frequently by Lakota, Dakota, and Nakota people. It is worn as a chaplet and as bracelets for purification by Sun Dancers. The herb is used to cover the floor of an Inipi (sweat lodge) and it is burned to clear away anger, fear, jealousy, and grief. The dried or fresh herb is also used as a physical and spiritual medicine as a tea and in baths (it is very effective for relieving the pain of arthralgias).

Palo Santo *(Bursera graveolens)* – is a tree native to Mexico and the Yucatan Peninsula, south to Guatemala, Honduras, Costa Rica, Argentina, Brazil, Columbia, Ecuador and Peru. The Spanish name means Holy Wood and the fragrant heartwood is burned as an incense to remove negative influences (mala energia) from people, homes and their personal possessions. Palo Santo can be used to clear negative thoughts, bad luck and evil spirits as well as to grow one's spirit. Due to its increasing popularity in North America, the tree is being overharvested. Only sustainably harvested Palo Santo should be used and this is a good example of why local, prolific or easy to grow herbs should be used for ritual use or medicine.

Sandalwood (*Santalum album*) – the white, highly scented wood is cultivated in northern India and Indonesia. The strong rot and insect resistant wood is still used for building, especially Hindu temples. It is also carved into mala beads used for prayer and protection. Incense made from Sandalwood is sacred to the god Vishnu and is burned at Hindu weddings to perfume the bride and groom. Sandalwood mixes well with Rose otto, and during a traditional Hindu ceremony in April a mixture of Rose water and Sandalwood essence is thrown on participants to wash away sins and allow everyone to begin the new year purified in body and soul. Sadly, Sandalwood has also been seriously overharvested and it is a highly threatened species. Only commercially grown Sandalwood should be used.

Sweet Grass (*Hierochloë odorata*) – There are several species of Sweet Grass that grow in the Northern Great Plains, Upstate New York, Maine, and the Georgia/South Carolina coast. All contain coumarins and when dried

have a lovely "vanilla" odor. Sweet Grass is often used by Iroquois and Penobscot basket makers, giving their baskets a delightful fragrance. It was also used as a perfume by many native peoples. Sweet Grass is usually braided and dried before burning, and among many people is burned after burning Cedar or Sage. The Cedar is used to clear anger or fear, the Sweet Grass "grows the spirit", promotes peacefulness, and calls Spirit when praying. Sweet Grass is also used in treating "spirit" sickness as a tea or by burning the herb.
In Cherokee tradition, this severe illness is known as uhisodi (the Blue) and it correlates to a deep depressive state where the victim loses their heart and the ability to care (Winston, 2001).

Baths – ritual baths or water treatments are a common practice in much of the world. In Caribbean, Central American, and African cultures, bathing in herb infused waters clears the effects of the evil eye (mal occhio), fear (susto), sadness (tristeza), or grief (peser). In NativeAmerican traditions, washing with herbs clears away the harmful influences associated with hunting (killing game and contact with blood), and death (funerals). In this tradition it is also common to have medicines blown on the patient to relieve illness caused by breaking taboos or by dreams.

Devil's Shoestring (*Tephrosia virginiana*) – southeastern native boys or men who want to be tireless runners or swift ballplayers in the game of Anetsa bathe their legs in a decoction of the tough rooted Devil's Shoestring. The idea that the root is tough, thus it can make the user's legs tough is known as homeopathic magic. In Cherokee medicine, this idea is commonly applied and used in herb formulas along with medicines that have a distinct physiological effect as well. The late Cherokee elder Edna Chekelelee often used 7 plants in a formula. 4 or 5 for their physical effect, 1 or 2 for their "personality" (homeopathic magical effect) and one to give the entire formula spiritual potency (see American Ginseng). In a very real sense this way of using herbs affects the body, mind, and spirit all at the same time.

Marigold (*Tagetes spp.*) – is a strong-smelling native of Africa that has become a common ornamental garden flower. Even though it is an introduced species it has been adapted by new world peoples. The Garinagu (Carib) people use a wash of Orange Peel and Marigold flowers to get rid of evil spirits and funeral attendants wash their hands in Marigold flower water to purify themselves (Arvigo & Balick, 1993). Maya priests wash their hands and faces with a decoction of the leaf and flower to enhance their ability to communicate with spirits (Arvigo & Balick, 1993).

Rue (*Ruta graveolens*) – is used in Mexican and European folk medicine, as well as in Mayan medicine as a bath to remove malign influences. According to Beatrice Waite, a traditional Maya healer, Rue baths or ceremonies utilizing Rue can clear all spiritual diseases including the effects of witchcraft, fright, and grief. Topical use of Rue can occasionally cause a rash or blistering, so caution is suggested in its use. In the Candomblé religion of Brazil, Rue is carried or pinned to clothing to ward off the evil eye (Voeks, 1997). Similarly, in the Afro-Cuban tradition of Santeria Rue is used to protect against the effects of witchcraft as well as to treat diseases caused by it (Brandon, 1991).

Sweet Birch (*Betula lenta*) – in several Southeastern native traditions Sweet Birch twigs or bark are chewed or made into a tea or bath to clear the harmful effects caused by coming into contact with powerful (i.e., possibly dangerous) forces. Women in their moon-time (menstruation) are very powerful and their energy is believed to be contrary to men's energy. Sweet Birch is used to clear the effects from men who have been negatively affected by menstrual blood. Other powerful energies including handling a corpse (death energy), coming in contact with ghosts (asgina) and the effects of war or prison are removed by bathing or washing with this medicine.

Amulets/talismans – another universal practice is the carrying of an herb or amulet to bring luck, protect against snakebite, to attract the opposite sex, or to strengthen the wearer. These "medicines" can be worn in a pouch around the neck, carried in the pocket (often in a small cloth or leather bag), or hung over a doorway or bed.

American Ginseng (*Panax quinquefolius*) – has long been used by native peoples as a powerful medicine and talisman. Beaded Ginseng roots are worn to give strength, courage, and stamina. Carrying a "remade" Ginseng root in one's pocket would attract wealth and good fortune, and make the holder popular. In some Southeastern native traditions, not only is Ginseng root used for its tonic properties, but the leaf is added to smoking mixtures and teas to give the formulas spiritual potency.

Asafoetida (*Ferula asafoetida*) – is also known as Food of the Gods and Devil's Dung. This strong-smelling oleo-resin has a long history of use as a medicine, flavor enhancer, and as a protective amulet. In Europe and especially in rural Appalachia "Asafedity" bags were worn around the neck to keep away sickness and malign influences. Whether it worked by keeping people away due to the unpleasant odor or it worked energetically is open to conjecture.

High John the Conqueror (*Ipomoea jalapa)* – is one of the most commonly used and powerful "medicines" in the African-American "root doctor" tradition. The root is carried in the pocket or in "mojo bags" to increase wealth, improve luck in gambling, and to promote sexual prowess and attraction. This fascinating tradition (mojo or root doctoring) still exists and most of the core beliefs and practices are holdovers from African traditions carried to the Americas by enslaved African people. The American Ipomoea is most probably a replacement for an unavailable African plant, but its use has persisted for over 300 years.

Red Buckeye (*Aesculus pavia*) – the shiny reddish seeds of this tree and other close relatives have a long history of ethnomedical use in North America and Europe. The Cherokee and later settlers in the Appalachian region have also carried the "nuts" in a pocket to ward off rattlesnakes, hemorrhoids, rheumatism, and to bring good luck (Hamel & Chiltoskey, 1975).

Rose (Rosa spp.) – have a long association with love, beauty, forgiveness and the Virgin Mary. Giving a loved one sweet smelling roses is a symbol of one's love and they are often offered after arguments as a token of forgiveness. The Greek goddess Aphrodite was adorned with Roses as a symbol of eternal love. Visions of Mary adorned or surrounded by Roses have occurred at Guadeloupe, Fatima, and Lourdes. The rosary beads used by Christians (Catholic, Coptic, and Eastern Orthodox) are named for a Rose garden, from the Latin rosarium. Special rosaries made from Rose petals and perfumed with Rose oil are available from the Shrine of Our Lady of Guadeloupe in Mexico City.

St. John's wort (*Hypericum perforatum*) – has become well known as the "depression" herb. Traditionally, herbalists have used it for melancholia, but it was more commonly used for nerve pain and nerve damage. The Latin name, Hypericum, is derived from Greek and means "over an apparition", referring to its ability to banish evil spirits. In Europe, bundles of the herb were hung over windows and doors to keep ghosts, sorcerers, and other agents of evil at bay.

Beverages and Teas – while most drinks or teas are taken for pleasure or medicinal effects, they also have ceremonial uses. In many traditional cultures they are also used as spiritual medicines to enhance dreaming, relieve grief or jealousy, and to strengthen the spirit. The ritual or magico-medical uses of teas are often difficult to differentiate from the ceremonial use of stimulant beverages (coffee, tea, kola nut, maté), relaxants (kava, beer, wine), and entheogens (peyote, ayahuasca). These substances are commonly used in their cultural milieus as not only something to drink but as social lubricants, enhancing feelings of well-being, calmness or alertness, and making visitors feel welcome.

Betony (*Stachys officinalis*) – is a commonly used medicinal herb in England and Europe. It is used as a nervine, mild antispasmodic, and bitter tonic. In Anglo-Saxon herbals the tea of the herb (as well as an amulet made from it) protects one against bad dreams, night terrors, delusions, and harmful spirits. Their belief in the sacredness of this herb was so great they even had a special ritual for gathering it. "The herb is very holy and it must be gathered in August without iron" [shovel, knife, or trowel] (Pollington, 2000).

Black Drink (*Ilex vomitoria*) – is widely used by the native peoples of the Southeastern U.S. This species of Holly is the only North American plant that contains caffeine. It is used as a purification tea, often with other added herbs (Gillenia, Eupatorium perfoliatum, Eryngo spp.) to cause vomiting. Even though Black Drink isn't an emetic itself, the tea combination is used ritually to clear "spoiled saliva" caused by bad dreams or disgusting smells or experiences. Black Drink was used by most Southeastern native peoples (Creek, Choctaw, Cherokee, Alabama, Timucua, Yuchi, Apalachee, Natchez) as a ritual beverage. Taking the tea made one pure and so it was used to indicate your intentions were friendly and peaceful (Hudson, 1979).

Coffee (Coffea arabica) – according to legend, herders discovered that goats eating the red coffee berries were very lively and active. They decided to try them and so the use of coffee as a stimulant began. In Ethiopia the coffee ceremony is an important ritual expressing friendship and respect to guests. This ceremony can last hours and the 3rd cup of coffee is believed to confer a blessing and bring about transformation of one's spirit.

Kava (*Piper methysticum)* – is or was an integral part of Polynesian, Melanesian, and Micronesian cultures, serving as a ceremonial and cultural beverage as well as a medicine. Ingestion of Kava promotes relaxation and sociability; offering a visitor Kava is a guarantee of welcome and peaceful intent. The use if Kava is so important that in many Pacific island cultures its use is thoroughly integrated into religious, economic, political, and social life (Lebot, 1992). Kava is used to resolve disputes, create cultural cohesion and in ancient times the use of this plant helped to transport users to the realms of the ancestors and gods. Unlike many entheogens, Kava is not hallucinogenic but is classified as a sedative hypnotic with significant muscle relaxing effects.

Lavender (*Lavendula angustifolia)* – has become a very popular fragrance used in perfumes, soaps, shampoos, and other cosmetics. The essential oil (inhalation) and/or the tea can be used to enhance mental clarity, relieve stagnant depression, and for "dream pillows" to promote dreaming. In most indigenous cultures, dreams are believed to be "real" or at least very important. Herbs to stimulate dreaming (Lavender, Mugwort, Rosemary, Bergamot, Damiana, Holy Basil) not only make for more vivid and colorful dreams, but enhance the dreamer's ability to experience this "other" world and its secrets.

Mugwort (*Artemisia vulgaris*) – has a long history of use throughout Europe and China. In the middle ages teas and beers made from Mugwort were used for medicinal and ritual uses. Mugwort was believed to enhance dreaming as well as digestion. Drinking the tea or wearing a sprig of Mugwort protected the user from disease, possession, misfortunes, fatigue, and evil spirits (Grieve, 1992).

Wine - one of the earliest wines was mead, made from fermented honey. It was used as an offering to the gods. Traces of wine made from grapes have been unearthed in ancient jars found in Iran (3500-2900 BC). In ancient Egypt, wine was reserved for the upper classes and it was buried with pharaohs to ensure an adequate supply in the afterlife. Dionysus was the Greek god of wine, winemaking and the grape harvest. Dionysusian rituals were an important part of early Greek religion, which celebrated wine drinking, joyful worship and ecstasy. In the Roman Catholic and Eastern Orthodox churches, taking consecrated wine and bread is a sacrament known as the eucharist. Once consecrated, the wine and bread are transformed into the "most precious body and blood of Christ". Many other Christian denominations, including Anglican/ Episcopalian and Lutherans, also use wine to celebrate the eucharist.

Mind Altering Plants – or entheogens, play an important role in many ritual practices. Some indigenous cultures, especially in South and Central America, used a large number of entheogens. North American, European, and Australian peoples seem to have used only a very limited number of such plants. Ancient peoples had discovered most of the plants capable of altering consciousness and developed methods of safely and effectively using these substances to gain knowledge and power. Through the use of such substances, individuals were sometimes given visions revealing their true names, their guardian spirits, life purpose, or personal songs. Medicine people used these plants for diagnosing illness, to discover the intent of enemies, to locate game, and to foresee the future. In most cultures these powerful medicines were greatly respected and used only under the guidance of well-trained medicine people. They were not used habitually or for recreational purposes. These "conjuring plants" could heal or harm the user and in many cases they were only used at pivotal moments in one's life.

Ayahuasca (*Banisteriopsis caapi or B. inebrians*) – the "vine of the soul" is a very important psychic medicine to the native peoples of the Northwestern Amazon. Ayahuasca, or Caapi, is actually a mixture of one of the two Banisteriopsis species and most commonly plants of either the Psychotria, or Brugmansia genus. It is believed that Ayahuasia can free the soul from corporal confinement, allowing it to wander free and return to the body at will. This permits the user to experience non-ordinary realities where he or she can communicate with spirits or their ancestors (Shultes & Hofmann, 1979). Medicine men use this "great medicine" to diagnose illness, to protect against enemies, to foretell the future, and to heal the body, mind, and soul. Traditional Ayahauscieros (Shamans trained to use this medicine) know all the songs necessary to invoke different animal visions and they require all people who are going to take this medicine to undergo long periods of strict fasting (no meat, salt, alcohol or sex).

Peyote (*Lophophora williamsii*) – is sacred to the Huichal Indians who are the "original Peyote people" and it is central to their mythology, ceremonies and healing rituals. Grandfather Peyote is also revered as a powerful sacrament in the Native American church and is often placed on top of or next to the Bible at Tipi meetings. A common perception is that such ceremonies are full of people experiencing wild hallucinations due to the mescaline alkaloids found in Peyote. Nothing could be further from the truth. Even though church members often consume significant amounts of Peyote buttons or Peyote tea, the atmosphere is one of worship with an intensity and focus rarely found in more conventional churches. The Native American church has many members rescued from chronic alcoholism, drug abuse, depression, spirit sickness, and grief by the power of this spiritual medicine.

Psilocybin mushroom (*Psilocybe spp.*) – the traditional use of the "little flowers of the gods" has only been reported in Mexico and Guatemala, even though various species of this mushroom are found in North and South America and Europe. Archeological evidence (mushroom stones) of an ancient mushroom religion suggest that use of these hallucinogenic fungi once ranged from Northern Mexico to South America. The best documentation of recent ceremonial use was of the Mazatec healer Maria Sabina. R. Gordon Wassen was allowed to take photographs and make sound recordings of her healing ceremonies. She was also interviewed and several books have been published with translations of her songs from her night long ceremonies (Veladas). The mushrooms are used to give visions, for divination and diagnosis, and to heal disease, especially of the mind and soul.

Tobacco (*Nicotiana rustica*) – is one of the most sacred plants for North American native peoples. It was a gift from spirit and, used properly, it enhances prayer, calms the mind, protects against ghosts/evil doers, and is used in divination. Archeological evidence attests to its importance. Tobacco was probably the first plant domesticated by the people of the western hemisphere (Winter, 2000). Native tobacco is smoked, chewed, burned, carried in pouches as protection, and offered to plants (before harvesting) and spirits as a sacred gift. In South America tobacco is commonly used (smoked, chewed, or as snuff) along with hallucinogenic plants (Yopo/Anadenanthera, Brugmansia, Coca) to enhance visions and spiritual power.

Paints and Perfumes – in many Native American traditions, red is the color of success. To paint one's face red using herbs or hematite showed your clan and the people that you were serious and dedicated to achieving success, whether in gambling, love, or war. Indigenous peoples have painted themselves for war (Woad), for marriage, for coming of age ceremonies, and in death (the red paint culture of Northeastern North America and Northwestern Europe). Today's use of cosmetics (rouge, eyeliner, kohl, and lipstick) by many women are remnants of an ancient tradition. Anointing oneself with fragrant oils and perfumes is still a common practice, the purpose today to attract the other sex, to cover body odors, are similar to ancient uses. In addition, in many ancient cultures people were (and sometimes still are) anointed with perfumes before praying to make one holy, to please the gods, and to stimulate the memory, concentration, and the intellect.

Bloodroot (Sanguinaria canadensis) – the red/orange root of Sanguinaria (mixed with animal fat) has been used by Cherokee people to ready themselves for war, playing the ballgame (Anetsa), or gambling. Painting one's face or clothes red signified a profound level of intensity, commitment, and seriousness to the job at hand. While few modern-day Cherokees paint themselves red, the root of this plant is still used for dyeing baskets, woodcarvings, and occasionally cloth.

Henna (*Lawsonia inermis*) - was first used in the late Neolithic period (7000 B.C.) and is believed to have been a part of the rituals surrounding early wheat domestication. It's use spread throughout the Mediterranean, Northern African, the Middle East, and India. Ancient clay tablets from Northwest Syria mention the use of henna by the goddess Anath, who was a goddess of fertility and battle. She adorned herself with henna before battle, while women painted their hands before marriage. The connection between battle (struggle) and marriage still exists in today's culture. The use of henna is enjoying renewed popularity in the west and its use in Middle Eastern and Southeast Asian countries has never waned. In Islamic, Sephardic Jewish, Hindu, and Buddhist wedding ceremonies its use is thought to enhance beauty and bring good luck to the marriage.

Jasmine (*Jasminum officinale v. grandiflorum*) – flowers are sacred to the Hindu god Vishnu and are used as offerings in religious ceremonies. In Borneo women put jasmine flowers in their hair to attract their lovers. The Indian god of love, Kama, has a bow and 5 arrows, each tipped with fragrant flowers, one of which is jasmine. Jasmine oils have long been used as aphrodisiacs. One of its common names "Mistress of the Night" suggests its ability to enhance love making as well as its increased odor at night when blooming. One source claims that anointing with Jasmine penetrated to the deepest levels of the soul and allowed full expression of love and passion.

Myrrh (*Commiphora spp.*) – was used in the ancient world in two forms – a liquid oil of myrrh for perfumery and the crystalline "pure myrrh". It is extracted from several Commiphora spp. that grow in Ethiopia, Somalia, and Southern Arabia. In ancient Egypt, Myrrh was used to anoint and embalm the dead. When the pharaoh Tutankhamen's tomb was opened in 1922, the smell of Myrrh was still noticeable (Langenheim, 2003). In biblical times Myrrh was used to prepare "the oil of holy ointment" (Exodus 30:23-25), as well as for perfuming the body and clothes, and as an incense (Dayagi-Mendals, 1989).

Ceremonial Foods - the ritual use of sacred foods is another universal phenomena. No matter if we are looking at a Creek Indian Green Corn ceremony, food offered to feed and placate the ancestors, or the Jewish use of unleavened bread (Matzah), people have, and in some cases still do, honor their "staff of life" (wheat, barley, corn, rice). In many cultures ceremonies that mark the availability of important foods such as corn, maple syrup, strawberries and beans are still vibrant rituals.

Corn (*Zea mays*) – in the Cherokee culture Selu, the first woman, became corn. Every year the corn is ritually planted, tended and harvested as the first woman is reborn. The Green Corn (corn on the cob) is her milk, which nourishes us as did our mother's milk, bringing us back to health and wholeness. Many southeastern native people (Cherokee, Yuchi, Creek, Natchez, Seminole, Choctaw) still celebrate the Green Corn ceremony, which is a yearly ritual of renewal, forgiveness and thanksgiving. In the American southwest, the Dené (Navajo) use sacred corn pollen as a prayer offering and for blessing participants in ceremonies (Raitt, 1987).

Chocolate (*Theobroma cacao*) – the cacao bean was used as a food, medicine and ritual offering by the Aztecs. It was the Europeans who eventually mixed the bitter cacao bean with sugar and milk to create the confection we now know as chocolate. Not only is chocolate one of the most popular confections and foods in the world, it has been shown (especially dark chocolate) to have mood elevating, antioxidant and antiinflammatory activity. Chocolate has become a traditional gift in many cultures and countries. On Valentine's day it is an essential gift to one's lover, children are given chocolate bunnies and eggs at Easter, and Jewish children are given milk chocolate coins at Hanukkah.

Dates (*Phoenix dactylifera*) – the Muslim prophet Muhammad ate 3 dates to break his fast. Today dates are often eaten at the Iftar, the meal to break the fast at Ramadan in remembrance. Palm sap is fermented and made into Palm wine. This alcoholic beverage is used by the Ibo people of Nigeria as an offering at weddings, funerals and births.

Wheat (*Triticum spp.*) – was the "staff of life" for the fertile crescent and is now the number one food crop in the world. It's importance is seen in both Christianity and Judaism. The Eucharist wafer, which is transubstantiated into the body of Christ, is made from wheat. In Jewish tradition, a wheat egg bread known as Challah, symbolizes the manna that fed the Israelites as they wandered in the desert for 40 years. The interwoven strands of the bread are reminders of the connection of family, love, truth, peace, creation and unity. Matzo (or unleavened bread) is eaten by Jewish people on the holy days of Passover, commemorating their exodus from Egypt and slavery. Consuming this cracker-like bread is said to remind those eating it of humility and the blessing of freedom.

Bibliography

Arvigo, R., Epstein, N., Spiritual Bathing: Healing Rituals and Traditions From Around the World, Celestial Arts, 2004

Arvigo, R., Balick, M, Rainforest Remedies-One Hundred Healing Herbs of Belize, Lotus Press, Twin Lakes, WI, 1993

Andoh, A., The Science and Romance of Selected Herbs Used in Medicine and Religious Ceremony, North Scale Institute, San Francisco, 1986

Bennett, J., Lilies of the Hearth, the Historical Relationship Between Women & Plants, Camden House, Ontario, 1991

Bothwell, D. & P., Food in Antiquity, F. Praeger Pub., NY, 1969

Brandon, G., The Uses of Plants in Healing in an Afro-Cuban Religion, Santeria, J Black Stud, 1991 Sep;22(1):55-76

Cartwright-Jones, C., A Brief History of Henna, http://www.hennapage.com/henna/history/index.html

Crow, D., Sacred Smoke: The Magic and Medicine of Palo Santo, Floracopoeia, 2012

Dayagi-Mendels, M., Perfumes and Cosmetics in the Ancient World, The Israel Museum, Jerusalem, 1989

Furst, P., Flesh of the Gods: The Ritual Use of Halllucinogens, Waveland Press, Prospect Heights, IL 1990

Genders, R., A History of Scent, Hanish Hamilton, London, 1972

Grieve, M., A Modern Herbal, Dorset Press, New York, 1992

Hamel, P., Chiltoskey, M., Cherokee Plants, Their Uses – A 400 Year History, Herald Publishing Co., Sylva, NC, 1975

Hudson, C. [Ed.], Black Drink-A Native American Tea, University of Georgia Press, Athens, 1979

Kavasch, B., American Indian Earth Sense – Herbaria of Ethnobotany and Ethnomycology, IAIS, Washington, CT, 1996

Kilpatrick, J.F. & A.G., Run Towards the Nightland, Magic of the Oklahoma Cherokees, Southern Methodist University Press, Dallas, 1967

Langenheim, J., Plant Resins; Chemistry, Evolution, Ecology and Ethnobotany, Timber Press, Portland, 2003

Lebot, V., et al, Kava, the Pacific Drug, Yale University Press, New Haven, 1992

Pieroni, A., Ritual Botanicals Against Evil-Eye in Tuscany Italy, Econ Bot, 2002:56(2):201-3

Pollington, S., Leechcraft, Early English Charms, Plantlore, and Healing, Anglo-Saxon Books, Norfolk, England, 2000

Prance, G., Nesbitt, M. [Eds.], The Cultural History of Plants, Routledge, NY 2005

Quiroz, D., Sosef, M., et al, Why Ritual Plant Use Has Ethnopharmacological Relevance, J Ethnopharmacol, 2016 Jul 21;188:48-56

Raitt, T.M., The Ritual Meaning of Corn Pollen Among the Navajo Indians, Religious Studies 1987;23(4):523-30

Ronnei, J., Zawi Chemi Shanider, http://maxpages.com/ribbentrop/zawi_chemi-shanider-iraq

Schultes, R.E., Hofmann, A., Plants of the Gods, Origins of Hallucinogenic Use, Alfred van der March Editions, New York, 1979

Simoons, F.J., Plants of Life, Plants of Death, University of Wisconsin Press, Madison, 1998

Snow, L.F., Walkin' Over Medicine, Westview Press, Boulder, 1993

Staub, P.O., Geck, M.S., et al, Incense and Ritual Plant Use in Southwest China: A Case Study Among the Bai in Shaxi, J Ethnobiol Ethnomed, 2011;7:43:n.p.

Stross, B., Mesoamerican Copal Resins, [circa 1993], http://www.utexas/courses/stross/papers/copal.html

Voeks, R.A., Sacred Leaves of Candomblé, African Magic, Medicine, and Religion in Brazil, University of Texas Press, Austin, 1997

Winston, D., Nvwoti; Cherokee Medicine and Ethnobotany, DW-CHS, Washington, NJ 2001

Winter, J.C., Tobacco Use by Native North Americans, University of Oklahoma Press, Norman, 2000

TREATMENT OF BACTERIAL MDR (MRSA, VRE)
WITH BOTANICAL THERAPIES
©2008 updated 2016 David Winston, RH(AHG)

What is Multiple Drug Resistance (MDR)?

All organisms including plant, animal and human cells, as well as bacteria, amoebas, and even cancer cells, have methods to eliminate cellular toxins. These detoxification mechanisms help to maintain the health of the organism or cell. In the case of bacteria and cancer cells, various biological pathways including enzymatic inactivation of chemicals, and activation of cellular efflux pumps reduce cellular concentrations of antibiotics, chemotherapeutic agents, or environmental poisons.

Some of these cellular efflux pumps act on specific chemicals, while others can excrete a wide range of compounds. Those that can excrete a number of unrelated substances are known as multiple drug resistance pumps (MDR pumps). These MDR pumps are effectively used by microbes and cancer cells to reduce the cellular concentration of a wide range of medications which prevents antibiotics and chemotherapeutic drugs from being effective. In the case of bacteria this "learned" resistance can be passed on to future generations of bacteria and even "shared" with unrelated species of bacteria via packets of genetic information called plasmids. A large number of gram-negative and gram-positive bacteria have become resistant to many once effective antibiotics and some are now resistant to all available antibiotics. Resistant bacteria include common human pathogens such as Staphylococcus aureus (MRSA, PRSA), Escherichia coli, Salmonella typhimurium, Enterococcus faecalis (VRE), E. faecium (VRE), Streptococcus pneumoniae, Hemophilus influenzae, Moraxella catarrhalis, Pseudomonas aeruginosa, and Salmonella enterica. The phenomena of drug resistance was first noted during the 1950's. In the late 1980's cancer researchers were the first to understand the very significant role of cellular MDR efflux pumps in creating resistant cells. The steady growth of this problem has created a serious worldwide healthcare crisis. In the early 21st century, as healthcare authorities have sounded warnings, finally the public and the media have discovered this "new" danger. According to the CDC there were approximately 94,360 serious MRSA infections in 2005 and of these, 18,650 people died due to these infections (CDC, 2007). The statistics reveal that 85% of infections were associated with healthcare (although 2/3 occurred out of hospitals and 1/3 during hospitalization) and about 14% had no obvious exposure to healthcare. Infection rates were highest in patients older than 65, African Americans, and men.

What are the causes of MDR?

Medical causes
- inappropriate use of antibiotics, i.e. given for viral infections
- prophylactic use of antibiotics
- inadequate hygiene in medical settings
- patients discontinuing use of antibiotics prematurely

Environmental causes
- amalgam fillings/mercury – promotes bacterial mutation
- pesticide and other toxin exposure – promotes bacterial mutation
- industrial chemical exposure (triclosan) – promotes bacterial mutation
- pharmaceutical medications (clofibrate, ethacrynic acid) – promote bacterial mutation
- naturally occurring bacterial evolution (survival methods of bacteria include MDR pumps, inactivating enzymes, biofilm production, target modification and bacterial immunity)

Agricultural causes
- widespread use of antibiotics in factory farming
- use of antibiotics to enhance animal growth
- antibiotic foliant sprays for combating bacterial plant diseases

Other risk factors include old age, transplant patients, people with IV ports, immunosuppressive medications, immunosuppressive diseases (HIV/AIDS, cancer, Lyme disease, CFIDS), patients in intensive care and on ventilators or with nasogastric feeding tubes.

Prevention of MDR bacterial infections
- wash hands thoroughly with soap and hot water after being in crowded environments, hospitals, or the gym – avoid using "antibacterial" soaps
- take antibiotics only when necessary, finish the prescription
- good diet and good nutrition enhance immune function and resistance
- cook meats well and avoid eating perishable foods that have been left out without proper refrigeration
- get adequate sleep, which enhances immune function and resistance
- use immune enhancing herbs (Maitake, Reishi, Eleuthero, Astragalus, Schisandra, American Ginseng, etc.) and immunopotentiating supplements (probiotics, whey powder, vitamins A, C and D, etc.)

The difference between bacterial persistence and MDR

Bacteria have a second survival strategy that can help them to survive toxic medications and even some herbs. This phenomenon is known as bacterial persistence. Persister bacteria do not necessarily mutate and pass on resistance traits to future generations of bacteria. Persisters create bacterial colonies that produce biofilms (slimy bacterial films or layers) which protect bacteria from toxins. Certain bacteria such as Helicobacter pylori and Streptococcus pyrogenes are well known for this trait. A few studies claim that some herbs can induce MDR, but further research suggests this is not accurate and persister bacteria may play a role in those reports (Yarnell & Abascal, Feb., 2003). Some herbs, such as Catnip, Roman Chamomile and Queens Crape Myrtle fruit (Lagerstroemia speciosa) have been shown to inhibit biofilm production in some bacterial species (Nostro, et al, 2001; Kazemian, et al, 2015; Singh, et al, 2012). They do this through the anti-quorum sensing activity (see page 10). The evidence suggests that anti-quorum sensing activity can significantly inhibit biofilm production and bacterial virulence and does not promote bacterial resistance.

Can herbs be a useful therapy for MDR?

Many herbs, as well as honey and clay, have a long history of being used topically and orally to treat infections. A significant number of herbs have clinical trials showing they have active antibacterial (as well as antiinflammatory, antiviral, and antifungal) activity. Herbs can be useful dealing with the issue of MDR in several ways. Firstly, for mild to moderate topical or internal infections, herbs which do not contribute to MDR (see bacterial persistence above) should be considered as a first choice of therapy. Raw garlic is highly effective for antibiotic-resistant pneumonia, Sage tea is effective for sore throats, Uva Ursi or Pipsissewa can treat many cases of cystitis, and Goldenseal or Coptis can be used for conjunctivitis, periodontal disease, cervicitis, or gastric ulcers.

In addition to reducing the overuse of antibiotics, research suggests that some herbs can inhibit the MDR pumps, allowing antibiotics to regain efficacy, other herbs directly kill or interfere with bacterial metabolism and some enhance antibiotic efficacy by either stimulating the immune system, creating a biological synergy or other unknown mechanisms. Most of the research cited in this paper are in-vitro studies and human or animal clinical trials are mostly lacking. Still, when you combine the long history of use of many of these plants for topical or internal infections with this preliminary data, it suggests herbs may be a useful adjunct to treating this growing problem.

Possible Herbal Therapies For Inhibiting MDR

Atractylodes/Cang Zhu root (*Atractylodes lancea*) – red Atractylodes contains compounds that powerfully inhibited MDR in-vitro (Abascal & Yarnell, 2002). In Chinese medicine, Cang Zhu is used to treat diarrhea, head colds, and upper respiratory tract infections.

Baical Scullcap/Huang Qin root *(Scutellaria baicalensis), possibly other Scutellaria species, including S. lateriflora, S. galericulata* – as well as the flavonoid Baicalin (a second flavonoid, Baicalein, also found in this herb also has activity, see Thyme) strongly reduced the MIC's of penicillin against both MRSA and PRSA. In addition, this flavonoid also enhanced the bacteriocidal activity of ampicillin, amoxycillin, benzylpenicillin, methicillin, and cefotaxime (Liu, et al, 2000). An alcohol extract of the whole herb improved activity of 4 different antibiotics against several strains of MRSA (Yang, et al, 2005). Huang Qin is commonly used in TCM for damp/heat infections such as infectious hepatitis, dysentery, tonsillitis, urinary tract infections, pneumonia, and bacterial infections with high fevers.

Barberry root and leaf *(Berberis spp.)*, also **Coptis root** *(Coptis chinensis),* **Goldenseal root** (*Hydrastis canadensis),* **Oregon Grape Root** (*Mahonia aquifolium, M. repens*) – isolated Berberine inhibits MRSA, but its efficacy can be inhibited by biofilms and by the MDR efflux pumps in bacteria (this is not true for Berberine containing herbs). Two flavolignans found in Barberry leaves (5-Methoxyhydrocarpin-D and Pheophorbide A) acted synergistically with Berberine to inhibit bacterial MDR pumps and enhance the activity of the Berberine (Stermitz, et al, 2000). All of the Berberine containing herbs are used for treating gum disease, conjunctivitis, sinus infections, sore throats, gastritis and gastric ulcers, urinary tract infections, and bacterial vaginosis.

Black Pepper fruit (*Piper nigrum),* **Pippali Long Pepper** (*P. longum)* **unripe fruit** – both of these pepper species (and possibly P. cubeba) contain Piperine, which enhances the accumulation of ciprofloxacin in MRSA (Stavri, et al, 2007).

Garlic bulb (*Allium sativum)* – this common food/herb creates an inhibitory synergy when it is combined with vancomycin for vancomycin-resistant enterococci (VRE). The dose given equaled a single raw clove of garlic taken on an empty stomach (Harris, et al, 2001). Mice given garlic were protected against laboratory-induced MRSA infections (Tsao, et al, 2003). In World War II, garlic was used as a wound dressing and I use fresh garlic as an effective treatment for antibiotic resistant pneumonia. Garlic has been shown to be effective (in-vitro) for Pseudomonas, E. coli, Clostridium, Proteus, Klebsiella, Staphylococcus aureus, Salmonella, as well as many fungi (Abascal & Yarnell, 2002).

Green Tea leaf (*Camellia sinensis)* – phenolic metabolites found in green and black tea such as the catechin gallates have been found to reverse methicillin-resistance in MRSA (Stavrik, etal, 2007). Epigallocatechin gallate has also been found to enhance the effects tetracycline in Tet (K) resistant Staphylococci (Stavri, et al, 2007). In an unpublished Egyptian study (Kassam, et al, 2008), Green tea enhanced bactericidal effects of all tested antibiotics including chloramphenicol, cephalosporin, tetracycline and ß-lactam antibiotics. In laboratory studies, Green Tea extract also had direct antibacterial activity against MRSA and PRSA (Radji, et al, 2013). Tea extracts have also been found effective in inhibiting Yersinia, Vibrio cholerae, Shigella, and dermal fungi (Abascal & Yarnell, 2002). Tea extracts also enhanced activity of ampicillin in-vitro (Aqil, et al, 2005).

Gotu Kola herb (*Centella asiatica)* – extracts of Gotu Kola showed in-vitro activity against 3 strains of resistant S. enterica (Stavri, et al, 2007). The MDR pumps found in these strains can cause resistance to tetracycline, flavoquinolones, and chloramphenicol. A methanol extract of this herb also inhibited MRSA (Zaidan, et al, 2005). Gotu Kola is indicated in traditional herbal practice for skin or connective tissue that is red, hot, and inflamed. It has also been used for treating bacterial erysipelas.

Honeysuckle flower (*Lonicera japonica)* – this common weedy plant contains hydrocarpin, a compound that has shown a significant ability to inhibit MDR pumps (Abascal & Yarnell, 2002). In TCM, Honeysuckle is frequently used for damp/heat respiratory, genito-urinary, and gastro-intestinal infections.

Licorice root/rhizome (*Glycyrrhiza glabra, G. uralensis)* - extracts of Licorice showed in-vitro activity against 3 strains of resistant S. enterica (Stavri, et al, 2007). The MDR pumps found in these strains can cause resistance to tetracycline, fluoroquinolones, and chloramphenicol. Licorice has antiinflammatory, antiviral, immune amphoteric, and adaptogenic activity and is traditionally used to heal gastritis, gastric ulcers, and sore throats. Phenolic compounds found in Licorice (glicophenone, glicoisoflavone) also strongly inhibited MRSA and another compound, licoricidin, decreased several MRSA strains' resistance to oxacillin (Hatano, et al, 2000).

Milk Thistle seed (*Silybum marianum)* – the flavanolignan silybin was found to be an effective bacterial MDR pump inhibitor in-vitro (Stermitz, et al, 2000). In a case I am familiar with, a patient with a life-threatening illness was hospitalized and eventually stabilized. While in the hospital, the patient acquired a serious MRSA infection. Only after adding Milk Thistle (standardized extract) to the antibiotic regimen, was the infection finally eliminated.

Myrrh gum resin (*Commiphora myrrha, C. molmol)* – extracts of Myrrh showed in-vitro activity against 3 strains of resistant S. enterica (Stavri, et al, 2007). The MDR pumps found in these strains can cause resistance to tetracycline, fluoroquinolones, and chloramphenicol. Myrrh has a long history of use for treating gum disease, sore throats, topical infections, gastritis, and gastric ulcers.

Orange Peel (*Citrus spp.)* – extracts of Orange Peel showed in-vitro activity against 3 different strains of resistant S. enterica (Stavri, et al, 2007). The MDR pumps found in these strains can cause resistance to tetracycline, fluoroquinolones, and chloramphenicol. In Middle Eastern medicine, Orange Peel is used to treat gastric ulcers, respiratory tract infections, and bacteria diarrhea.

Plantain leaf *(Plantago spp.)* – contains Baicalin (see Scullcap) which has strong activity against MRSA & PRSA. Plantain leaf has substantially more of this flavonoid then does Scullcap (Abascal & Yarnell, 2002).   This weedy herb has a long history of use for topical infections, gum disease, gastric ulcers, and venomous insect bites.

Prickly Ash bark *(Zanthoxylum clava-herculis)* – an alkaloid extract (and especially the alkaloid chelerythrine) from this shrubby tree strongly inhibited MDR efflux pumps in MRSA (Gibbons, et al,

2003). Laboratory studies have found that Prickly Ash increased S. aureus sensitivity to several antibiotics including erythromycin, norfloxacin and sulfamethazine (Parlato, 2011).

Rhubarb root *(Rheum spp.)* – a major constituent of Rhubarb, Rhein, strongly inhibited bacterial MDR, especially in S. aureus, B. megaterium, E. coli, and Salmonella enterica (Tegos, et al, 2002). In TCM Rhubarb is commonly used to treat bacterial infections of the GI and GU tracts. In a Chinese study Rhubarb also enhanced antibiotic activity against MRSA (Yang, et al, 2005).

Rosemary herb *(Rosmarinus officinalis)* – a Rosemary extract and several isolated diterpenes (carnosic acid, carnosol, etc.) had antibacterial and MDR inhibiting effects against MRSA and other resistant strains of S. aureus (Oluwateryi, et al, 2004). Rosemary also contains high levels of antibacterial essential oils and has been used for topical infections, and sore throats.

Thyme herb *(Thymus vulgaris)* - Baicalein (also see Baical Scullcap), a flavone found in the leaves of this common spice, is believed to inhibit several different MDR pumps as well as possibly damage the integrity of bacterial cell walls. Baicalein when used with tetracycline or ß-lactam antibiotics (oxacillin, cefmetazole, ampicillin) significantly reduced the MIC of these drugs needed to kill MRSA Stavri, et al, 2007). Thyme also contains significant amounts of essential oil, especially the compound thymol, which is a powerful antibacterial, antifungal, and antiviral agent. Thyme has a long history of use for treating respiratory tract and topical infections. In a laboratory study, the EO strongly inhibited clinical strains of multi-drug resistant Staphylococcus, Enterococcus, E. coli and Pseudomonas (Sienkiewica, et al, 2012).

Herbs and other natural substances that inhibit/kill MRSA and other antibiotic resistant bacteria

Amla fruit *(Emblica officinalis)* – this Indian fruit is rich in vitamin C and polyphenols. It had broad spectrum antibacterial activity against resistant Staph aureus and Salmonella paratyphi (Ahmed & Beg, 2001).

Andrographis herb *(Andrographis paniculata)* – studies (in vitro) showed water extracts of Andrographis had significant inhibitory activity toward S. aureus and MRSA, as well as Pseudomonas aeruginosa (Zaidan, et al, 2005). Andrographis is traditionally used in Chinese and Ayurvedic medicine for treating viral and bacterial infections including bacillary dysentery, bacterial diarrhea, bronchitis, tonsillitis, urethritis, hepatitis A, and enteritis.

Bai Zhi root *(Angelica dahurica)* – polyacetylenic compounds such as falcarindiol powerfully inhibited multidrug resistant and methicillin-resistant S. aureus (Lechner, et al, 2006). The root is traditionally used in TCM as a tea for sinusitis and Otitis media and topically for boils and other skin infections.

Cardamom seed *(Elettaria cardamomum)* – showed significant antibacterial activity against MRSA strains isolated from human wounds (Karthy, et al, 2009). The EO exhibited significant antibacterial activity against E. coli in an in vitro study (Naveed, et al, 2013). This common spice has a long history of use for treating bacterial diarrhea, gum disease and fungal infections.

Catnip herb *(Nepata cataria)* – this common member of the mint family inhibited MRSA in-vitro and reduced bacterial adherence of S. aureus by preventing biofilm formation (Nostro, et al, 2001). It has been used to treat children's fevers and colds as well as topically for red, painful swellings.

Cinnamon *(Cinnamomum verum)* – the EO of Cinnamon bark was shown in laboratory tests to strongly inhibit Salmonella and other multi-drug resistant bacteria (Naveed, et al, 2013). The other EOs tested (Cumin, Cardomom and Clove) all exhibited activity, but the Cinnamon EO was superior in activity. In another in vitro study, Cinnamon EO damaged the bacterial cell membrane of E. coli and it reversed resistance to piperacillin by altering cell membrane permeability and QS inhibition (Yap, et al, 2015).

Clay – a specific type of clay, "French Green Clay" was found to be very effective as a topical application for infections caused by Mycobacterium ulcerans, and S. aureus (including MRSA). It was also useful for inhibiting E. coli and Salmonella, two common causes of food poisoning. Interestingly, this green clay has been used to treat diarrhea and food poisoning for centuries (Williams, 2007).

Elecampane root *(Inula helenium)* – an in-vitro study found that Elecampane strongly inhibited over 300 strains of S. aureus including MRSA (O'Shea, 2009). The Eclectics used Inula to treat tuberculosis (along with injectable Echinacea) and it is effective for treating antibiotic resistant pneumonia and viral or bacterial bronchitis.

Eucalyptus leaf (*Eucalyptus globulus*) – this weedy native of Australia has long been used for respiratory and urinary tract infections. It has significant activity against resistant Staph aureus (Ahmed & Beg, 2001).

Flax seed *(Linum usitatissimum)* – Flax seed has a long history of oral use for treating diarrhea and topical use for relieving styes and boils. In an animal study, the seed was found to control bacterial diarrhea by reducing intestinal motility and secretions, as well as strongly inhibiting VRE, E. coli, Bacillus cereus, MRSA and Enterococcus faecalis (Palla, et al, 2015).

Forsythia fruit/Lian Qiao *(Forsythia suspensa)* - the fruit of this species of Forsythia is used in TCM to clear heat especially in the blood, lymph, respiratory, and genito-urinary tracts. It is frequently used with Isatis, Figwort, Coptis, or Lonicera for sore throats, lymphadenitis, mastitis, styes, erysipelas, cystitis, and nephritis. Studies show it has in-vitro activity against. S. aureus, Diplococcus pneumoniae, α & ß hemolytic strep, E. coli, Salmonella, B. proteus, Bacillus subtilis, Streptococcus mutans and Shigella.

Henna leaf *(Lawsonia inermis)* – dye made from this plant has a long history of use for creating beautiful body paintings in India and the middle east. Henna also has broad spectrum antibacterial activity especially against resistant Staph aureus, Salmonella paratyphi, and a yeast – Candida albicans (Ahmed & Beg, 2001).

Hochu-ekki-to/Bu-zhong-yi-qi-tang – this Kampo/TCM formula contains Astragalus, Atractylodes lancea, Ginseng root, Angelica root, Bupleurum root, Jujube date, Citrus peel, Licorice root, Sheng Ma/Chinese Black Cohosh root and Ginger. In a clinical trial with 34 patients, urinary MRSA was eradicated in 12, reduced to very low numbers in 10, and all patients had better outcomes than in control patients (Nishida, 2003).

Holy Basil herb *(Ocimum tenuifolium)* – this aromatic adaptogen showed significant in-vitro inhibitory activity against 3 strains of MRSA (Dahiya and Purkayastha, 2012; Aqil, et al, 2005). Holy Basil is rich in antibacterial essential oils and is used in India to treat diarrhea, gastric ulcers, bronchitis, and influenza. A new area of research known as microbial endocrinology also has found that high levels of stress hormones can make us more susceptible to infection. Holy Basil and other adaptogens (Licorice,

Schisandra, Panax spp., Eleuthero, etc.) can help prevent bacterial infections by reducing cortisol levels (Freestone, et al, 2008). By enhancing immune function adaptogens may help resolve infections as well.

Honey – the honey we put in our tea has a long history of topical use for skin infections. Manuka honey from New Zealand not only speeds wound and burn healing, but it is effective for treating topical MRSA infections (AP, 2007).

Japanese Knotweed root *(Fallopia japonica)* – has direct antibacterial activity against S. mutans and S. sobrinus in vitro at higher doses. Interestingly, very low doses strongly inhibited virulence factors in both bacteria (Song, et al, 2006). This herb is also a rich source of resveratrol, which inhibits bacterial MDR pumps (Tegos, et al, 2002). In TCM the root is used for treating enteritis, appendicitis, bronchitis, pneumonia, tonsillitis, boils, abscesses, and dysentery.

Jue Ming Zi seed *(Cassia tora)* – this Chinese herb contains naphthalenes and anthraquinones which actively inhibited 4 strains of MRSA in laboratory studies (Hatano, et al, 1999). Considering that these compounds are excreted via the bowel it may be of use for gastro-intestinal infections as well as for topical use.

Lemongrass *(Cymbopogon citriodora)* – the EO of this aromatic grass was found to be highly active at inhibiting clinical isolates of gram-positive bacteria, including MRSA and VRE (Warnke, et al, 2013).

Moringa seed *(Moringa oleifera)* – the seed of this tropical tree (it grows in arid tropical and semi-tropical regions, including zones 9-10 in the U.S.) has potent activity against MRSA. It is antibacterial, it inhibits MDR pumps, and was also able to restore efficacy of ß-lactam antibiotics against MRSA in vitro (Karthy, et al, 2009). Moringa leaf extracts also inhibited bacterial growth (E. coli, Pseudomonas aeruginosa, Staph aureus and Salmonella typhi) and enhanced the activity of antibiotics (Dzotam, et al, 2016).

Oak galls *(Quercus spp.)* – an ethanolic extract of Q. infectoria (probably most if not all concentrated Oak bark extracts would have similar activity) had strong in-vitro inhibitory activity against 35 strains of MRSA (Voravuthikunchai & Kitpipit, 2005). Aqueous extracts also inhibited MRSA in a laboratory study (Chusri & Voravuthikunchai, 2008) and had anti-biofilm activity (Chusri, et al, 2012). Tannins (also found in Rhatany, Wild Geranium, Alum root, Bayberry root bark, Indian Madder, etc.) possess significant topical and local antibacterial activity. Oak bark has a long history of topical use for treating wounds and cuts. It was also used orally for relieving diarrhea and dysentery.

Oregano *(Origanum vulgare)* – Proprietary Oregano oil products are widely available in the natural products marketplace. These products combine varying amounts of Oregano EO (5-30%) diluted in a carrier oil. These products are widely used as natural antimicrobials. Laboratory studies of the EO and ethanolic extracts of Oregano have found they strongly inhibit E. coli, K. pneumoniae, B. subtilis, S. aureus and P. vulgaris (Dahiya & Parkayastha, 2012).

Osha root *(Ligusticum porteri)* – the essential oil of Osha and its constituents potentiated the effects of Norfloxacin against MDR Staphyloccus aureus and it inhibited the Nor A MDR efflux transporter (Cegiela-Carlioz, et al, 2005). Osha is used by native and hispanic peoples in the southwest for treating lung infections, sore throats, and skin infections.

Peppermint EO *(Mentha piperita)* – in an in vitro study (Sandasi, et al, 2010) and an in vivo experiment (Rafoli, et al 2005), Peppermint oil strongly inhibited formation of biofilms by Streptococcus mutans, S. pyogenes and Listeria monoytogenes.

Pomegranate bark *(Punica granatum)* – ethanolic extracts of Pomegranate bark had significant in-vitro antibacterial activity against 35 strains of MRSA (Voravuthikunchai & Kitpipit, 2005). It also enhanced the effectiveness of tetracycline in vivo (Aqil, et al, 2005).

Propolis – bees use Propolis as a natural antimicrobial in their hives. Humans have used it for mummification and topically and orally for infections. Propolis (in an animal study) combined with Mupirocin was significantly more effective than Mupirocin alone in clearing nasal MRSA infections (Omen, et al, 2007).

Pulsatilla herb *(Anemone patens)* – a study done at the Cork Institute of Technology found Pulsatilla has strong in-vitro activity against MRSA (O'Shea, 2007). The Eclectic physicians used Pulsatilla topically for abcessed teeth and internally for sinusitis and otitis media with a thick yellow discharge.

Rose petals *(Rosa rugosa)* – The petals of the common beach Rose inhibited the growth of E. coli, S. aureus, Bacillus cereus, and Bacteroides vulgaris, but did not negatively affect normal bowel flora. Hycholyzable tannins such as rugosin D and tellimagradin II are through to be the active constituents (Kamijo, et al, 2008). Infusions of Rose petals have a long history of use for eye infections.

Rosemary herb/EO *(Rosmarinus officinalis)* – rich in essential oil compounds, Rosemary has long been used for treating colds, respiratory infections, topical infections, and gastritis. Studies confirm it has broad spectrum antibacterial, antiviral, and antifungal effects (Weckesser, et al, 2007; Lugman, et al, 2007). It also has been shown to inhibit Listeria monocytogenes (Sandasi, et al, 2010) and MRSA biofilms (Quave, et al, 2008).

St. John's wort flowering tops *(Hypericum perforatum)* – one of the active constituents of St. John's wort, hyperforin, had powerful antibacterial activity against both MRSA and PRSA (Abascal & Yarnell, 2002). St. John's wort infused oil (Hypericum oil) is used topically for painful infections, insect bites, and nerve pain. In Europe, the oil is used internally for treating gastric ulcers.

Sophora root *(Sophora flavescens)* – Ku Shen root is used in TCM for lowering fevers and reducing pain. A flavonoid extracted from the root, Kurarinone, had strong inhibitory (in-vitro) effects against MRSA and VRE (Chen, et al, 2005).

Soy (Glycine max) – a fermented soy milk broth was effective in eliminating VRE in a mouse model (65-80%) and in 99% of rats (Chin, et al, 2012). Both tempe and tofu have exhibited anti-adhesion activity against E. coli (Mo, et al, 2012).

Tea Tree EO *(Melaleuca alternifolia)* – the essential oil of the Tea Tree was able to inhibit MRSA (LaPlante, 2007) and was superior to chlorhexidine or silver sulfadiazine at clearing topical MRSA infections (Dryden, et al, 2004). Even though Melaleuca EO was effective for inhibiting MRSA (a gram-positive bacteria), it is even more active against gram-negative bacteria such as E. coli, Klebsiella or Pseudomonas (Warnke, et al, 2013).

Tea Tree is widely used topically for treating infections, boils, athlete's foot, and in mouthwashes for treating gum disease and sore throats. It has also been shown to inhibit Listeria monocytogenes biofilm production (Sandasi, et al, 2010).

Usnea lichen *(Usnea barbata and other spp.)* – Usnea has a long history of use for upper respiratory tract infections. In recent in vitro studies, it effectively inhibited growth of Staph aureus (including MRSA), Propionibacterium acnes, and Corynebacterium species (Weckesser, et al, 2007). It also inhibited yeast (it has been used as a bolus for treating vaginal yeast infections) and fungi.

Uva Ursi herb *(Arctostaphylos uva-ursi)* – an extract of Bearberry (Uva-Ursi) enhanced the activity of oxacillin and cefmetazole against MRSA. A constituent of this plant, corilagin, is synergistic with oxacillin, enhancing its antibacterial effects (Abascal & Yarnell, 2002). This herb is used for treating urinary tract (cystitis, urethritis, bacterial prostatitis, nephritis) infections in European and American herbal traditions.

White Sage leaf *(Salvia apiana)* - this California species of Sage is rich in essential oil, as well as antiinflammatory and antiviral/antibacterial flavonoids. It has a long history of ethnobotanical use as well as more recent use for strep throat, tonsillitis, gum disease, gastritis, bacterial diarrhea, as well as topically for infected wounds. While no modern research confirms these uses, it's relative garden Sage (which is milder) has been shown to potentiate gentamicin.

Wild Indigo herb/root *(Baptisia tinctoria)* – there are no modern studies confirming this herb's antibacterial activity, but its continued history of use by the Eclectics, Physiomedicalists and modern American herbalists gives credence to its reputation as a powerful antibacterial agent. Baptisia is indicated for tissue that looks and/or smells like rotting meat. The tissue has a leaden, dusky hue (impaired circulation) and is often necrotic. I use it very successfully to treat putrid sore throat (with Echinacea and Sage), purulent Otitis media, sinus infections, lymphadenitis, and cellulitis.

Witch Hazel leaf/bark *(Hamamelis virgiana)* – the flavonoid myricetin had potent antibacterial activity and inhibited MRSA (Liu, 1995). Hamamelis has a long history of use for treating cuts, abrasions and other topical infections.

Herbs that enhance antibiotic activity (this may be due to yet unrecognized MDR inhibition, herb-antibiotic synergy, immune enhancement, or anti-QS activity)

Barberry root and leaf *(Berberis spp.)*, also Coptis root *(Coptis chinensis),* Goldenseal root *(Hydrastis canadensis),* Oregon Grape Root *(Mahonia aquifolium, M. repens)* and other berberine containing herbs (Phellodendron, Xanthorrhiza, etc.) – isolated berberine reduced MRSA adhesion, inhibited all tested strains of MRSA, and it increased the effectiveness of ß-lactam antibiotics (ampicillin, oxacillin) against MRSA (Yu, et al, 2005). In a more recent study, isolated berberine also enhanced the in vitro antibacterial effects of azithryomycin and levofloxacin against MRSA (Zuo, et al, 2012). Many berberine-containing herbs have a long history of use for treating sore throats, gastritis, sinusitis, UTIs and skin infections.

Beleric myrobalans *(Terminalia belerica)* – this is one of the three herbs that make up the classic Ayurvedic formula Triphala. It had significant antibacterial activity and enhanced the effects of tetracycline in vivo (Aqil, et al, 2005).

Bugleweed herb *(Lycopus spp.)* – Lycopus diterpenes had no antibacterial activity, but strongly potentiated activity of tetracycline and erythromycin against MRSA (Gibbons, et al, 2003).

The Eclectic physicians used Lycopus for treating diarrhea, dysentery, gastritis, enteritis, chronic catarrhal conditions and hot/damp pneumonia.

207

Chebulic myrobalans *(Terminalia chebula)* - this is another of the three ingredients in the classic Ayurvedic formula Triphala. It had antibacterial activity and enhanced the effects of tetracycline in vivo (Aqil, et al, 2005).

Eleuthero bark *(Eleutherococcus senticosus)* – studies indicate that Eleuthero may enhance the efficacy and activity of monomycin and kanamycin (Winston & Maimes, 2007). It is an adaptogen and can enhance immune function as well (see Holy Basil for more on the benefits of adaptogens for infections).

Essential Oils – combinations of three essential oils (EO) and antibiotics created significant synergy, reducing b-lactam bacterial resistance and enhancing efficacy of the antibiotics against E. coli. A combination of EO of Peppermint and meropenem or piperacillin had greater efficacy, as did the combination of piperacillin and Cinnamon EO or piperacillin and Lavender EO (Yap, et al, 2013).

Hops strobiles *(Humulus lupulus)* – prominent Hops constituents lupulone, humulene, and anthohumol have been found to inhibit gram-positive bacteria and mycobacteria, as well as some protozoa. In a 2008 study, it was found these compounds also enhanced the antibacterial activity of neomycin, polymyxin B sulfate, ciprofloxacin, and tobramycin (Natarajan, et al, 2008). The authors of this study speculate that these compounds could be added to antibiotic ointments for topical infections as well as lozenges for strep throat. In European folk medicine Hops poultices have been used to treat boils and red, hot infections.

Isatis leaf/root *(Isatis tinctoria, I. indigotica)* - Da Qing Ye (Isatis leaf), and Ban Lan Gen (Isatis root) are used in TCM to clear heat and detoxify fire poison (infections). Both are used for acute bacterial infections including strep throat, tonsillitis, sinusitis, boils, erysipelas, impetigo, acute enteritis, and urinary tract infections. The alcohol extract of the herb was effective at enhancing the effects of antibiotics against several strains of MRSA (Yang, et all, 2005).

Lavender essential oil *(Lavandula angustifolia)* – in a laboratory study, the EO was able to reverse bacteria resistance in E. coli to piperacillin (Yap, et al, 2015). It is believed to work by altering bacterial membrane permeability and inhibition of bacterial QS.

Passion Flower fruit *(Passiflora edulis)* – the peel (pericarp) of this species had widespread antibacterial activity and it enhanced the efficacy of tetracycline, ciprofloxacin, norfloxacin, chloramphenicol, erythromycin and kanamycin (Dzotam, et al, 2016).

Rose petals *(Rosa canina, R. rugosa, R. damascena))* – a polyphenol isolated from Roses, tellimegrandin I, was able to powerfully reduce the minimum inhibitory concentration (MIC) of ß-lactam antibiotics needed to treat MRSA (Shiota, et al, 2004). A Rose petal extract had in vitro antibacterial activity against Bacillus cereus, Staphylococcus epidermidis, S. aureus and Pseudomonas aeruginosa (Tofighi, et al, 2015). In an earlier in vitro study, it inhibited many of the same bacteria as well as Bacillus subtilis, Micrococcus luteus, E. coli, Klebsiella pneumoniae and Proteus mirabilis as well as 2 strains of Candida (Nowak, et al, 2015).

Sage herb *(Salvia officinalis)* – crude Sage extracts and the diterpenoid carnosol strongly potentiated gentamicin and other aminoglycosides in treating VRE/vancomycin-resistant enterococci (Horluchi, et al, 2007). Sage tea is very effective for treating sore throats (including strep throat) and it has been used for gastric ulcers as well.

Turmeric root/rhizome *(Curcuma longa)* – an ethyl-acetate extract of Turmeric decreased intracellular invasion by MRSA, was active as an antibacterial agent and enhanced efficacy of beta-lactam antibiotics (ampicillin & oxacillin) against MRSA (Kim, et al, 2005). Curcumin extracted from Turmeric root strongly inhibited virulence factors, including biofilm production, in Pseudomonas aeruginosa (Rudrappa & Bais, 2008). Turmeric has long been used in southeast Asia for treating gastritis, gastric ulcers, sore throats, and infectious hepatitis, as well as topically for infected cuts.

Uva Ursi leaf *(Arctostaphylos uva-ursi)* – a polyphenol isolated from Uva Ursi, known as corilagin, had a very significant ability to reduce the MIC (minimum inhibitory concentration) of ß-lactam antibiotics needed to treat MRSA (Shiota, et al, 2004). Uva Ursi is a well-known urinary tract antiseptic used to treat cystitis, urethritis and nephritis.

Anti-Quorum Sensing and Anti-biofilm Herbs

Bacteria communicate via a stimuli and response system using various signaling molecules. This system is triggered by bacterial population density and is known as quorum sensing (QS). QS determines gene regulation of virulence factors, biofilm production and antibiotic resistance. Many plants, essential oils and phytochemicals have been found to possess anti-quorum sensing activity which can inhibit bacterial virulence and prevent biofilm production. Certain phytochemicals especially plant phenolics (gallotannins, flavonoids, stilbenes, proanthocyanandins, coumarins and phenylpropoanoids), terpenes (monoterpenes, diterpenes, sesquiterpenes and triterpenes) and organosulpher compounds from Garlic have significant levels of activity.

Burdock root *(Arctium lappa)* – has been shown to inhibit bacterial quorum sensing and biofilm production in the urinary pathogens E. coli, Proteus mirabilis and Serratia marcescens (Rajasekharan, et al, 2015).

Clove essential oil *(Syzygium aromaticum)* – showed significant anti-QS activity against Chromobacterium violaceum and Pseudomonas aeruginosa (Khan, et al, 2009).

Cranberry *(Vaccinium macrocarpon)* – has long been used to inhibit bacterial adhesion of E. coli in the urinary tract and H. pylori in the stomach. The proanthocyanadin extract combined with cirproflaxin significantly enhanced the anti-QS effects of both compounds and exhibited improved anti-virulence activity (Vadekeetil, et al, 2016).

Garlic *(Allium sativum)* – in both in vivo and in vitro studies Garlic has been shown to inhibit renal bacteria counts (P. aeruginosa) and protected the kidney from infection-induced damage (Harjai, et al, 2010). It has direct antibacterial activity as well as significantly inhibiting virulence factors and quorum-sensing signals.

Lavender EO *(Lavandula angustifolia)* – see herbs that enhance antibiotic activity.

Peppermint EO *(Mentha piperita)* – and its constituent menthol, exhibited strong anti-QS activity in P. aeruginosa and Aeromonas hydrophila. Both inhibited acyl homoserine lactone (AHL) regulated virulence factors and biofilm formation (Husain, et al, 2015). In a related in vivo study, menthol enhanced survival times in nematodes via broad-spectrum anti-QS effects.

Roman Chamomile *(Chamaemelum nobile)* – has a long history of use for GI inflammation and bacterial inflammation and bacterial diarrhea, as well as topical infections. In this laboratory study samples of Pseudomonas aeruginosa were taken from wounds, septicemia and UTIs.

In all cases the Roman Chamomile had some antibacterial activity, but even stronger anti-biofilm effects (Kazemian, et al, 2015).

Queen's Crape Myrtle *(Lagerstroemia speciosa)* – the fruit of this southeast Asian tree has been shown to inhibit QS in Pseudomonas aeruginosa. It reduced bacterial virulence factors, inhibited biofilm production, and enhanced bacterial susceptibility to tobramycin (Singh, et al, 2012).

Rosemary EO *(Rosmarinus officinalis)* – the herb has been used for treating GI, GU, skin and respiratory tract infections. The EO has been shown in in vitro research to strongly inhibit QS signals in E. coli reducing virulence, biofilm production and bacterial resistance.

Turmeric *(Curcuma longa)* – the isolated extract Curcumin has been shown to inhibit virulence factors and biofilm production in Pseudomonas aeruginosa, which is sometimes resistant to anti-QS activity. The Curcumin is believed to work by affecting iron homeostasis and the oxidative stress response of the bacteria (Sethupathy, et al, 2016). In another study, Curcumin exhibited anti-QS activity against four different uropathogens (E. coli, P. aeruginosa, Proteus mirabilis and Serratia marcescens) and it sensitized them to the effects of antibiotics (Packiavathy, et al, 2014).

Bibliography

Abascal, K., Yarnell, E., Herbs and Drug Resistance, Part I – Herbs and Microbial Resistance to Antibiotics, Alt Comp Ther, August, 2002, 8(4):237-41

Abascal, K., Yarnell, E., Herbs and Drug Resistance, Part I – Herbs and Microbial Resistance to Antibiotics, Alt Comp Ther, Oct. 2002, 8(5):284-90

Aqil, F., Khan, M.S., et al, Effect of Certain Bioactive Plant Extracts on Clinical Isolates of Beta-lactamase Producing Methicillin Resistant Staphylococcus aureus, J Basic Microbiol., 2005;45(2):106-14

Ahmed, I., Beg, A., Antimicrobial and Phytochemical Studies on 45 Indian Medicinal Plants Against Multi-Drug Resistant Human Pathogens, Jr. Ethnopharm, 2001:74(2):113-23

Anonymous, Invasive MRSA, CDC Fact Sheet, 2007, www.cdc.gov/ncidod/dhqp/ ar_mrsa_ invasive_FS.html#

Anonymous, Honey Makes Medical Comeback, 2007, Associated Press, www.msnbc. msn.com/id/ 22398921

Anonymous, Staph Germ Undermines Body's Defenses, 2007, Associated Press, www.intelihealth. com/ IH/ihtPrint/EMIHC267/333/29758/650243.html

Cegiela-Carlioz, P., Bessiere, J-M, et al, Modulation of Multi-Drug Resistance (MDR) in Staphylococcus aureus by Osha (Ligusticum porteri L. Apiaceae) Essential Oil Compounds, Flav. Frag. Jrl, 2005;20(6):671-5

Chen, J., Chen, T., Chinese Medical Herbology and Pharmacology, Art of Medicine Press, City of Industry, CA, 2004

Chen, L., Qingyi, L., et al, Inhibition of Growth of Streptococcus mutans, Methicillin-Resistant Staphylococcus aureus, and Vancomycin-Resistant Enterococci by Kurarinone, A Bioactive Flavonoid Isolated From Sophora flavescens, Jrl. Clin. Micro. 2005, 43 (7):3574-5

Chin, Y.P., Tsui, K.C., et al, Bactericidal Activity of Soymilk Fermentation Broth by In Vitro and Animal Models, J Med Food, 2012 Jun;15(6):520-6

Chusri, S., Phatthalung, P.N., et al, Anti-Biofilm Activity of Quercus infectoria G. Olivier Against Methicillin-Resistant Staphylococcus aureus, Lett Appl Microbiol, 2012 Jun;54(6):511-7

Chusri, S., Voravuthikunchai, S.P., Quercus infectoria: A Candidate for the Control of Methicillin-Resistant Staphylococcus aureus Infections, Phytother Res, 2008 Apr;22(4):560-2

Dahiya, P., Purkayastha, S., et al, Phytochemical Screening and Antimicrobial Activity of Some Medicinal Plants Against Multi-Drug Resistant Bacteria From Clinical Isolates, Indian J Pharm Sci, 2012 Sep-Oct;74(5):443-50

Dryden, M.S., Dailly, S., et al, A Randomized, Controlled Trial of Tea Tree Topical Preparations Versus a Standard Topical Regimen For The Clearance of MRSA Colonization, J Hosp Infect, 2004, Apr;56(4):283-6

Dzotam, J.K., Touani, F.K., et al, Antibacterial and Antibiotic-Modifying Activities of Three Food Plants (Xanthosoma mafaffa Lam., Moringa oleifera (L.) Schott and Passiflora edulis Sims) Against Multi-Drug Resistant (MDR) Gram-Negative Bacteria, BMC Complementary and Alter Med, 2016;16(9):8 pp

Felter, H.W., Lloyd, J.U., King's American Dispensatory, Eclectic Medical Publications, Sandy, OR, 1984

Freestone, P.P., Sandrini, S.M., et al, Microbial Endocrinology: How Stress Influences Susceptibility to Infection, Trends in Microbiology, 2008: 16(2):55-64

Gibbons, S., Leimkugel, J., et al, Activity of Zanthoxylum clava-herculis Extracts Against Multi-Drug Resistant Methicillin-Resistant Staphylococcus aureus (MDR-MRSA), Phytother Res, 2003 Mar; 17 (3):274-5

Gibbons, S., Oluwatuyi, M., et al, Bacterial Resistance Modifying Agents From Lycopus europaeus, Phytochem, 2003, Jan;62(1):83-7

Grieve, M., A Modern Herbal, Dorset Press, New York, 1992

Guz, N.R., Stermitz, F.R., et al, Flavonolignan and Flavone Inhibitors of a Staphylococcus aureus Multidrug Resistance Pump: Structure-Activity Relationships, J Med. Chem., 2001;44(2):261-8

Harjai, K., Kumar, R., et al, Garlic Blocks Quorum Sensing and Attenuates the Virulence of Pseudomonas aeruginosa, FEMS Immunol Med Microbiol, 2010 Mar;58(2):161-8

Harris, J.C., Cottrell, S.L., et al, Antimicrobial Properties of Allium sativum (Garlic) Appl. Microbiol. Biotechnol, 2001:57(3):282-6

Hatano, T., Uebayashi, H., et al, Phenolic Constituents of Cassia Seeds and Antibacterial Effect of Some Naphthalenes and Anthraquinones on Methicillin-Resistant Staphylococcus aureus, Chem Pharm Bull (Tokyo), 1999, Aug;47(8):1121-7

Hatano, T., Shintani, Y., et al, Phenolic Constituents of Licorice. VIII. Structures of Glicophenone and Glicoisoflavanone, and Effects of Licorice Phenolics on Methicillin-Resistant Staphylococcus aureus, Chem Pharm Bull (Tokyo), 2000, Sep;48(9):1286-92

Haydel, S.E., Williams, L.B., Broad-Spectrum In Vitro Antibacterial Activities of Clay Minerals Against Antibiotic-Susceptible and Antibiotic Resistant Bacterial Pathogens, 2007, Geological Society of America Annual Meeting

Horiuchi, K., Shiota, S., et al, Potentiation of Antimicrobial Activity of Aminoglycosides by Carnosol From Salvia officinalis, Biol Pharm Bull, 2007, Feb;30(2):287-90

Husain, F.M., Ahmad, I., et al, Sub-MICs of Mentha piperita Essential Oil and Menthol Inhibits AHL Mediated Quorum Sensing and Bioflim of Gram-Negative Bacteria, Front Microbiol, 2015 May 13;6:420

Huycke, M., Sahm, D., et al, Multiple-Drug Resistant Enterococci: The Nature of the Problem and an Agenda for the Future, Emerg. Infec. Dis., 1998:4(2):239-49

Kamijo, M., Kanazawa, Funaki, M., Effects of Rosa rugosa Petals on Intestinal Bacteria, Biosci Biotech Biochem, 2008, 72, 706450I-5

Karthy, E.S., Ranjitha, P., et al, Antimicrobial Potential of Plant Seed Extracts Against Multidrug Resistant Methicillin Resistant Staphylococus aureus (MDR-MRSA), Inter J Biol, 2009;1(1):34-40

Kassam, M., Fanaki, N., et al, Green Tea Shows Superbug-Battling Potential, www.nutraingredients-usa.com/new/printNewsBis.asp?id=84356

Kazemian, H., Ghafourian, S., et al, Antibacterial, Anti-Swarming and Anti-Biofilm Formation Activities of Chamaemelum nobile Against Pseudomonas aeruginosa, Rev Soc Bras Med Trop, 2015 Jul-Aug;48(4):432-6

Khan, M.S., Zahin, M., et al, Inhibition of Quorum Sensing Regulated Bacterial Functions by Plant Essential Oils With Special Reference to Clove Oil, Lett Appl Microbiol, 2009 Sep;49(3):354-60

Kim, K.J., Yu, H.H., et al, Antibacterial Activity of Curcuma longa L. Against Methicillin-Resistant Staphylococcus aureus, Phytother Res., 2005, Jul:19(7):599-604

Klevins, R.M., Morrison, M., et al, Invasive Methicillin-Resistant Staphylococcus aureus Infections in the United States, JAMA, 2007;298(15):1763-71

Koh, C-L, Sam, C-K, et al, Plant-Derived Natural Products as Sources of Anti-Quorum Sensing Compounds, Sensors, 2013;13:6217-28

Langeveld, W.T., Veldhuizen, E.J., et al, Synergy Between Essential Components and Antibiotics: A Review, Critical Rev Microbiol, 2014;40(1):76-94

LaPlante, K.L, In Vitro Activity of Lysostaphin, Mupirocin, and Tea Tree Oil Against Clinical Methicillin-Resistant Staphylococcus aureus, Diagn Microbiol Infect Dis, 2007, Apr;57(4):413-8

Lechner, D., Stavri, M., et al, The Anti-staphylococcal Activity of Angelica dahurica (Bai Zhi), Phytochemistry, 2004, Feb;65(3):331-5

Liu, C-S, Cham, T-M, et al, Antibacterial Properties of Chinese Herbal Medicine Against Nosocomial Antibiotic Resistant Strains of Pseudomonas aeruginosa in Taiwan, 2010, 35(6):1047-60

Liu, I.X., Durhan, D.G., Baicalin Synergy With Beta-Lactam Antibiotics Against Methicillin-Resistant Staphylococcus aureus and Other Beta-Lactam-Resistant Strains of S. aureus, J. Pharm. Pharmacol., 2000:52(3):361-6

Liu, M., Matsuzak, S., Antibacterial Activity of Flavonoids Against Methicillin-Resistant Staphylococcus aureus (MRSA), Dokkyo Jrl. Med. Sci. 1995:22:253-61

Lugman, S., Dwivedi, G.R., et al, Potential of Rosemary Oil to be Used in Drug Resistant Infections, Altern Ther Health Med., 2007 Sep-Oct;13(5):54-9

Mo, H., Zhu, Y., et al, In Vitro Digestion Enhances Anti-Adhesion Effect of Tempe and Tofu Against Escherichia coli, Lett Appl Microbiol, 2012 Feb;54(2):166-8

Moussaoui, F, Alaoui, T., Evaluation of Antibacterial Activity and Synergistic Effect Between Antibiotic and the Essential Oils of Some Medicinal Plants, Asian Pacific J Trop Biomed, 2015;6(1):32-7

Muluye, R.A., Bian, Y., et al, Anti-Inflammatory and Antimicrobial Effects of Heat-Clearing Chinese Herbs: A Current Review, J Tradit Complement Med, 2014 Apr-Jun;4(2):93-8

Natarajan, P., Katta, S., et al, Positive Antibacterial Co-Action Between Hop (Humulus lupulus) Constituents and Selected Antibiotics, Phytomedicine, 2008;15:194-201

Naveed, R., Hussain, I., et al, Antimicrobial Activity of the Bioactive Components of Essential Oils From Pakistani Spices Against Salmonella and Other Multi-Drug Resistant Bacteria, BMC Complement Alter Med, 2013;13:265

Nayak, B.S, Isitor, G., et al, The Evidence Based Wound Healing Activity of Lawsonia inermis Linn., Phytother Res, 2007, Sep;21(9):827-31

Nishida, S., Effect of Hochu-ekki-to On Asymptomatic MRSA Bacteriuria, J Infect. Chemother. 2003;9:58-61

Nostro, A. Cannatelli, A.M., The Effect of Nepata cataria Extract on Adherence and Enzyme Production of Staphylococcus aureus, Int. Jrl. Antimicrob. Agents, 2001:18(6):583-5

Nowak, R., lech, M., et al, Cytotoxic, Antioxidant, Antimicrobial Properties and Chemical Composition of Rose Petals, J Sci Food Agric, 2014 Feb;94(3):560-7

Oluwatuyi, M., Kaatz, G.W., et al, Antibacterial and Resistance Modifying Activity of Rosmarinus officinalis, Phytochem., 2004, Dec;64(24):3249-54

Onlen, Y., M.D., Duran, N., et al, Antibacterial Activity of Propolis Against MRSA and Synergism with Topical Mupirocin, Jrl. Alt. Comp. Med., Medicine, 2007, 13 (7):713-8

O'Shea, S., Lucey, B., et al, In Vitro Activity of Inula helenium Against Clinical Staphylococcus aureus Strains Including MRSA, Br J Biomed Sci, 2009;66(4):186-9

Packiavathy, I.A., Priya, S., et al, Inhibition of Biofilm Development of Uropathogens by Curcumin-An Anti-Quorum Sensing Agent From Curcuma longa, Food Chem, 2014 Apr 1; 1;148:453-60

Palla, A.H., Khan, N.A., Pharmacological Basis for the Medicinal Use of Linum usitatissimum (Flaxseed) in Infectious and Non-Infectious Diarrhea, J Ethnopharmacol, 2015 Feb 3;160:6108

Parlato, S.M., Antimicrobial Sensitivity and Resistance Development Caused by Nutraceuticals, Rutgers University, 2011, http://M883.libraries.rutgers.edu/dir/tmp/rutgers-lib_31151-PDF-1.pdf

Quave, C.L., Plano, L.R., et al, Effects of Extracts From Italian Medicinal Plants on Planktonic Growth, Biofilm Formation and Adherence of Methicillin-Resistant Staphylococcus Aureus, J Ethnopharmacol, 2008, Aug 13:118(3):418-28

Radji, M., Agustama, R.A., et al, Antimicrobial Activity of Green Tea Extract Against Isolates of Methicillin-Resistant Staphylococcus aureus and Multi-Drug Resistant Pseudomonas aeruginosa, Asia Pac J Trop Biomed, 2013 Aug;3(8):663-7

Rajasekharan, S.K., Ramesh, S., et al, Burdock Root Extracts Limit Quorum-Sensing-Controlled Phenotypes and Biofilm Architecture in Major Urinary Tract Pathogens, Urolithiasis, 2015 Feb;43(1):29-40

Rasooli, L., Sayegh, S., et al, Phytotherapeutic Prevention of Dental Biofilm Formation, Phytother Res., 2008, Sept:22(9):1162-7

Rouveix, B., Clinical Implications of Multiple Drug Resistance Efflux Pumps of Pathogenic Bacteria, Jrl. of Antimicro. Chemo., 2007. 59(6):1208-9

Rudrappa, T., Bais, H.P., Curcumin, a Known Phenolic From Curcuma longa, Attenuates the Virulence of Pseudomonas aeruginosa PA01 in Whole Plant and Animal Pathogenicity Models, J Ag Food Chem, 2008, 56: 1955-62

Samy, R.P., Manikandan, H., et al, Evaluation of Aromatic Plants and Compounds Used to Fight Multidrug Resistant Infections, Evid-Based Complement Altern Med, 2013;2013:525613, 17 pp.

Sandasi, M., Leonard, C.M., et al, The in Vitro Antibiofilm Activity of Selected Culinary Herbs and Medicinal Plants Against Listeria Monocytogenes, Lett Appl Microbiol, 2010;50(1):30-5

Sethupathy, S., Prasath, K.G., et al, Proteomic Analysis Reveals Modulation of Iron Homeostasis and Oxidative Stress Response in Pseudomonas aeruginosa PAO1 by Curcumin Inhibiting Quorum Sensing Regulated Virulence Factors and Biofilm Production, J Proteomics, 2016 Aug 11;145:112-26

Shiota, S., Shimuizu, M., et al, Mechanisms of Action of Corilagin and Tellimagrandin I That Remarkably Potentiate the Activity of Beta-Lactams Against Methicillin-Resistant Staphylococcus aureus, Microbiol Immunol, 2004;48(1):67-73

Sienkiewicz, M., Lysakowska, M., et al, The Antimicrobial Activity of Thyme Essential Oil Against Multidrug Resistant Clinical Bacterial Strings, Microb Drug Resist, 2012 Apr;18(2):137-48

Singh, B.N., Singh, H.B., et al, Lagerstroemia speciosa Fruit Extract Modulates Quorum Sensing-Controlled Virulence Factor Production and Biofilm Formation in Pseudomonas aeruginosa, Microbiology, 2012 Feb;158(Pt 2):529-38

Skrinjar, M.M., Nemet, N.T. , Antimicrobial Effects of Spices and Herbs Essential Oils, APTEFF:2009;40:195-209

Smith, E., Williamson, E., et al, Isopimaric Acid From Pinus nigra Shows Activity Against Multidrug-Resistant and EMRSA Strains of Staphylococcus aureus, Phytother Res., 2005 Jun;19(6):538-42

Sokovic, M., Glamoclija, J., et al, Antibacterial Effects of the Essential Oils of Commonly Consumed Medicinal Herbs Using an In Vitro Model, Molecules, 2010, 15:7532-46

Song, J.H., Kin, S.K., et al, In Vitro Inhibitory Effects of Polygonum cuspidatum on Bacterial Viability and Virulence Factors of Streptococcus mutans and Streptococcus sobrinus, Arch Oral Biol, 2006, Dec;51(12):1131-40

Stafford, L., Using Essential Oils Against Drug-Resistant Bacteria; New Treatment Possibilities For a Global Health Priority, Herbalgram, 2010;88:32-45

Stavri, M., Piddock, et al, Bacterial Efflux Pump Inhibitors From Natural Sources, J. Antimicrob. Chemother., 2007, 59:1247-60

Stermitz, F.R., Tawara-Matsuda, J., et al, 5-Methoxyhydnocarpin-D and Pheophorvide A: Berberis Species Components That Potentiate Berberine Growth Inhibition of Resistant Staphylococcus aureus, J Nat Prod, 2000, 63 (8):1146-9

Subramaniyan, S., Divyasree, S., et al, Phytochemicals as Effective Quorum Quenchers Against Bacterial Communication, Recent Pat Biotechnol, 2016;10(2):153-66

Szabo, M.A., Varga, G.Z., et al, Inhibition of Quorum-sensing Signals by Essential Oils, Phytother Res, 2010 May;24(5):782-6

Ta, C.A., Arnason, J.T., Mini Review of Phytochemicals and Plant Taxa With Activity as Microbial Biofilm and Quorum Sensing Inhibitors, Molecules, 2016;21(29):26 pp

Tegos, G., Stermitz, F.R., et al, Multidrug Pump Inhibitors Uncover Remarkable Activity of Plant Antimicrobials, Atimic Agent Chem, 2002:46(10):3133-41

Tofighi, Z., Molazem, M., et al, Antimicrobial Activities of Three Medicinal Plants and Investigation of Flavonoids of Tripleurospermum disciforme, Iran J Pharm Res, 2015 Winter;14(1):225-31

Tsao, S.M., Hsu, C.C., et al, Garlic Extract and Two Diallyl Sulphides Inhibit Methicillin-Resistant Staphylococcus Aureus Infection in BALB/cA Mice, J Antimicrob Chemother, 2003;52(6):974-80

Vadekeetil, A., Alexandar, V., et al, Adjuvant Effect of Cranberry Proanthocyanidin Active Fraction on Antivirulent Property of Ciprofloxacin Against Pseudomonas aeruginosa, Microb Pathog, 2016 Jan;90:98-103

Voravuthikunchai, S.K Kitpipit, L., Antibacterial Activity of Crude Extracts of Thai Medicinal Plants Against Clinical Isolates of Methicillin-Resistant Staphylococcus aureus, Songklanakarin Jrl Sci. Tech., 2005, 27:525-34

Warnke, P.H., Lott, A.J., et al, The Ongoing Battle Against Multi-Resistant Strains: In-Vitro Inhibition of Hospital-Acquired MRSA, VRE, Pseudomonas, ESBL E. coli and Klebsiella Species in the Presence of Plant-Derived Antispectic Oils, J Craniomaxillofac Surg., 2013 Jun;41(4):321-6

Weckesser, S., Engle, K., et al, Screening of Plant Extracts for Antimicrobial Activity Against Bacteria and Yeasts With Dermatological Relevance, Phytomedicine, 2007, Aug;14(7-8):508-16

Williams, S.C., Clay That Kills: Ground Yields Antibacterial Agents, www.sciencenews.org/scripts/printthis. asp?ckip=$2Farticles%2F20071003%2Fclip%5Ffob4%2Easp

Winston, D., Maimes, S., Adaptogens: Herbs For Strength, Stamina, and Stress Relief, Healing Arts Press, Rochester, VT, 2007

Winston, D., Winston's Botanical Materia Medica, DWCHS, Washington, NJ, 2016

Wright, G.D., Q&A: Antibiotic Resistance: Where Does It Come From and What Can We Do About It?, BMC Biology, 2010;8:123

Yang, Z.C., Wang, B.C., et al, The Synergistic Activity of Antibiotics Combined With Eight Traditional Chinese Medicines Against Two Different Strains of Staphylococcus aureus, Colloids Surf B Biointerfaces, 2005, Mar 25;41(2-3):79-91

Yap, P.S., Krishnan, T., et al, Membrane Disruption and Anti-Quorum Sensing Effects of Synergistic Interaction Between Lavandula angustifolia (Lavender Oil) in Combination With Antibiotic Against Plasmid-Conferred Multi-Drug-Resistant Escherichia coli, J Appl Microbiol, 2014 May;116(5):1119-28

Yap, P.S., Krishnan, T., et al, Antibacterial Mode of Action of Cinnamomum verum Bark Essential Oil, Alone and in Combination With Piperacillin, Against a Multi-Drug-Resistant Escherichia coli Strain, J Microbiol Biotechnol, 2015 Aug;25(8):1299-306

Yap, P.S., Lim, S.H., et al, Combination of Essential Oils and Antibiotics Reduce Antibiotic Resistance in Plasmid-Conferred Multidrug Resistant Bacteria, Phytomedicine, 2013 Jun 15;20(8-9):710-3

Yarnell, E., Abascal, K., The Complicated Web of Toxins, Drug Resistance, and Herbs, Alt Comp Ther, 2003:9(1)16-8

Yu, H.H., Kim, K.J., et al, Antimicrobial Activity of Berberine Alone and in Combination With Ampicillin or Oxacillin Against Methicillin-Resistant Staphylococcus aureus, J Med Food, 2005 Winter;8(4):454-61

Zaidan, M.R., Noor Rain, A., et al, In Vitro Screening of Five Local Medicinal Plants for Antibacterial Activity Using Disc Diffusion Methods, Trop Biomed, 2005, Dec; 22(2):165-70

Zuo, G.Y., Li, Y., et al, Antibacterial and Synergy of Berberines With Antibacterial Agents Against Clinical Multi-Drug Resistant Isolates of Methicillin-Resistant Staphylococcus aureus (MRSA), Molecules, 2012 Aug 29;17(9):10322-30

Botanical and Nutritional Protocols for Diabetes Mellitus
©2002, revised 2016 David Winston, RH(AHG)

Basics of Diabetes Mellitus (DM)

Diabetes Mellitus is a metabolic condition characterized by hyperglycemia caused by impaired insulin secretion and/or effectiveness. This condition, especially non-insulin-dependent diabetes (NIDDM) is increasingly common among Americans and is the fourth leading cause of death in the U.S. In addition to early mortality, risks associated with diabetes include retinopathy, nephropathy, peripheral and autonomic neuropathies, peripheral arterial disease, and athero-sclerosis. It is estimated that over 13 million Americans suffer from DM and over 6.5 million of them remain undiagnosed. Early warning signs of DM include constant thirst (polydipsia), tingling in the heels, fatigue, frequent urination (polyuria), excessive hunger (polyphagia), poor wound healing, skin tags in men, vaginal itching in women, and Acanthosis nigricans, also known as dirty neck/arm syndrome. Non-fasting blood sugar consistently over 200 mg/dL is diagnostic of diabetes, as is a fasting blood glucose over 126.

The major clinical types of Diabetes Mellitus are:

INSULIN-DEPENDENT DM (IDDM, TYPE I DM)

Is an autoimmune disease where the beta cells in the pancreas are severely damaged or destroyed causing total insulin deficiency. Patients are insulin dependent and most often less than 30 years old when diagnosed. 10-15% of DM cases are IDDM. A number of possible causes for IDDM have been proposed including childhood viral diseases such as mumps, rubella, mononucleosis, and coxsackie virus. Another potential cause is childhood consumption of cow's milk, which has been causally associated with higher risk of developing IDDM. The theory suggests that the immune system reacts to the bovine insulin in the milk and then targets the insulin-secreting cells (beta cells) in the pancreas. Studies have also shown introduction of grains into an infant's diet before 3 months increases the risk of developing IDDM by 4 times. Vitamin D deficiency has also been found to correlate to higher levels of type 1 DM (Bener, et al, 2009). Herbs, exercise, diet, and nutritional supplements can be useful adjuncts to insulin therapy but cannot replace it.

NON-INSULIN-DEPENDENT DM (NIDDM, TYPE II DM)

Is defined as chronic hyperglycemia with relative insulin deficiency or insulin resistance. NIDDM patients are usually over 30 years old, have a previous history of hyperinsulinemia (Metabolic Syndrome) and insulin resistance. Diet, exercise, herbs and nutritional supplements can offer an often effective alternative or adjuncts to standard medical therapies for this condition. There are two types of NIDDM, non-obese NIDDM (10% of NIDDM patients) is associated with insulin deficiency, while obese NIDDM (90% of NIDDM patients) is associated with an overweight population who also usually have hyperlipidemia (especially triglycerides), do little or no exercise and eat a typical western diet with excessive calories, carbohydrates and poor quality fats. Genetics also plays a significant role in this disease, as is seen in certain ethnic populations such as the Tohono O'odham people of the Southwest who have the highest rates of NIDDM in the world. Familial NIDDM is also commonly seen and hyperinsulinemia due to insulin resistance and Metabolic Syndrome are common precursors to full blown NIDDM. Patients with insulin resistance have elevated cortisol levels, hyperlipidemia (elevated triglycerides, decreased HDL cholesterol), abdominal obesity, a tendency toward hypertension, atherosclerosis, polycystic ovarian syndrome, and in 15-20% of cases develop NIDDM. Estimates vary but some studies suggest that between 30 and 50% of the U.S. population suffers from insulin resistance.

GESTATIONAL DIABETES MELLITUS (GDM)

Is associated with pregnancy and occurs in 4-8% of pregnant women. Risk factors include a family history of diabetes, obesity, older maternal age and ethnicity (Native and African American or Hispanic). During pregnancy, all women tend to experience some degree of glucose intolerance. By the 3rd trimester higher levels of cortisol, progesterone, human placental lactogen (HPL), prolactin, estradiol as well as increased adipose tissue cause insulin resistance. Most women are asymptomatic and GDM is usually discovered in routine screenings.

Uncontrolled GDM can increase birth weight of the fetus, lead to higher rates of cesarean section and induced labor as well as a greater chance of the child developing childhood obesity and NIDDM later in life. Women with GDM have a much greater likelihood of developing NIDDM over the 5-10 years after their pregnancy then women who do not have it. Treatment for GDM includes dietary changes (low glycemic index/load diet, increasing chromium, B vitamins, magnesium and selenium intake) and increased exercise. In some cases oral glycemic agents or insulin are utilized.

Diabetic patients (especially IDDM) need to carefully monitor blood sugar levels as dietary changes, exercise, supplements and herbs may alter the need for insulin, or in NIDDM patients, other medications such as Sulfonylureas or Biguanides.

Orthodox Treatment of NIDDM

There are several types of FDA approved medications for treating NIDDM. All of them help control blood sugar levels, some enhance insulin production or sensitivity. In many cases more than one medication is needed to effectively regulate blood glucose. The following list are the most commonly used medications with a brief summary of how they work and possible adverse effects:

Biguanides (metformin/Glucophage®) – are derived from guanidine compounds first isolated from Goat's Rue (Galega officinalis). This drug inhibits glycogenesis in the liver, reducing blood glucose levels. It also reduces insulin resistance and is used for both type I and type II DM. There are claims that this drug is also beneficial for reducing weight, preventing cardiovascular disease and treating polycystic ovarian syndrome (Knorr, 2001). While this may be true, this medication can cause diarrhea and digestive upset in up to 30% of people taking it. It can also cause lactic acidosis and so is contraindicated in people with renal insufficiency.

Sulfonylureas (gliclazide, glipizide, glyburide, glibenclamide, etc.) - work by increasing secretion of insulin from the pancreatic beta cells. There is also evidence that these drugs sensitize beta cells to glucose and inhibit lipolysis and insulin clearance by the liver. Adverse effects associated with these drugs include hypoglycemia, weight gain, gastric upset, headache and they may increase beta cell loss in the pancreas. The FDA has required these medications to carry warnings about increased risk of myocardial infarction and they cannot be taken during pregnancy or by women who may become pregnant.

Thiazolidinediones (rosiglitazone/Avandia®, pioglitazone/Actos®) – this class of medication increases utilization of glucose by the cells, muscle tissue and fat and reduces hepatic glucogenesis. They enhance glycemic control and lower HbA1c levels. Side effects from these medications include headaches, water retention, sore throat, back pain, cold symptoms, shortness of breath, chest pain and nausea/gastric upset. People with congestive heart failure should not take this drug and they may increase risk of heart attacks.

Meglitinides (repaglinide/Prandin®, nateglinide/Starlix®) - also work by stimulating the beta cells to secrete insulin. They are taken before meals because the medicine is rapidly excreted. Combining them with sulfonylureas can cause blood sugar levels to drop too low and cause hypoglycemia. Other adverse effects include weight gain and joint pain.

Alpha-glycosidase inhibitors (acarbose/Prelose®, meglitol/Glyset®) – inhibit digestion of carbohydrates by inhibiting production of enzymes needed to metabolize them. This helps to control post prandial-blood sugar levels in both type I and type II diabetics. Common side effects include flatulence, GI upset, and diarrhea. Several herbs have been shown to have the ability to inhibit α-amylase (carbohydrate digesting enzyme) similar to this class of drugs. Maitake powder (Grifola frondosa) has been found to do this, as have Bilberry leaves and Tamarind leaves, which were similar in strength to Acarbose (Funke & Melzig, 2006). Several other herbs had significant activity but were less active than Acarbose, including Lemon Balm, Bean pods, Rosemary and Green Tea.

SGLT2 inhibitors (canagliflozin/Invokana®, dapaggliflozin/Forxgia®) – Sodium-glucose transporter 2 is a protein in the kidney which causes either excretion or reabsorption of glucose. SGLT-2 inhibitors prevent reabsorption, decreasing blood sugar levels and increasing glucose levels in the urine. They may also increase insulin sensitivity, decrease gluconeogenesis and enhance insulin release from the beta cells. The increase in glucose in the urine can cause an increase in UTIs and yeast infections. Several recent studies also suggest this class of drug can cause hypotension, dizziness and possibly increased risk of stroke.

DPP (dipeptidyl peptidase)-4 inhibitors (sitagliptin/Janevia®, betagliptin/Onglyza®, linagliptin/Tradjenta®) – work by inhibiting the breakdown of GLP-1, a naturally occurring substance that decreases blood sugar levels. This causes a decrease in serum glucose and HbA1c levels. Adverse effects of these drugs include headaches, nausea, hypertension, dizziness, nasopharyngitis and possibly pancreatitis. Berberine (Goldenseal, Chinese Coptis) and lupeol (Red Alder bark, Mulberry bark) are both naturally occurring DPP-4 inhibitors.

Bile acid sequestrants (BAS) - such as colesevelam/ Welchol®, lower cholesterol and blood sugar levels. They bind bile acids, causing the body to use up cholesterol to replace it. Because this medicine is not absorbed into the blood stream it does not cause liver problems. The mechanism by which it lowers blood sugar is not clearly understood. While this medicine is useful, taking it is similar to drinking liquid sandpaper. It can irritate the throat and cause significant constipation and gas.

Treatment - Diet

- Calorie restriction can significantly reduce blood sugar levels. Weight loss has a pronounced effect on NIDDM and in some cases diet and weight loss alone can effectively control this condition.

- Consume low glycemic index/load foods and eat good quality protein and fats such as game meats, deep-sea fish, nuts (almonds, walnuts, hickory nuts, Brazil nuts, filberts), seeds and olive oil. Other good food sources include most green vegetables, sea vegetables, some fresh fruits (blueberries, plums, pears), and legumes. Regular consumption of whole almonds at breakfast decreased blood glucose levels in people with impaired glucose tolerance (Mori, et al, 2011).

- Avoid simple carbohydrates (fruit juices, alcohol, sodas, white flour, sugar, honey, molasses, and white rice) and poor quality fats (trans fats, saturated fats and polyunsaturated fats such as canola, corn and soy oils). Recent research also suggests that non-caloric sweeteners such as saccharin, aspartame or acesulfame-K can increase insulin levels, increase insulin resistance and stimulate appetite.

- High soluble fiber foods such as guar gum, pectin, oats, barley, slippery elm and psyllium powder slow down digestion of carbohydrates and glucose release. Diabetic patients (IDDM) taking 14 to 26 grams of guar gum per day needed less insulin and experienced less glycosuria. A meta-analysis of studies examining the use of fiber for diabetes found that regular use reduced blood sugar and HbA1c levels (Post, et al, 2012).

- Increase dietary potassium sources. Potassium increases insulin sensitivity and reduces the effects of excess sodium in the diet. Foods rich in this essential nutrient include avocado, cantaloupe, lima beans, parsnips, sardines, soy, and broccoli.

- Dietary antioxidants/antiinflammatories are very useful to help prevent some of the oxidative damage caused by DM. Foods rich in OPCs include green tea, blueberries, rosemary, sage, turmeric, red wine, elderberries, blackberries, garlic, beets, cherries, black beans and red or purple grapes.

- Eat raw garlic (1-2 cloves per day) and/or onions (1 onion per day). Research has shown both can modestly reduce blood sugar levels (Grover, et al, 2002).

- Consumption of large amounts of unsweetened coffee (7 cups per day!) was associated with a 45% reduction in risk of developing diabetes. This is thought to be due to its polyphenol and magnesium content (Hu, et al, 2006). Drinking Guarana, the South American beverage tea, was associated with reduced blood pressure and lower levels of advanced oxidation protein products (AOPP) in diabetics (da Costa, et al, 2011). Regular consumption of green or black tea was found to reduce oxidative stress in diabetics, lower C-reactive protein levels and enhance glutathione levels (Neyestani, et al, 2010). Yerba Mate was also found to reduce blood sugar and HbA1c in diabetics (Rios, et al, 2015).

Supplements for NIDDM

- Alpha Lipoic Acid (ALA) - 200-600 mg per day can significantly reduce or prevent diabetic neuropathies (Ibrahimpasic, 2013). It is a powerful antioxidant helping to prevent inflammatory damage including atherosclerosis and diabetic retinopathy. Preliminary research suggests ALA combined with acetyl-l-carnitine has a synergistic effect and decreases insulin resistance (Shen, et al, 2008).

  In a human study of adolescents with type 1 diabetes, ALA (along with an antioxidant diet) improved endothelial dysfunction (Scaumuzza, et al, 2015). In another study ALA but itself increased peripheral insulin sensitivity (Kamennova, 2006). Some research suggests the R-lipoic acid (RLA) is the most effective form of this supplement, but in clinical practice I achieve better results with ALA than RLA.

- Evening Primrose oil - with its high level of prostaglandin E1, has shown the ability to improve diabetic neuropathy and potentiate insulin's effects.

- Co-enzyme Q-10 (ubiquinone) – is often deficient in people with diabetes mellitus, especially if taking oral hypoglycemic agents. Several small clinical trials found that CO-Q-10 improved blood sugar control, peripheral glucose utilization and reduced blood pressure (Kamennova, 2006; Mayorou, et al, 2005; Hollgson, et al, 2002). Other studies have failed to find similar results, but noted it may reduce DM-induced oxidative stress (Moazen, et al, 2015). Any person taking statin drugs or Red Yeast Rice should supplement Co-Q-10 (dose: 200-600 mg per day).

- Grape Seed extract, pine bark extracts, quercetin or other flavonoid-rich products are powerful antioxidants/antiinflammatories which stabilize cell membranes, prevent capillary leakage and production of inflammatory cytokines. They may be of benefit for Diabetes Mellitus-induced circulatory problems, such as leg ulcers and retinopathies.

- B complex vitamins – Thiamine, or B1, is an important nutrient for glucose metabolism. B-6 has shown substantial activity for treating diabetic neuropathy and for inhibiting platelet aggregation (50 mg. BID). Biotin (up to 16 mg. per day) is a cofactor for the enzyme glucokinase, which breaks down glucose. Inadequate glucokinase can contribute to developing or worsening of diabetes mellitus.

- Vitamin C – is often low in diabetic patients, and lack of vitamin C contributes to capillary permeability and circulatory problems. Inadequate vitamin C is also linked to decreased cellular transport of insulin and increased blood lipids (dose: 1-2 grams per day).

- Vitamin D – has been found to play a role in insulin synthesis and secretion in humans and animals (Mathien, et al, 2005). Low levels of this vitamin/prohormone are linked to increased insulin resistance and glucose intolerance and a higher risk of developing both type I and type II DM. In clinical trials, high dose vitamin D (50,000 i.u. every 2 weeks) reduced insulin resistance and serum insulin levels in women with GDM (Zhang, et al, 2016) and it improved insulin sensitivity and HbA1c levels in people with T2DM (Jehle, et al, 2014). In another RCT, cholecalciferol improved the suppressive capacity of regulatory T-cells (Treg) in young people with recent onset type 1 diabetes (Treber, et al, 2015)

- Vitamin E - due to increased oxidative damage caused by diabetes, antioxidants such as Vitamin E (mixed tocopherols and tocotrienols) are important to prevent inflammatory damage. They also help increase HDL cholesterol levels and improve fatty acid metabolism (dose: 200 i.u. daily).

- Inositol (myo-inositol) has been found to reduce the incidence of GDM in women with a family history of type 2 diabetes (D'Anna, et al, 2013). There was also a reduction in fetal macrosomnia (big baby syndrome).

- Vitamin K (phylloquinone) – higher levels of dietary K1 are associated with a significant reduction in the risk of developing T2DM (Ibarrola-Jurado, et al, 2012).

- Calcium – higher levels of calcium and dairy consumption are associated with reduced risk of developing DM. Several large epidemiological studies indicate that the combination of adequate calcium and vitamin D helps to regulate glucose metabolism and inhibit insulin resistance (Pittas, et al, 2007).

- Chromium - is an essential nutrient that helps the body metabolize glucose. Chromium in the form of chromium picolinate, chromate™, and high chromium yeast has shown the ability to improve glucose tolerance, decrease fasting glucose levels, improve insulin sensitivity and improve blood lipid profiles (Pavia, et al, 2015). A study combining chromium picolinate (600 mcg) with biotin (2 mg) found that it improved glucose tolerance by 15% in obese people with DM (Singer & Geokas, 2006).

- Magnesium - magnesium deficiency is common with DM. It is essential for normal functioning of the insulin receptors, it reduces the risk of cardiovascular disease, helps to increase HDL cholesterol levels and decreases platelet aggregation. In a RCT women with GDM who took magnesium had reduced fasting plasma glucose, serum insulin, triglycerides and C-reactive protein levels. While it decreased insulin resistance, it also improved beta-cell function and pregnancy outcomes (Asemi, et al, 2015) (dose: 500-750 mg per day)

- Selenium – supplementation of this trace element in women with GDM reduced fasting plasma glucose, serum insulin, insulin resistance, hs-CRP, while improving insulin sensitivity and antioxidant status (Asemi, et al, 2015).

- Vanadium – this trace element has been found to enhance insulin sensitivity, glycemic control and HbA1c levels in type 2 diabetic patients (Dey, et al, 2002; Cusi, et al, 2001) and it decreased blood sugar levels in type I diabetics (Soveid, et al, 2013) (dose: 150 mcg. per day).

- Zinc - adequate zinc levels are essential to normal insulin metabolism. Zinc protects the beta cells in the pancreas, and improves insulin synthesis, secretion and utilization as well as glucose tolerance. Supplementing zinc in women with GDM lowered fasting blood glucose, serum insulin, insulin resistance, triglycerides and VLDL-C levels, while improving beta-cell function (Karamali, et al, 2015) (dose: 25-40 mg. per day).

Lifestyle

- Increase exercise as it decreases insulin resistance and improves circulation and cardio-vascular health.

- Avoid smoking as it increases oxidative stress on the circulatory system, depletes Vitamin C and decreases blood O_2 levels.
- Chronic stress contributes to Syndrome X by elevating cortisol and adrenaline levels which increases blood sugar levels and insulin resistance. Lack of sleep is a major stressor and studies show that inadequate sleep increases the risk of obesity, hypertension and diabetes. In a 2009 study researchers found lack of sleep led to insulin resistance and reduced glucose tolerance (Nedeltcheva, et al, 2009). Adequate sleep (8 hours per night), stress reduction techniques such as meditation, Tai Qi, or Qi Gong and herbs including adaptogens and nervines can reduce cortisol levels, insulin resistance and obesity.

Why Do Herbs and Foods Benefit Diabetes?
What are the Mechanisms of Their Activity?

Many herbs, foods and nutrients have been shown to reduce blood sugar levels and inhibit the oxidative damage caused by T2DM (some also have benefits for T1D). They do this via multiple mechanisms, which we will briefly outline:

Inhibition of glucose in the intestine – several plants have been found to inhibit α-glucosidase or α-amylase, enzymes which convert starches into sugars. This inhibits postprandial blood glucose levels and is the way the pharmaceutical acarbose works (acarbose unfortunately creates significant GI issues for many people). Several herbs have been found to have α-glucosidase and α-amylase, inhibitory effects including Sage, Fenugreek and Runner Bean pods, Green Tea, Rosemary, Kudzu, Triphala, Shan Yao, Arjuna bark, Aegle marmelos leaf, Blueberry leaf, Lemon Balm, Tamarind, Bitter Melon and possibly Andrographis (Crios, et al, 2015; Ghoshi, et al, 2014). The "active constituents" seem to be primarily polyphenols.

Increased glucose uptake and transport – various transporter molecules can affect blood sugar levels. GLUT-4 (glucose transporter type-4) is a protein in fat and muscle tissue (skeletal and cardiac) that moves glucose into the cells. Increasing GLUT-4 expression reduces blood sugar levels and enhances muscle storage of glucose as glycogen. Herbs that have been found to up-regulate GLUT-4 include Guduchi, Fenugreek, Bitter Melon, Banaba leaf, Andrographis, Cinnamon and Nettle leaf (Rios, et al, 2015). Another transporter molecule is PPARγ (Peroxisome proliferator activated receptor-gamma). This nuclear receptor regulates fatty acid storage, stimulates the secretion of GLUT-4 and it promotes insulin sensitivity (by increasing adiponectin release and inhibiting resistin) and glucose homeostasis. Many herbs have been shown (in laboratory and animal research) to upregulate PPARγ, including Guduchi, Magnolia, bark, Sage, Licorice, Rosemary, Pomegranate, Fenugreek, Rehmannia, Dioscorea, Agaricus blazei and Aronia berry (Rios, et al, 2015).

Herbs that increase insulin secretion and/or pancreatic β-cell function – when we eat food containing glucose and fat, GI hormones known as incretins are secreted. They stimulate pancreatic insulin release. Specifically, there are two "incretin" hormones, GIP (glucose-dependent insulinotropic polypeptide) and GLP-1 (glucagon-like peptide-1). Both are short-lived in their activity and are quickly deactivated by an enzyme DPP-4 (dipeptidyl peptidase-4). Herbs have been found to affect this process in two ways. There are some herbs/foods that act as GLP-1 analogs (inulin-type fructose found in Chicory, Jerusalem Artichoke, Burdock root or Dandelion root) and others that inhibit DPP-4 (Indian Malabar bark, Jambol seed). Several plants have been shown in animal studies to either promote pancreatic beta cell proliferation and/or protect against beta cell damage. Preliminary studies suggest that Gymnema and Indian Malabar bark may be able to do this.

Antioxidant/Antiinflammatory activity – Diabetes is an inflammatory disease and much of the damage caused by chronically elevated blood sugar (atherosclerosis, NAFLD, AMD, peripheral neuropathy) can be reduced or prevented by the use of antioxidant/antiinflammatory herbs. Herbs such as Turmeric, Amla, Green Tea, Rosemary, Garlic, Lycium fruit, Milk Thistle, Schisandra, Coffee, Cocoa, Blueberries and Pomegranate have a modest ability to lower blood sugar levels but a very significant effect for reducing the damage caused by T1 or T2 DM.

BOTANICALS FOR TREATING DM

Aloe gel (Aloe vera) – has been shown in animal and human studies to reduce fasting blood glucose and triglycerides (Huseini, et al, 2012; Dey, et al 2002; Grover, et al, 2002) as well as insulin resistance, total weight and body fat % (Choi, et al, 2013).

Banaba leaf (Lagerstroemia speciosa) – has been used in the Philippines for millennia to treat diabetes and kidney disease. In animal and human studies, this plant has been found to lower blood sugar and cholesterol levels, as well as reduce weight (Klein, et al, 2007; Yoshio, et al, 1999).
Dose: tea – 2 tsp. dried herb, 8 oz hot water, steep 45 minutes, take 4-8 oz. BID/TID
        capsule (12:1 extract, standardized to 1.5% corosolic acid) – 1-2 per day

Berberine-containing herbs – various herbs that contain the isoquinoline alkaloid berberine (Chinese Coptis, Indian Barberry, Goldenseal) and berberine itself, have been found to modestly reduce serum glucose levels. While this alkaloid and herbs that contain it are not adequate as stand-alone treatments for diabetes, they do have some significant benefits and a long history of safe use. The famed American herbalist Dr. Christopher recommended the use of Goldenseal (rich in berberine) in his diabetes formulas. In TCM Chinese Coptis is often combined with Scutellaria baicalensis to lower blood sugar levels (Liu, et al, 2013). The Indian herb Berberis aristata has also been used to treat diabetes and a combination of a standardized extract of this herb (1000 mg./day) with standardized Milk Thistle (210 mg./day) was more effective than berberine alone (Di Pierro, et al, 2013). The phytopharmaceutical combination improved fasting glucose, LDL cholesterol, triglycerides, liver enzymes and HbA1c in people with suboptimal glycemic control. In a clinical study, isolated berberine or Metformin was given to people newly diagnosed with NIDDM. Both berberine and Metformin significantly decreased fasting blood sugar, HbA1c, post-prandial blood glucose and triglycerides (Yin, et al, 2008). In a second study people with poor controlled diabetes given berberine had similar improvements of blood sugar metabolism, along with reduced insulin resistance (Yi, et al, 2008).

Bitter Melon unripe fruit (Momordica charantia) - has long been used in China and throughout Southeast Asia as well as the Caribbean to treat IDDM and NIDDM. It is a powerful hypoglycemic agent and patients using this herb should proceed slowly and carefully monitor blood sugar levels. The plant contains an insulin-like chemical and oral consumption of the tea lowered blood sugar levels and improved glucose tolerance (Welihinda, et al, 1986). It also reduced metabolic syndrome in both men and women (Tsai, et al, 2012).
Dose: juice - 1-4 oz. per day
        powder - 100 mg. TID
        tincture - fresh unripe fruit (1:2) 30 gtt. TID

Bitters - such as Artichoke leaf, Chicory root, Red Alder bark, and Gentian root all help to modestly improve glucose tolerance and blood lipid profiles while promoting digestion and elimination.
Dose: tincture (1:5) - .5-1 mL before meals

Blueberry leaf (Vaccinium corymbosum and other spp.) - although Blueberry, Bilberry or Huckleberry leaf has a long history of use in diabetes, its effects are limited and excessive long-term use may cause hydroquinone-induced liver damage. Michael Moore clearly states that the appropriate use of Blueberry leaf is for IDDM patients to extend the hypoglycemic effects of their insulin shots. He notes that the early morning hyperglycemia (dawn phenomenon) that can wake up diabetics and prevent a return to sleep can be lessened by taking 4 oz. of Vaccinium tea in the late afternoon. Blueberry and Bilberry fruits also seem to reduce blood sugar levels (Grace, et al, 2009) and can help prevent diabetic retinopathy.
Dose: tincture (1:5) - 1-2 mL TID
        tea - 1/2 tsp. dried leaves, 8 oz. hot water, steep 30 minutes, take 4 oz. BID

Bugleweed herb (Lycopus virginicus) – was an Eclectic treatment for IDDM, it reduces excessive urination but it is not known if it affects blood sugar levels. The specific indication is Diabetes Mellitus with constant thirst passing large quantities of clear urine.
Dose: fresh tincture (1:2.5) - 1 mL QID

Cinnamon bark (Cinnamomum verum, C. cassia) - has been shown to increase the utilization of endogenous insulin, lower fasting blood glucose, triglyceride and HbA1c levels, while reducing fat mass (Sahib, 2016; Vafa, et al, 2012; Davis & Yokoyama, 2011). It also improves digestion and peripheral circulation, making it appropriate for IDDM and NIDDM patients.
Dose: tea – ¼ - ½ tsp. ground bark, 8 oz. hot water, steep 15-20 minutes, take 4 oz. TID
        tincture (1:5) - 1.5-2 mL TID
        powder – 1 g per day

Dandelion root (Taraxacum officinalis) - the bitter tasting root of Dandelion acts as an aperient, cholagogue, and mild hypoglycemic agent. It is useful as part of a treatment protocol for NIDDM patients who have a long transit time, poor digestion, trouble digesting fats and elevated blood lipids.
Dose: tincture (1:2) - 2-4 mL TID
>   tea - 1-2 tsp. dried root, 8 oz. hot water, decoct 10 minutes, steep 40 minutes, take 2-3 cups per day

Devil's Club bark (Oplopanax horridum) – is used for NIDDM patients with insulin resistance, obesity, a mild elevation of blood pressure and elevated blood lipids, especially triglycerides. This herb seems to work especially well for "butterball" types, people who are short and wide, as well as people of color (Native Americans, Hispanics, and African Americans).
Dose: tincture (1:5) - 1-1.5 mL TID
>   tea - 1 tsp. dried root bark, 8 oz. hot water, steep 1 hour, take 4 oz. TID

Fenugreek seed (Trigonella foenum-graecum) – is an excellent source of soluble fiber, and it binds endotoxins in the gut. It lowers total cholesterol, VLDL-C and triglyceride levels while improving HDL cholesterol levels. It has also been found to improve insulin sensitivity and glycemic control (Gupta, et al, 2001) while reducing fasting blood sugar levels and HbA1c (Rafraf, et al, 2014; Kassalan, et al, 2009).
Dose: tea - 2 tsp. seeds, 10 oz. water, decoct 10 minutes, steep 40 minutes, take 2-3 cups per day
>   powdered seeds - 20-30 g. BID

Fragrant Sumac bark (Rhus aromatica) – was an Eclectic remedy used for IDDM that probably works more on the kidneys than the pancreas.
The specific indications are Diabetes Mellitus with pale urine, the person is debilitated and has constant thirst. The fruit powder of Sumac (R. coriaria) was shown in a RCT to reduce serum glucose, HbA1c and ApoB in people with T2DM (Shidfar, et al, 2014). The powder (3 g per day) also enhanced total antioxidant capacity (TAC) and Apolipoprotein A-1 levels.
Dose: tincture (1:5) - .25-1.5 mL every 3 hours.

French Runner bean pods (Phaseolus vulgaris) – are a traditional European hypoglycemic agent used as a tea to lower blood sugar levels and insulin requirements. The pods inhibit α-amylase and reduce the breakdown of carbohydrates (Helmstadter, 2010).
Dose: tea - a handful of dried bean pods (no beans), 10 oz. water, decoct 20 minutes, drink 2-3 cups per day

Fringe Tree root bark (Chionanthus virginicus) – the Eclectics used this herb for treating Diabetes Mellitus with weight loss, no appetite, listlessness, and glucosuria. The person may also have liver involvement with pain in the right hypochondrium and clay-colored stools.
Dose: fresh root bark tincture (1:2) – 5- .75 mL QID

Fu Ling fungus (Wolfiporia cocos) – is a potassium-sparing diuretic (aquaretic), nervine, and hypoglycemic agent, used in TCM. Fu Ling also reduces total cholesterol, especially LDL and VLDL cholesterol. In an animal study Poria was found to reduce post-prandial blood glucose levels, as well as enhancing insulin sensitivity (Li, et al, 2011). It can be used as part of a protocol for mild NIDDM along with Ophiopogon, Codonopsis, Ginseng, Chinese Dioscorea or Astragalus.
Dose: tea - 1 tsp. dried fungus, 12 oz. water, decoct slowly for 30 minutes, steep 30 minutes, take 4 oz. TID

Ginseng root (Panax ginseng) - modestly lowers blood sugar levels in NIDDM patients (Vuksan, et al, 2008). It acts as an adaptogen, helping to normalize endocrine function via the HPA axis. It is used in TCM along with Codonopsis, Astragalus, Chinese Dioscorea and other herbs to control insulin resistance and early stage DM. American Ginseng (Panax quinquefolius) has also been found to modestly reduce blood sugar levels.
Dose: tincture (1:5) - 1-2 mL TID/QID
          tea - 1 tsp. dried root, 12 oz. water, decoct slowly 15-20 minutes, then steep 1 hour,
          take 4 oz. TID

Goat's Rue herb (Galega officinalis) – contains two compounds, known as guanidine and galegine, which were the basis for the biguanide medication Metformin. The herb has a history of use in Europe for inhibiting the profuse urination caused by DM, for promoting lactation and for lowering fevers. Dr. R. Weiss, in his classic text, Herbal Medicine, combined Goat's Rue herb and seed with Bean pods, Bilberry leaves and Peppermint as a tea for controlling blood sugar. He cautions guandine compounds do not directly lower blood sugar levels, but work via hepatic glycogenesis and can have adverse effects with long-term usage.
tincture - 1-2 ml , 2-3 times per day
tea - 1 tsp dried herb, 8oz hot water, let steep 15-20 minutes, take 2 cups per day

Gymnema herb (Gymnema sylvestre) -A unique herb that has been utilized in Ayurvedic medicine to treat IDDM and NIDDM for millennia. The Indian name "Gurmar" means sugar destroyer because the herb diminishes the ability to taste sweet things. Unlike most simple hypoglycemic agents, Gymnema seems to be able to regenerate the beta cells in the pancreas.
While definitive studies on this are lacking, animal and human trials do show decreased insulin requirements in IDDM patients. In these studies, participants had reduced fasting blood glucose, glycosylated hemoglobin, and glycosylated plasma protein levels (Shanmugasundaram, et al, 1990). Gymnema given to people with NIDDM had increased insulin levels and decreased blood sugar levels, HbA1c, polyphagia and insulin resistance (Kumar, et al, 2010; Baskaren, et al, 1990).
Dose: tincture (1:3) - 2-4 mL. TID
          tea - 1 tsp. dried herb/root, 8 oz. water, decoct 10 minutes, steep 30 minutes,
          take 4 oz. QID

Hibiscus flower (Hibiscus sabdariffa) – this tart, red tea is used in the Caribbean to treat NIDDM. Animal studies show that it lowers blood sugar levels and human studies have found drinking the tea can enhance HDL cholesterol levels, while decreasing LDL and triglyceride levels (Mozaffari-Khosravi, et al, 2009). Patients also had modest improvement in blood pressure and a reduction in insulin resistance (Gurrola-Diaz, et al, 2010).
Dose: tea: 1-2 tsp. dried flowers, 8 oz. hot water, steep for 20 minutes, take 2-3 cups per day
          tincture (1: 2 or 1:5): 2-4 mL TID

Holy Basil herb (Ocimum sanctum) – is one of the prominent rasayana or rejuvenative remedies in Ayurvedic medicine. In addition to being a mild adaptogen, carminative, antioxidant and antidepressant, Tulsi has been found in multiple animal studies and a human study (Agarwal, et al, 1996) to modestly lower blood sugar levels. In this study, fasting blood sugar was reduced 17.6% and post-prandial blood glucose fell by 7.3%.
Dose: tea: 1 tsp. dried leaf, 8 oz. hot water, steep, covered, 15-20 minutes, take 4 oz. 3x/day
          tincture (1:5 or 1:2): 2-3 mL TID/QID

Indian Malabar bark/Vijayasar (Pterocarpus marsupium) – the wood and bark of this Indian tree have been used to treat diabetes for millennia. Numerous animal studies show that it reduces blood glucose levels and isolated constituents have been found to promote pancreatic beta cell regeneration and insulin release. In a human clinical trial 69% of NIDDM patients were able to control blood glucose levels with this herb (Grover, et al, 2002). In a RCT, 72% of diabetics were able to control blood sugar levels using 3 g. per day of Pterocarpus (ICMR, 2005).
Dose: 300 mg. capsule BID

Ivy Gourd leaf (Coccinia grandis, syn. C. cordifolia or C. indica) – is a member of the Curcubitaceae family and is related to Bitter Melon. The young fruits are edible and the leaves are traditionally used in Ayurvedic and Siddha medicine. One of the major uses of the leaf is to treat diabetes. Numerous animal studies (rats and dogs), as well as several small human studies indicate that this traditional use of the leaf has some validity. In a study with newly detected diabetic patients, Coccinia reduced fasting and post-prandial blood glucose levels (16% and 18%), as well as HbA1c (Kuriyan, et al, 2008). In another study of poorly controlled diabetics, 10 of the 16 showed significant improvements in glucose tolerance, while none of the control subjects did (Azadkhan, et al, 1980). In a third study of healthy people, Ivy Gourd leaf also reduced post-prandial blood sugar levels, suggesting the herb works by inhibiting glucose-6-phosphatase, a liver enzyme that plays a key role in hepatic gluconeogenesis. People with hypoglycemia should avoid using this herb.
Dose: 2-250 mg. tablets BID

Jambul seed/bark (Syzygium cumini) – is used to treat Diabetes Mellitus with fatigue, thirst, nosebleeds, leg cramps and peripheral neuropathy. In addition, the person excretes copious amounts of urine with little sugar present. In animal studies this herb mostly seems to be effective for lowering blood glucose levels. In human studies it has not been shown to be effective (Teixeira, et al, 2006 & 2004).
Dose: tincture (1:5): 1-2 mL TID

Liuwei Dihuang/Rehmannia 6 formula – is one of the great traditional formulas of Chinese medicine. It is comprised of processed Rehmannia, Chinese Dogwood fruit, Chinese Dioscorea root (See Shan Yao), Poria (see Fu Ling), Water Plantain root and Tree Peony bark. It is used to treat many conditions, and can be an important part of a protocol for treating type I or II diabetes and preventing diabetic complications. The formula modestly lowers blood sugar levels and significantly reduces the inflammatory damage that causes diabetic nephropathy, neuropathy and encephalopathy (Liu, et al, 2013; Poon, et al, 2011).

Mai Men Dong tuber (Ophiopogon japonicus) – is a hypoglycemic agent and yin tonic commonly used in TCM. It is used in formulas for mild NIDDM. The best-known formula is the Ophiopogon and Tricosanthes combination, Mai Men Dong Yin Zi, which contains Ophiopogon, Licorice, unprocessed Rehmannia, Schisandria, Ginseng, Trichosanthes root, Bamboo leaves, Fu Ling and Kudzu root
Dose: tea - 1 tsp. dried tubers, 8 oz. water, decoct 15 minutes, steep 1 hour, take 4 oz. TID

Neem seed (Azadirachta indica) – in a human study, Neem seed reduced blood sugar levels in patients with NIDDM and when given concurrently with hypoglycemic medication it enhanced the efficacy of the drug (Waheed, et al, 2006).
Dose: tincture (1:5) - .5–1 mL BID/TID
        capsules (4:1) - 150-250 mg TID

Nettle leaf (Urtica dioica) – in Europe there is a tradition of using Nettle leaf (Stinging Nettles) to reduce blood sugar levels. In laboratory and animal studies, Urtica leaf has been shown to have insulin secretagogue, PPARγ agonistic and α-glucosidase inhibitory effects (it blocks carbohydrate absorption in the intestines). In a RCT, Nettle leaf extract (500 mg, every 8 hours) reduced fasting glucose, postprandial glucose and HbA1c in diabetics to a much greater degree than pharmaceutical drugs alone or placebo (Kianbakht, et al, 2013) given with conventional oral hypoglycemic medication.
Dose: tincture (1:5) - 3-5 mL TID/QID
> tea - 1-2 tsp. dried leaf, 8 oz. hot water, steep for 1 hour, take 3-4 cups/day
> capsules - 2(00) capsules BID/TID

Prickly Pear Cactus juice/fruit (Opuntia spp.) - the juice or fruit of this cactus produces a substantial decrease in blood sugar levels and can be used for IDDM and NIDDM patients (Frati-Munari, et al, 1989).
In a second clinical trial, consuming Prickly Pear with food reduced post-prandial blood glucose and serum insulin levels in people with type 2 diabetes (Lopez-Romero, et al, 2014).
Dose: juice - 1 oz. TID

Prodigiosa bark (Brickellia grandiflora) – this southwestern plant used by Hispanic and native peoples was also introduced to a wider audience by the late iconic herbalist, Michael Moore.
He used it as a daily treatment for NIDDM with insulin-resistance, a tendency to obesity, elevated triglycerides, and a high-stress lifestyle.
Dose: tincture (1:5) – 1.5-2 mL QID
> tea - 1 tsp. dried herb to 8 oz. hot water, steep 40 minutes, 2-4 oz. BID (morning and afternoon)

Sage leaf (Salvia officinalis) – in a RCT, 500 mg TID of Sage leaf extract taken for 3 months significantly reduced fasting glucose, HbA1c, total cholesterol, triglycerides and LDL-C levels in diabetic patients (Kianbakht & Dabaghian, 2013).
Dose: tincture (1:5) – 1-2 mL TID/QID
> tea - 1 tsp. dried herb, 8 oz. hot water, steep covered for 20-30 minutes, take 4 oz. 3 times per day

Shan Yao root (Dioscorea bulbifera, D. alata, D. opposita), as well as **Japanese Wild Yam** (D. nipponica, D. japonica) – have long been used as part of several classic formulas to treat diabetes and prevent or inhibit diabetic complications. The phytochemical diosgenin as well as the herb has been shown to inhibit α-amylase and α-glucosidase (Ghosh, et al, 2014), both of which are needed to convert starches into sugar. In animal studies, Dioscorea reversed insulin resistance (Gao, et al, 2007) and reduced blood sugar levels (Sato, et al, 2014). In a human clinical trial, Shan Yao was more effective than fosinopril for lowering blood sugar levels, blood pressure, LDL cholesterol and diabetic nephropathy (Singh, et al, 2013). Dioscorea extracts have also been shown to improve diabetic neuropathy in animal studies (Jin, et al, 2013).
Dose: tincture (1:4 or 1:5): 2-3 mL TID/QID
> tea: 1-2 tsp. dried root, 12 oz. water, decoct 30 minutes, steep 1 hour, take 1 cup 2-3x/day

Trichosanthes root/Gua Lou Gen (Tricosanthes kirilowii, T. dioica) - the root, fruit and seed of this plant are used in TCM to treat thirsting and wasting syndrome, which often describes diabetes. There are many animal studies showing that this herb lowers blood sugar levels. Human studies are lacking. It is often used in a formula known as Jiang Tang Jia Pian or reducing sugar pill, which contains Astragalus, Chinese Solomon's Seal, Trichosanthes root, Prince Seng and Processed Rehmannia. In a

Chinese study, 76.5% of people taking this formula had improved glucose tolerance (Dharmananda, 1996).
Dose: tea – 2 tsp. dried root to 12 oz. water, decoct 20 minutes, steep ½ hour, take 4 oz. TID

Triphala (the fruits of Phyllanthus emblica, Terminalia chebula and Terminalia belerica) - this traditional Ayurvedic formula improves bowel function, reduces blood lipids, acts as an antioxidant, decreases carbohydrate absorption and slows glucose release. In an animal study Triphala inhibited lipid peroxidation and lowered blood sugar levels (Sabu & Kuttan, 2002). In a small human study, people taking Triphala for 45 days had a reduction in blood sugar levels (Rajan & Antony, 2008).
Dose: powder - 1-2 tsp. in juice or water BID

HERBS /SUPPLEMENTS TO PREVENT OXIDATIVE DAMAGE CAUSED BY DIABETES

To prevent and inhibit diabetic retinopathy
    Amla fruit (Phyllanthes emblica)
    Buddleia flower (Buddleia officinalis)
    Blueberry/Bilberry fruit (Vaccinium spp.)
    Cassia tora/Jue Ming Zi seed (Cassia tora)
    Elderberry (Sambucus nigra)
    Ginkgo standardized extract (Ginkgo biloba)
    Lutein and zeaxanthin-found in Calendula, Spinach, Chrysanthemum flowers, Dandelion
     flowers and Kale
    Lycium fruit (Lycium chinense or L. barbarum)
    Pycnogenol® (Pinus pinaster)
    Triphala (Terminalia chebula, T. belerica and Phyllanthus emblica)
    Turmeric (Curcuma longa)

To prevent and inhibit atherosclerosis
    Amla fruit (Phyllanthes emblica)
    Garlic (Allium sativum)
    Green Tea (Camellia sinensis)
    Grape Seed extract (Vitis vinifera)
    Hawthorn (Crataegus spp.)
    Horsetail (Equisetum arvense)
    Pycnogenol® (Pinus pinaster)
    Rosemary (Rosmarinus officinalis)

For peripheral neuropathy
    Alpha lipoic acid or R-Lipoic Acid
    Blueberry/Bilberry fruit (Vaccinium spp.)
    Cinnamon (Cinnamomum cassia)
    Ginkgo standardized extract (Ginkgo biloba)
    L-carnitine (N-acetyl-carnitine)
    Lycium fruit (Lycium chinense or L. barbarum)
    Prickly Ash bark (Zanthoxylum clava-herculis)
    St. John's wort (Hypericum perforatum)

For diabetic erectile dysfunction

      Ginkgo standardized extract (Ginkgo biloba)
      Lycium fruit (Lycium chinense or L. barbarum)
      Red Ginseng (Panax ginseng)
      L-arginine
      Rhodiola (Rhodiola rosea)
      Vitamin E (with Sildenafil/Viagra)
      Yin Yang Huo herb (Epimedium grandiflorum)

For hyperlipidemia

      Bitters-i.e., Artichoke leaf, Dandelion root, Gentian root, etc.
      Garlic (Allium sativum)
      Gum Guggul (Commiphora mukul)
      L-carnitine (N-acetyl carnitine)
      Plant Sterols/Stanols – Octocosanol
      Red Yeast Rice (Monascus purpureus)
      Soluble fiber (Fenugreek powder, psyllium, flax, oats, etc.)
      Almonds (Prunus dulcis)
      Water Plantain (Alisma orientalis)
      Hawthorn (Crataegus spp.)
      Asian White Ginseng (Panax ginseng)
      Dan Shen (Salvia miltiorrhiza)
      Avocado (Persea americana)
      Sage (Salvia officinalis)

BIBLIOGRAPHY

Agarwal, P., Rai, V., et al, Randomized Placebo-Controlled, Single Blind Trial of Holy Basil Leaves in Patients with Noninsulin-Dependent Diabetes Mellitus, Int J Clin Pharmacol Ther, 1996 Sep;34(9):406-9

Al-Rowais, N.A., Herbal Medicine in the Treatment of Diabetes Mellitus, Saudi M J, 2002;23(11):1327-31

Andrade-Cetto, A., Effects of Medicinal Plant Extracts on Gluconeogenesis, Botanics: Targ Ther;2012;2:106

Asemi, Z., Karamali, M., et al, Magnesium Supplementation Affects Metabolic Status and Pregnancy Outcomes in Gestational Diabetes: A Randomized, Double-Blind, Placebo-Controlled Trial, Am J Clin Nutri, 2015a Jul;102)1):222-9

Asemi, Z., Jamilian, M., et al, Effects of Selenium Supplementation on Glucose Homeostasis, Inflammation, and Oxidative Stress in Gestational Diabetes: Randomized, Double-Blind, Placebo-Controlled Trial, Nutrition, 2015b Oct;31(10):1235-42

Baskaran, K., Ahamath, B.K., et al, Antidiabetic Effect of a Leaf Extract From Gymnema sylvestre in Non-Insulin-Dependent Diabetes Mellitus Patients, J Ethnopharmacol, 1990 Oct;30(3):295-300

Batchelder, H.J., Allopathic Specific Condition Review: Diabetes Mellitus, Prot J Bot Med, 1996;1(3):79-84

Bener, A., Alsaied, A., et al, High Prevalence of Vitamin D Deficiency in Type I Diabetes Mellitus and Healthy Children, Acta Diabetol, 2009 Sep;46(3):183-9

Bone, K., Clinical Applications of Ayurvedic and Chinese Herbs, Phytotherapy Press, Queensland, 1996

Cefalu, W.T., Stephens, J.M., et al, Diabetes and Herbal (Botanical) Medicine, Herbal Medicine in Benzie, I.F.F., Wachtel-Galor, S. [Eds] Biomolecular and Clinical Aspects, 2nd ed., Boca Raton FL, CRC Press, 2011

Cefalu, W.T., Ye, J., et al, Efficacy of Dietary Supplementation with Botanicals on Carbohydrate Metabolism in Humans, Endocr Metab Immune Disord Drug Targets, 2008;8:78-81

Chang, C.L.T., Lin, Y., et al, Herbal Therapies for Type 2 Diabetes Mellitus: Chemistry, Biology, and Potential Application of Selected Plants and Compounds, Evid Based Complement Alternat Med, 2013;2013:378657

Chauhan, A., Sharma, P.K., et al, Plants Having Potential Antidiabetic Activity: A Review, Der Pharmacia Lettre, 2010;2(3):369-87

Chiva-Blanch, G., Urpi-Sarda, M., et al, Effects of Red Wine Polyphenols and Alcohol on Glucose Metabolism and the Lipid Profile: A Randomized Clinical Trial, Clin Nutr, doi: 10.1016/j.clnu.2012.08.022

Choi, H.C., Kim, S.J., et al, Metabolic Effects of Aloe Vera Gel Complex in Obese Prediabetes and Early Non-Treated Diabetic Patients; Randomized Controlled Trial, Nutrition, 2013 Sep;29(3):1110-4

Costa Krewer, C., Ribeiro, E.E., et al, Habitual Intake of Guarana and Metabolic Morbidities: An Epidemiological Study of an Elderly Amazonian Population, Phytother Res, 2011 Feb 22 [ePub ahead of print]

Cusi, K., Cukier, S., et al, Vanadyl Sulfate Improves Hepatic and Muscle Insulin Sensitivity in Type 2 Diabetes, J Clin Endocrinol Metab, 2001 Mar;86(3):1410-7

D'Anna, R., Scilipoti, A., et al, Myo-Inositol Supplementation and Onset of Gestational Diabetes Mellitus in Pregnant Women With a Family History of Type 2 Diabetes: A Prospective, Randomized, Placebo-Controlled Study, Diabetes Care, 2013 Apr;36(4):854-7

Davis, P.A., Yokoyama, W., Meta-Analysis Demonstrates That Cinnamon Lowers Fasting Blood Glucose, J Med Food, 2011 [ePub ahead of print]

Derosa, G., Limas, C.P., et al, Dietary and Nutraceutical Approach to Type 2 Diabetes, Arch med Sci, 2014;10(2):336-44

Dey, L., Attele, A.S., et al, Alternative Therapies for Type 2 Diabetes, Alt Med Rev, 2002;7(1):45-58

Dharmananda, S., Treatment of Diabetes with Chinese Herbs, 1996, www.itmonline.com

Di Pierro, F., Putignano, P., et al, Preliminary Study About the Possible Glycemic Clinical Advantage in Using a Fixed Combination of Berberis aristata and Silybum marianum Standardized Extracts Versus Only Berberis aristata in Patients With Type 2 Diabetes, Clin Pharmacol, 2013 Nov 19;5:167-74

Frati-Munari, A.C., Del Valle-Martinez, L.M., et al, Hypoglycemic Action of Different Doses of Nopal (Opuntia streptacantha Lemaire) in Patients with Type II Diabetes Mellitus [in Spanish], Arch Invest Med (Mex), 1989 Apr-Jun;20(2):197-201

Funke, I., Melzig, M., Traditionally Used Plants in Diabetes Therapy-Phytotherapeutics as Inhibitors of α-amylase Activity, Braz J Pharmacog, 2006 Jan/Mar;16(1):1-5

Gao, X., Li, B., et al, Dioscorea opposite Reverses Dexamethasone Induced Insulin Resistance, Fitoterapia, 2007 Jan;78(1):12-5

Ghosh, S., More, P., et al, Diosgenin From Dioscorea bulbifera: Novel Hit for Treatment of Type II Diabetes Mellitus With Inhibitory Activity Against α-Amylase and α-Glucosidase, PLoS One, 2014 Sep 12;9(3):e106039

Grace, M.H., Ribnicky, D.M., et al, Hypoglycemic Activity of a Novel Anthocyanin-Rich Formulation From Lowbush Blueberry, Vaccinium angustifolium Aiton, Phytomedicine, 2009 May;16(5):406-15

Grover, J.K., Yadav, S., et al, Medicinal Plants of India with Anti-Diabetic Potential, J Ethnopharmacol, 2002;81:81-100

Gupta, A., Gupta, R., et al, Effect of Trigonella foenum-graecum (Fenugreek) Seeds on Glycemic Control and Insulin Resistance in Type 2 Diabetes Mellitus: A Double Blind Placebo Controlled Study, J Assoc Phys, 2001;49:1057-61

Gurrola-Diaz, C.M., Garcia-Lopez, P.M., et al, Effects of Hibiscus sabdariffa Extract Powder and Preventive Treatment (Diet) on the Lipid Profiles of Patients with Metabolic Syndrome (MeSy), Phytomedicine, 2010 Jun;17(7):500-5

Hariharan, R.S., Venkataraman, S., et al, Efficacy of Vijayasar (Pterocarpus marsupium) in the Treatment of Newly Diagnosed Patients With Type 2 Diabetes Mellitus: A Flexible Dose Double-Blind Multicenter Randomized Controlled Trial, Diabetol Croat, 2005;34-1:13-20

Helmstadter, A., Beans and Diabetes: Phaseolus vulgaris Preparations as Antihyperglycemic Agents, J Med Food , 2010;13(2):251-4

Hodgson, J.M., Watts, G.F., et al, Coenzyme Q10 Improves Blood Pressure and Glycaemic Control: A Controlled Trial in Subjects With Type 2 Diabetes, Eur J Clin Nutr, 2002 Nov;56(11):1137-42

Hui, H., Tang, G., et al, Hypoglycemic Herbs and Their Action Mechanisms, Chin Med, 2009;4:11, www.cmjournal.org/content/4/1/11

Huseini, H.F., Kianbakht, S., et al, Anti-Hyperglycemic and Anti-Hypercholesterolemic Effects of Aloe vera Leaf Gel in Hyperlipidemic Type 2 Diabetic Patients: A Randomized Double-Blind Placebo-Controlled Clinical Trial, Planta Med, 2012 Mar;78(4):311-6

Ibarrola-Jurado, N., Salas-Salvado, J., et al, Dietary Phylloquinone Intake and Risk of Type 2 Diabetes in Elderly Subjects at High Risk of Cardiovascular Disease, Am J Clin Nutr, 2012 Nov;96(5):1113-8

Ibrahimpasic, K., Alpha Lipoic Acid and Glycaemic Control in Diabetic Neuropathies at Type 2 Diabetes Treatment, Med Arch, 2013;67(1):7-9

Jehle, S., Lardi, A., et al, Effect of Large Doses of Parenteral Vitamin D on Glycaemic Control and Calcium/Phosphate Metabolism in Patients With Stable Type 2 Diabetes Mellitus: A Randomised, Placebo-Controlled, Prospective Pilot Study, Swiss Med Wkly, 2014 Mar 20;144:w13942

Jin, H.Y., Kim, S.H., et al, Therapeutic Potential of Dioscorea Extract (DA-9801) in Comparison With Alpha Lipoic Acid on the Peripheral Nerves in Experimental Diabetes, J Diabetes Res, 2013;2013:631218

Kamenova, P., Improvement of Insulin Sensitivity in Patients With Type 2 Diabetes Mellitus After Oral Administration of Alpha-Lipoic Acid, Hormones (Athens), 2006 Oct-Dec;5(4):251-8

Karamali, M., Heidarzadeh, Z., et al, Zinc Supplementation and the Effects on Metabolic Status in Gestational Diabetes: A Randomized, Double-Blind, Placebo-Controlled Trial, J Diabetes Complications, 2015 Nov-Dec;29(8):1314-9

Kassaian, N., Azadbakht, L., et al, Effect of Fenugreek Seeds on Blood Glucose and lipid Profiles in Type 2 Diabetic Patients, Int J Vitam Nutr Res, 2009 Jan;79(1):34-9

Kianbakht, S., Dabaghian, F.H., Improved Glycemic Control and Lipid Profile in Hyperlipidemic Type 2 Diabetic Patients Consuming Salvia officinalis L. Leaf Extract: A Randomized Placebo. Controlled Clinical Trial, Complement Ther Med, 2013 Oct;21(5):441-6

Kianbakht, S., Khalighi-Sigaroodi, F., et al, Improved Glycemic Control in Patients With Advanced Type 2 Diabetes Mellitus Taking Urtica dioica Leaf Extract: A Randomized Double-Blind Placebo-Controlled Clinical Trial, Clin Lab, 2013;59(9-10):1071-6

Klein, G., Kim, J., et al, Antidiabetes and Anti-Obesity Activity of Lagerstroemia speciosa, Evid Based Complement Alternat Med, 2007 Dec;4(4):401-7

Kochhar, A., Nagi, M., Effect of Supplementation of Traditional Medicinal Plants on Blood Glucose in Non-Insulin-Dependent Diabetics: A Pilot Study, J Med Food, Winter 2005;8(4):545-9

Knorr, J., The Multiple Benefits of Metformin, LifeExtension, 2001 Sep;7(9):36-41

Kuhn, M. & Winston, D., Winston & Kuhn's Herbal Therapy and Supplements, A Scientific and Traditional Approach, 2nd ed., Lippincott, Philadelphia, PA, 2008

Kumar, S.N., Mani, U.V., et al, An Open Label Study on the Supplementation of Gymnema sylvestre in Type 2 Diabetes, J Diet Suppl, 2010 Sep;7(3):273-82

Kuriyan, R., Rajendran, R., et al, Effect of Supplementation of Coccinia cordifolia Extract on Newly Detected Diabetic Patients, Diabetes Care, 2008 Feb;31(2):216-20

Li, S., Chen, X., et al, Effects of Acetyl-L-Carnitine and Methylcobalamin for Diabetic Peripheral Neuropathy: A Multicenter, Randomized, Double-Blind, Controlled Trial, J Diabetes Investig, 2016 Sep;7(5):777-85

Li, W.L., Zheng, H.C., et al, Natural Medicines Used in the Traditional Chinese Medical System for Therapy of Diabetes Mellitus, J Ethnopharmacol, 2004;92:1-21

Liu, S.Z., Deng, Y.X., et al, Antihyperglycemic Effect of the Traditional Chinese Scutellaria-Coptis Herb Couple and its Main Components in Streptozotocin-Induced Diabetic Rats, J Ethnopharmacol, 2013 Jan 30;145(2):409-8

Liu, J.P., Feng, L., et al, Neuroprotective Effect of Liuwei Dihuang Decoction on Cognition Deficits of Diabetic Encephalopathy in Streptozotocin-Induced Diabetic Rat, J Ethnopharmacol, 2013 Oct 28;150(1):371-81

López,-Romero, P., Pichardo-Ontiveros, E., et al, The Effect of Nopal (Opuntia ficus indica) on Postprandial Blood Glucose, Incretins, and Antioxidant Activity in Mexican Patients With Type 2 Diabetes After Consumption of Two Different Composition Breakfasts, J Acad Nutr Diet, 2014 Nov;114(11):1811-8

Marz, R, ND, Medical Nutrition From Marz, Omni Press, Portland, OR, 1999

Mathieu, C., Gysemans, C., et al, Vitamin D and Diabetes, Diabetologia, 2005 Jul;48(7):1247-57

Meletis, L., ND & Bramwell, B., Natural Approaches to the Prevention and Management of Diabetes Mellitus, in Alt Comp Ther, 2001;7(3):132-7

Mentreddy, S.R., Mohamed, A.I., et al, Medicinal Plants with Hypoglycemic/Anti-hyperglycemic Properties: A Review, Proceedings AAIC, 2005;20:341-53

The Merck Manual of Diagnosis and Therapy, 17th edition, Merck & Co., Rahway, NJ, 1999

Mirmiran, P., Bahadoran, Z., et al, Functional Foods-Based Diet as a Novel Dietary Approach for Management of Type 2 Diabetes and its Complications: A Review, World J Diabetes, 2014 June 15;5(3):267-81

Mitri, J., Muraru, M.D., et al, Vitamin D and Type 2 Diabetes: A Systematic Review, Eur J Clin Nutr, 2011 Sep;65(9):1005-15

Moazen, M., Mazloom, Z., et al Effect of Coenzyme Q10 on Glycaemic Control, Oxidative Stress and Adiponectin in Type 2 Diabetes, J Pak Med Assoc, 2015 Apr;65(4):404-8

Modak, M., Dixit, P., et al, Indian Herbs and Herbal Drugs Used for the Treatment of Diabetes, J Clin Biochem Nutr, 2007;40:163-73

Moore, M., Medicinal Plants of the Desert and Canyon West, Museum of New Mexico Press, Santa Fe, NM, 1989

Moore, M., Medicinal Plants of the Pacific West, Red Crane Books, Santa Fe, NM, 1993

Mori, A.M., Considine, R.V., et al, Acute and Second-Meal Effects of Almond Form in Impaired Glucose Tolerant Adults: A Randomized Crossover Trial, Nutr Metab (Lond), 2011;8(1):6

Mozaffari-Khosravi, H., Jalali-Khanabadi, B.A., et al, Effects of Sour Tea (Hibiscus sabdariffa) on Lipid Profile and Lipoproteins in Patients With Type II Diabetes, J Altern Complement Med, 2009 Aug;15(8):899-903

Munasinghe, M.A.A.K., Abeysena, C., et al, Blood Sugar Lowering Effect of Coccinia grandis (L.) J. Voigt: Pathy for a New Drug for Diabetes Mellitus, Experiment Diab Res, 2011;2011:978762

Murray, M., ND & Pizzorno, J., ND, A Textbook of Natural Medicine, Churchill Livingstone, Edinburgh, 1999

Nedeltcheva, A.V., Kessler, L., et al, Exposure to Recurrent Sleep Restriction in the Setting of High Caloric Intake and Physical Inactivity Results in Increased Insulin Resistance and Reduced Glucose Tolerance, J Clin Endocrinol Metab, 2009 Sep;94(9):3242-50

Neyestani, T.R., Shariatzade, N., et al, Regular Daily Intake of Black Tea Improves Oxidative Stress Biomarkers and Decreases Serum C-Reactive Protein Levels in Type 2 Diabetic Patients, Ann Nutr Metab, 2010;57(1):40-9

Paiva, A.N., Lima, J.G., et al, Beneficial Effects of Oral Chromium Picolinate Supplementation on Glycemic Control in Patients With Type 2 Diabetes: A Randomized Clinical Study, J Trace Elem Med Biol, 2015 Oct;32:66-72
Pittas, A.G., Lau, J., et al, The Role of Vitamin D and Calcium in Type 2 Diabetes. A Systematic Review and Meta-Analysis, J Clin Endocrinol Metab, 2007 Jun; 92(6):2017-29

Poon, T.Y., Ong, K.L., et al, Review of the Effects of the Traditional Chinese Medicine Rehmannia Six Formula on Diabetes Mellitus and its Complications, J Diabetes, 2011 Sep;3(3):184-200

Post, R.E., M.D., King, D.E., M.D., Dietary Fiber for the Treatment of Type 2 Diabetes Mellitus: A Meta-Analysis, JABFM, 2012 Jan-Feb;25(1):16-23

Rafraf, M., Malekiyan, M., et al, Effect of Fenugreek Seeds on Serum Metabolic Factors and Adiponectin Levels in Type 2 Diabetic Patients, Int J Vitam Nutr Res, 2014;84(3-4):196-205

Rajan, S.S., Antony, S., Hypoglycemic Effect of Triphala on Selected Non-Insulin Dependent Diabetes Mellitus Subjects, Anc Sci Life, 2008 Jan;27(3):45-9

Rhodes, J.M., Jewell, D.P., et al, Treatment of Diabetes Mellitus With Coccinia indica, Brit Med J, 1980 Apr:1044
Rios, J.L., Francini, F., et al, Natural Products for the Treatment of Type 2 Diabetes Mellitus, Planta Med, 2015;81:975-94

Sabu, M.C., Kuttan, R., Anti-Diabetic Activity of Medicinal Plants and its Relationship with Their Antioxidant Property, J Ethnopharmacol, 2002 Jul;81(2):155-60

Sahib, A.S., Anti-Diabetic and Antioxidant Effect of Cinnamon in Poorly Controlled Type-2 Diabetic Iraqi Patients: A Randomized, Placebo-Controlled Clinical Trial, J Intercult Ethnopharmacol, 2016 Feb 21;5(2):108-13

Sato, K., Fujita, S., et al, Acute Administration of Diosgenin or Dioscorea Improves Hyperglycemia With Increases Muscular Steroidogenesis in STZ-Induced Type 1 Diabetic Rats, J Steroid Biochem Mol Biol, 2014 Sep;143:152-9

Scaramuzza, A., Giani, E., et al, Alpha-Lipoic Acid and Antioxidant Diet Help to Improve Endothelial Dysfunction in Adolescents With Type 1 Diabetes: A Pilot Trial, J Diabetes Res, 2014;2015:474561

Sham, T-T, Chan, C-O, et al, A Review on the Traditional Chinese Medicinal Herbs and Formulae With Hypolipidemic Effect, BioMed Res Intern;2014;2014:925302

Shane-McWhorter, L., Biological Complementary Therapies: A Focus on Botanical Products in Diabetes, Diab Spec, 2001;14(4):199-208

Shanmugasundaram, E.R., Rajeswari, G., et al, Use of Gymnema sylvestre Leaf Extract in the Control of Blood Glucose in Insulin-Dependent Diabetes Mellitus, J Ethnopharmacol, 1990 Oct;30(3):281-94

Shen, W., Liu, K., et al, R-Alpha-Lipoic Acid and Acetyl-L-Carnitine Complementarily Promote Mitochondrial Biogenesis in Murine 3T3-L1 Adipocytes, Diabetologia, 2008;51:165-74

Shidfar, F., Rahideh, S.T., et al, The Effect of Sumac (Rhus coriaria, L.) Powder on Serum Glycemic Status, ApoB, ApoA-1 and Total Antioxidant Capacity in Type 2 Diabetic Patients, Iran J Pharm Res, 2014 Fall;13(4):1249-55

Singer, G.M. Geohas, J., The Effect of Chromium Picolinate and Biotin Supplementation on Glycaemic Control in Poorly Controlled Patients with Type-2 Diabetes Mellitus: A Placebo-Controlled, Double-Blinded, Randomized Trial, Diabetes Technol Ther, 2006 Dec;8(6):636-43

Singh, R.G., Rajak, M., et al, Comparative Evauaution of Fosinopril and Herbal Drug Dioscorea bulbifera in Patients of Diabetic Nephropathy, Saudi J Kidney Dis Transpl, 2013 Jul;24(4):737-42

Soveid, M., Dehghani, G.A., et al, Long-Term Efficacy and Safety of Vanadium in the Treatment of Type 1 Diabetes, Arch Iran Med, 2013 Jul;16(7):408-11

Teixeira, C.C., Syzygium cumini (L.) Skeels in the Treatment of Type 2 Diabetes: Results of a Randomized, Double-Blind, Double-Dummy, Controlled Trial, Diabetes Care, 2004 Dec;27(12):3019-20

Teixeira, C.C., The Efficacy of Folk Medicines in the Management of Type 2 Diabetes Mellitus: Results of a Randomized Controlled Trial of Syzygium cumini (L.) Skeels, J Clin Pharm Ther, 2006 Feb;31(1):1-5

Treiber, G., Prietl, B., et al, Cholecalciferol Supplementation Improves Suppressive Capacity of Regulatory T-Cells in Young Patients With New-Onset Type 1 Diabetes Mellitus-A Randomized Clinical Trial, Clin Immunol, 2015 Dec;161(2):217-24

Tsai, C.H., Chen, E.C., et al, Wild Bitter Gourd Improves Metabolic Syndrome: A Preliminary Dietary Supplementation Trial, Nutr J, 2012 Jan 13;11:4

Tzu-Hsuan, L., Chia-Chung, H., et al, Anti-Hyperglycemic Properties of Crude Extract and Triterpenes From Poria cocos, Evid-Based Complemen Alt Med, 2011, www.hindawi.com/ journals/ ecam/2011/128402

Waheed, A., Miana, G.A., et al, Clinical Investigation of Hypoglycemic Effect of Seeds of Azadirachta-Indica in Type-2 (NIDDM) Diabetes Mellitus, Pak J Pharm Sci, 2006 Oct;19(4):322-5

Wang, Z., Wang, J., et al, Treating Type 2 Diabetes Mellitus With Traditional Chinese and Indian Medicinal Herbs, Evid Based Complement Alternat Med, 2013;2013:343594

Xie, W., Zhao, Y., et al, Traditional Chinese Medicines in Treatment of Patients with Type 2 Diabetes Mellitus, Evid Based Complemen Alt Med, 2011 March 17:726723

Weiss, R.F., MD, Herbal Medicine Classic Edition, Thieme, Stuttgart, 2000

Welihinda, J., Karunanayake, E.H., et al, Effect of Momordica charantia on the Glucose Tolerance in Maturity Onset Diabetes, J Ethnopharmacol, 1986;17:277-82

Winston, D., Herbal Therapeutics-Specific Indications For Herbs and Herbal Formulas, Herbal Therapeutics Research Library, Washington, NJ 2013

Vuksan, V., Sievenpiper, J., Herbal Remedies in the Management of Diabetes: Lessons Learned From the Study of Ginseng, Nutr Metab Cardio Dis, 2005;15:149-60

Vuksan, V., Sung, M.K., et al, Korean Red Ginseng (Panax Ginseng) Improves Glucose and Insulin Regulation in Well-Controlled, Type 2 Diabetes: Results of a Randomized, Double-Blind, Placebo-Controlled Study of Efficacy and Safety, Nutr Metab Cardiovasc Dis, 2008 Jan;18(1):46-56

Yarnell, E., Abascal, K., Herbs for Diabetes, Altern Complement Ther, 2014 December;20:6:328-33

Yeh, G.Y., MD, Eisenberg, D.M, MD, et al, Systematic Review of Herbs and Dietary Supplements for Glycemic Control in Diabetes, Diab Care, 2003 April;26(4):1277-94

Yin, J., Xing, H., et al, Efficacy of Berberine in Patients With Type 2 Diabetes Mellitus, Metabolism, 2008 May;57(5):712-7

Yoshio, I., Chen, J-T., et al, Effectiveness and Safety of Banabamin Tablet Containing Extract From Banaba in Patients with Mild Type 2 Diabetes [in Japanese], J Pharmacol Ther, 1999;27(5):829-35

Zhang, Q., Cheng, Y., et al, Effect of Various Doses of Vitamin D Supplementation on Pregnant Women With Gestational Diabetes Mellitus: A Randomized Controlled Trial, Exp Ther Med, 2016 Sep;12(3):1889-95

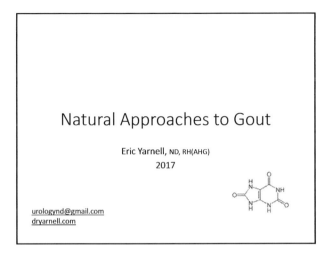

Natural Approaches to Gout

Eric Yarnell, ND, RH(AHG)
2017

urologynd@gmail.com
dryarnell.com

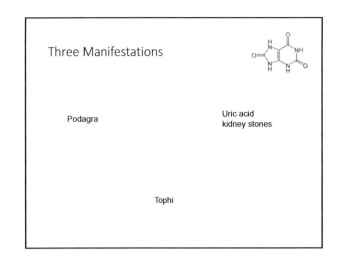

Three Manifestations

Podagra

Uric acid
kidney stones

Tophi

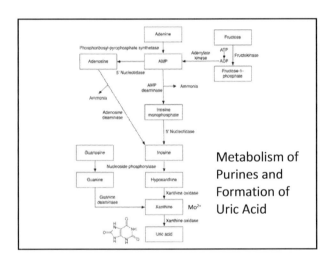

Metabolism of Purines and Formation of Uric Acid

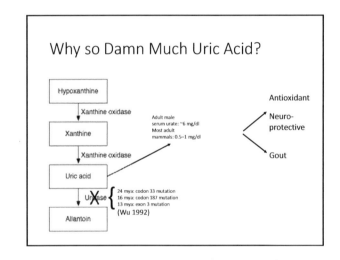

Why so Damn Much Uric Acid?

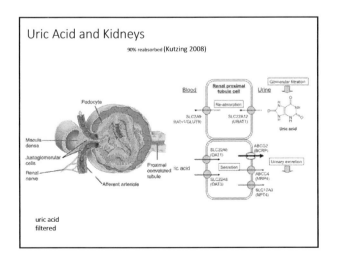

Uric Acid and Kidneys

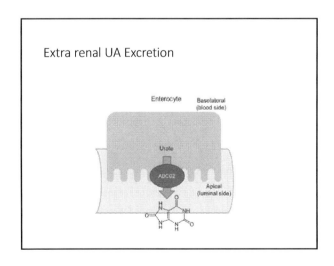

Extra renal UA Excretion

Two Types

TYPE	PROBLEM AREA	FREQUENCY	CAUSES
Under excretors	Kidneys (Torres 2014): 1. Excessive re-absorption 2. Impaired secretion	90%	Genetic + high purine, salt, fructose, etoh diet
Over producers	Tissue destruction	10%	Chemotherapy; hemolytic diseases

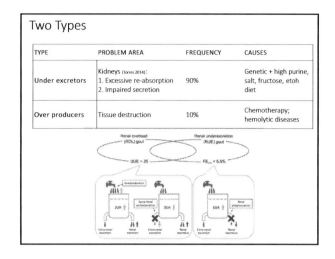

Drugs for Gout

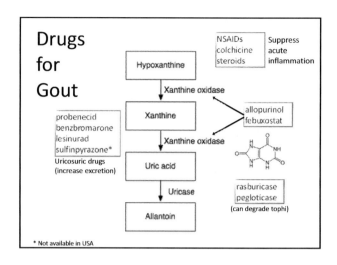

* Not available in USA

Usual Doses

DRUG	USUAL ADULT DOSE	MONITORING	RENAL SAFETY
Lesinurad (must be used with XOI)	200 mg po qd	CrCl (quarterly)	Medium (CrCl>45)
Benzbromarone	25–50 mg po qd initial (max 200 mg)	Serum transaminases (monthly)	High (CrCl >20)
Probenecid	250 mg po bid initial (increase by 250/dose q2wk, max 1 g bid)	CrCl (quarterly)	Medium (CrCl >50)
Febuxostat	40–80 mg po qd	Serum transaminases (annually)	High
Allopurinol	100–300 mg po qd	None	Low (titrate does to CrCl)
Rasburicase	0.15-0.2 mg/kg IV qd in 50 ml 0.9% NaCl over 30 min	None	High

Serum uric acid levels are monitored with all these drugs.

Uricosuric Targets

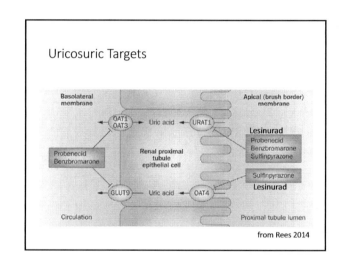

from Rees 2014

Comparative trials

TRIAL	N	COMPARATORS	OUTCOMES
Schepers 1981	6	benzbromarone 100 mg qd, probenecid 500 mg bid, allopurinol 300 mg qd	benzbromarone > probenecid > allopurinol for ↓ serum UA
Reinders 2009	56	benzbromarone 200 mg qd, probenecid 1000 mg bid	benzbromarone > probenecid ↓ serum UA (mean 64% vs. 50%)
Xu 2015	504	febuxostat 40 or 80 mg qd, allopurinol 300 mg qd	febuxostat 80 mg > others for ↓ serum UA, no diff. in gout flares
Schumacher 2008	1,072	febuxostat 40, 80 or 240 mg qd, allopurinol 100 or 300 mg qd	febuxostat > allopurinol ↓ serum UA (48% vs. 22% reached <6 mg/dl)

Mutations and Gout

GENE	PROTEIN	NOTES
SLC22A12	URAT1	rs11231825 associated with gout (Torres 2014)
SLC2A9	GLUT9	rs16890979, rs11942223, and rs5028843 strong risk in all Polynesians, Europeans (Phipps-Green 2010; Hollis-Moffat 2009) rs6855911 associated with ↓UA (Li 2007) Other SNPs account for up to 5% of genetic risk for gout (Vitart 2008)
ABCG2	ABCG2	rs2231142 "normoexcretor" phenotype (Torres 2014) rs2231142 associated with gout in Western Polynesians (Phipps-Green 2010)
SLC22A11	OAT4	SNPs associated with diuretic-induced gout (McAdams-DeMarco 2013)

Genes with no reported SNPs associated with gout:
SLC22A6 (OAT1), SLC22A8 (OAT3), ABCC4 (MRP4)

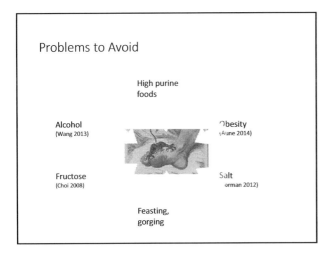

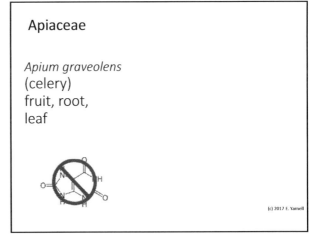

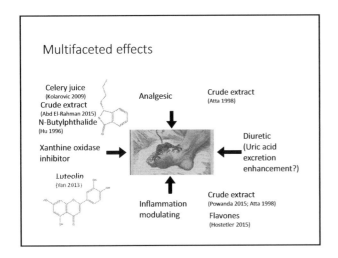

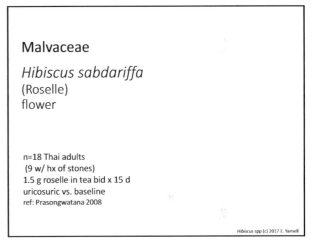

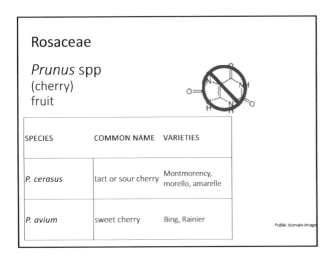

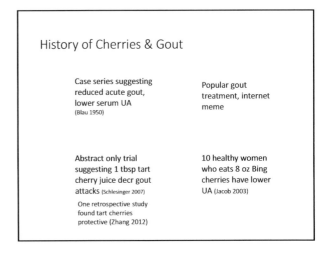

Rubiaceae

Coffea arabica
(coffee)
seed

(c) 2017 E. Yarnell

Coffee and Gout

- Meta-analysis of 11 epidemiologic studies (Zhang 2016):
  - No effect on serum UA
  - Decreased gout incidence in dose-dependent fashion
- Meta-analysis of 9 epidemiologic studies (Park 2016):
  - Did decrease serum UA (1–3 cups/d in men, 4–6 cups/d in women)
  - Decreased gout incidence in dose-dependent fashion

Roasting Chemistry

chlorogenic acid

3-caffeoylquinic-1,5-lactone

pyrogallol → pH>7 → purpurogallin

- Chlorogenic acids are XOI in green coffee beans (Gawlik-Dziki 2017)
- Chlorogenic acid lactones are XOI in roasted coffee (Honda 2014)
- Pyrogallol key metabolite of these that is active in roasted coffee (Honda 2016)
- Purpurogallin formation in alkaline body fluids important for XOI activity of pyrogallol (Honda 2017)

Colchicaceae

Colchicum autumnale
(autumn crocus)
bulb

Public domain image

Colchicine

- Discovery: 1820 by Caventou & Pelletier
- Pseudoalkaloid
- Inhibits:
  - microtubule polymerization
  - mitotic spindles
  - inflammatory pathways

Dose and Problems

- Colchicine dose: 1 mg then 0.5 mg q2–6h (max 2.5 mg qd)
- Even at this dose, some patients get nausea
  - Do not use higher doses, they cause universal GI problems (diarrhea, vomiting)
- Tincture (1:5) dose: 5 gtt bid (per Bill Mitchell, ND)
- Efficacy review (van Echteld 2014)

二妙散 Èr Miāo Sǎn
Two Marvel Powder

6–12 g
(often prepared
with ginger juice)

▨ Original source: 丹溪心法 Dàn Xī Xīn Fǎ (Essential Teaching of Zhu Danxi) by Zhū Dān-Xī, 1481 CE

▨ Atractylodes chinensis
蒼朮 cāng zhú and huáng bǎi XOI; effective at ↓ serum UA (Kong 2004); huáng bǎi alkaloids and obaculactone main XOI compounds (Li 2014)

▨ Formula but not isolated ingredients inflam. mod. (Chen 2014)

▨ Two trials combining the formula with other herbs effective for acute gout in humans, equivalent to drugs (Zhou 2014)

9–12 g

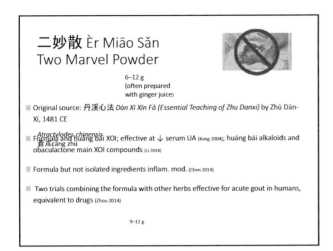

※Original source: 成方便讀 Chéng Fāng Biàn Dú (Convenient Reader of Established Formulas) by Zhāng Bǐng-Chéng, 1904 CE
※Variant of Two Marvel Teapill
※In a clinical trial in 207 pt with acute gout, each of three different versions of four marvel tea pill outperformed drugs for sx relief (Shi 2008)

四妙丸 sì miào wán
Four Marvel Tea pill

LATIN NAME	CHINESE NAME
Atractylodes chinensis	蒼朮 cāng zhú
Phellodendron amurense	黃栢 huáng bǎi
Achyranthes bidentata	牛膝 niú xī
Coix lachryma-jobi var ma-yuen	薏苡仁 yì yǐ rén

Equal parts, 6–9 g tid

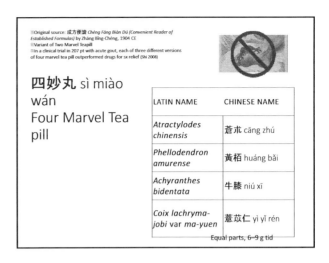

Acute Uric Acid Kidney Stones

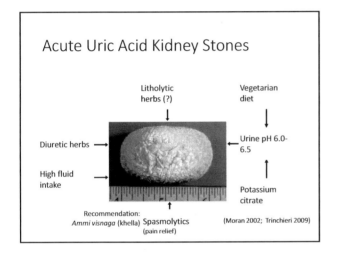

Litholytic herbs (?)

Vegetarian diet

Diuretic herbs →

Urine pH 6.0-6.5

High fluid intake

Potassium citrate

Recommendation: Ammi visnaga (khella) Spasmolytics (pain relief)

(Moran 2002; Trinchieri 2009)

Glossary

ABC = ATP-binding cassette transporter
MRP = multidrug resistance-associated protein
OAT = organic anion transport
SLC = solute carrier
SNP = single nucleotide polymorphism
UA = uric acid
URAT = urate transporter
XOI = xanthine oxidase inhibitor

References provided on following 3 pages.

References

Abd El-Rahman HSM, Abd-ELHak NAM. Xanthine oxidase inhibitory activity and antigout of celery leek parsley and molokhia. *Adv Biochem* 2015;3:40-50.

Atta AH, Alkofahi A. Anti-nociceptive and anti-inflammatory effects of some Jordanian medicinal plant extracts. *J Ethnopharmacol* 1998;60(2):117-24.

Aune D, Norat T, Vatten LJ. Body mass index and the risk of gout: a systematic review and dose-response meta-analysis of prospective studies. *Eur J Nutr* 2014;53(8):1591-601.

Blau LW. Cherry diet control for gout and arthritis. *Texas Rep Biol Med* 1950:8(3):309-11.

Chen G, Li KK, Fung CH, et al. Er-Miao-San, a traditional herbal formula containing Rhizoma Atractylodis and Cortex Phellodendri inhibits inflammatory mediators in LPS-stimulated RAW264.7 macrophages through inhibition of NF-κB pathway and MAPKs activation. *J Ethnopharmacol* 2014;154(3):711-718.

Choi HK, Curhan G. Soft drinks, fructose consumption, and the risk of gout in men: prospective cohort study. *BMJ*. 2008;336(7639):309-12.

Forman JP, Scheven L, de Jong PE, et al. Association between sodium intake and change in uric acid, urine albumin excretion, and the risk of developing hypertension. *Circulation* 2012;125(25):3108-16.

Gawlik-Dziki U, Dziki D, Świeca M, Nowak R. Mechanism of action and interactions between xanthine oxidase inhibitors derived from natural sources of chlorogenic and ferulic acids. *Food Chem* 2017;225:138-145.

Hollis-Moffatt JE, Xu X, Dalbeth N, et al. Role of the urate transporter *SLC2A9* gene in susceptibility to gout in New Zealand Māori, Pacific Island, and Caucasian case-control sample sets. *Arthritis Rheum* 2009;60(11):3485-92.

Honda S, Fukuyama Y, Nishiwaki H, et al. Conversion to purpurogallin, a key step in the mechanism of the potent xanthine oxidase inhibitory activity of pyrogallol. *Free Radic Biol Med* 2017;106:228-235.

Honda S, Masuda T. Identification of pyrogallol in the ethyl acetate-soluble part of coffee as the main contributor to its xanthine oxidase inhibitory activity. *J Agric Food Chem* 2016 Oct 10 [Epub ahead of print].

Honda S, Miura Y, Masuda A, Masuda T. Identification of crypto- and neochlorogenic lactones as potent xanthine oxidase inhibitors in roasted coffee beans. *Biosci Biotechnol Biochem* 2014;78(12):2110-6.

Hostetler G, Riedl K, Cardenas H, et al. Flavone deglycosylation increases their anti-inflammatory activity and absorption. *Mol Nutr Food Res* 2012;56(4):558-69.

Hu D, Huang XX, Feng YP. Effect of dl-3-n-butylphthalide (NBP) on purine metabolites in striatum extracellular fluid in four-vessel occlusion rats. *Yao Xue Xue Bao* 1996;31(1):13-7 [in Chinese].

Jacob RA, Spinozzi GM, Simon VA, et al. Consumption of cherries lowers plasma urate in healthy women. *J Nutr* 2003;133(6):1826-9.

Kolarovic J, Popovic M, Mikov M, et al. Protective effects of celery juice in treatments with doxorubicin. *Molecules* 2009;14(4):1627-38.

Kong LD, Yang C, Ge F, et al. A Chinese herbal medicine ermiao wan reduces serum uric acid level and inhibits liver xanthine dehydrogenase and xanthine oxidase in mice. *J Ethnopharmacol* 2004;93(2-3):325-330.

Kutzing MK, Firestein BL. Altered uric acid levels and disease states. *J Pharmacol Exp Ther* 2008;324:1-7.

Li S, Liu C, Guo L, et al. Ultrafiltration liquid chromatography combined with high-speed countercurrent chromatography for screening and isolating potential α-glucosidase and xanthine oxidase inhibitors from Cortex Phellodendri. *J Sep Sci* 2014;37(18):2504-2512.

Li SG, Sanna S, Maschio A, et al. The GLUT9 gene Is associated with serum uric acid levels in Sardinia and Chianti cohorts. *PLoS Genet* 2007;3(11): e194.

McAdams-DeMarco MA, Maynard JW, Baer AN, et al. A urate gene-by-diuretic interaction and gout risk in participants with hypertension: Results from the ARIC study. *Ann Rheum Dis* 2013;72(5):701-6.

Moran ME, Abrahams HM, Burday DE, Greene TD. Utility of oral dissolution therapy in the management of referred patients with secondarily treated uric acid stones. *Urology* 2002;59:206-10

Park KY, Kim HJ, Ahn HS, et al. Effects of coffee consumption on serum uric acid: Systematic review and meta-analysis. *Semin Arthritis Rheum* 2016;45:580-6.

Phipps-Green AJ, Hollis-Moffatt JE, Dalbeth N, et al. A strong role for the *ABCG2* gene in susceptibility to gout in New Zealand Pacific Island and Caucasian, but not Māori, case and control sample sets. *Human Molecular Gene* 2010;19(24):4813–9.

Powanda MC, Whitehouse MW, Rainsford KD. Celery seed and related extracts with antiarthritic, antiulcer, and antimicrobial activities. *Prog Drug Res* 2015;70:133-53.

Prasongwatana V, Woottisin S, Sriboonlue P, Kukongviriyapan V. Uricosuric effect of roselle (*Hibiscus sabdariffa*) in normal and renal-stone former subjects. *J Ethnopharmacol* 2008;117(3):491-5.

Rees F, Hui M, Doherty M. Optimizing current treatment of gout. *Nature Rev Rheumatol* 2014;10:271-82.

Reinders MK, van Roon EN, Jansen TL, et al. Efficacy and tolerability of urate-lowering drugs in gout: A randomised controlled trial of benzbromarone versus probenecid after failure of allopurinol. *Ann Rheum Dis* 2009;68(1):51-6.

Schepers GW. Benzbromarone therapy in hyperuricaemia; comparison with allopurinol and probenecid. *J Int Med Res* 1981;9(6):511-5.

Schlesinger N, Ron Y, Chen CC. Do cherries reduce acute gouty attacks in patients with gouty arthritis? *Ann Rheum Dis* 2007;67(suppl 3):iii0742.

Schumacher HR Jr, Becker MA, Wortmann RL, et al. Effects of febuxostat versus allopurinol and placebo in reducing serum urate in subjects with hyperuricemia and gout: A 28-week, phase III, randomized, double-blind, parallel-group trial. *Arthritis Rheum* 2008;59(11):1540-8.

Shi XD, Li GC, Qian ZX, et al. Randomized and controlled clinical study of modified prescriptions of Simiao Pill in the treatment of acute gouty arthritis. *Chin J Integr Med* 2008;14:17-22.

Torres RJ, de Miguel E, Bailén R, et al. Tubular urate transporter gene polymorphisms differentiate patients with gout who have normal and decreased urinary uric acid excretion. *J Rheumatol* 2014;41(9):1863-70.

Trinchieri A, Esposito N, Castelnuovo C. Dissolution of radiolucent renal stones by oral alkalinization with potassium citrate/potassium bicarbonate. *Arch Ital Urol Androl* 2009;81(3):188-91.

van Echteld I, Wechalekar MD, Schlesinger N, et al. Colchicine for acute gout. *Cochrane Database Syst Rev* 2014;(8):CD006190.

Vitart V, Rudan I, Hayward C, et al. SLC2A9 is a newly identified urate transporter influencing serum urate concentration, urate excretion and gout. *Nat Genet* 2008;40(4):437-42.

Wang M, Jiang X, Wu W, Zhang D. A meta-analysis of alcohol consumption and the risk of gout. *Clin Rheumatol* 2013;32(11):1641-8.

Wu X, Muzny DM, Lee CC, Caskey CT. Two independent mutational events in the loss of urate oxidase during hominoid evolution. *J Mol Evol* 1992;34:78-84.

Xu S, Liu X, Ming J, et al. A phase 3, multicenter, randomized, allopurinol-controlled study assessing the safety and efficacy of oral febuxostat in Chinese gout patients with hyperuricemia. *Int J Rheum Dis* 2015;18(6):669-78.

Yan J, Zhang G, Hu Y, Ma Y. Effect of luteolin on xanthine oxidase: inhibition kinetics and interaction mechanism merging with docking simulation. *Food Chem* 2013;141(4):3766-73.

Zhang Y, Neogi T, Chen C, et al. Cherry consumption and decreased risk of recurrent gout attacks. *Arthritis Rheum* 2012;64(12):4004-11.

Zhang Y, Yang T, Zeng C, et al. Is coffee consumption associated with a lower risk of hyperuricaemia or gout? A systematic review and meta-analysis. *BMJ Open* 2016;6:e009809.

Zhou L, Liu L, Liu X, Chen P, Liu L, Zhang Y, et al. Systematic review and meta-analysis of the clinical efficacy and adverse effects of Chinese herbal decoction for the treatment of gout. *PLoS One* 2014;9: e85008.

COMMONLY MISPRESCRIBED DRUGS AND WHAT TO DO ABOUT THEM

Eric Yarnell, ND, RH(AHG)
2017

urologynd@gmail.com
dryarnell.com

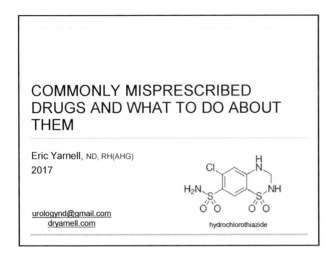

hydrochlorothiazide

SCOPE OF MISPRESCRIBING

MISPRESCRIBING AND THE ELDERLY

- The problem is huge

- Comprehensive review found that 21% of community-dwelling elderly on at least one inappropriate drug (Liu 2002)

- Extremely conservative review, using very strict criteria, found that 1 inappropriate drug was prescribed in 16.7 million physician visits in 2000 in the USA (Goulding 2004)

PRESCRIBING CASCADE

Ref: Rochon 1997

Drug 1 given	New adverse effect	New adverse effect
etc.	Drug 2 given	Misdiagnosed as new medical problem

Examples:
Metoclopramide→Parkinsonism→L-DOPA/carbidopa
Antihistamines, amitriptyline→constipation→laxatives (Monane 19
NSAIDs→hypertension→anti-hypertensive drugs (Rochon 1995)
β-blocker→depression→antidepressant (Avorn 1986)

PRESCRIBING CASCADE 2

Ref: Everitt 1990

Scenario One:

Patient presents with insomnia

65% → Sleep medicines prescribed → Treatable causes!

35% → More questioning → Drinking lots of coffee, actually getting 7 h sleep

Scenario Two:

Patient presents with abd. irritation

65% → Antiacid drug prescribed → Treatable causes!

35% → More questioning → Taking aspirin, coffee, smoking, under stress

DEATH AND MISPRESCRIBING

- Properly prescribed drugs are a major cause of death (Lazarou 1998)

- This meta-analysis looked only at hospitalized patients (where reporting is better)

- Still found >100,000 deaths/yr in the US alone in this population

- What if we included community deaths?

THIAZIDE PROBLEMS

- Worsen glucose tolerance (secondary to lowered K^+ levels; Shafi 2008)

- Worsen LDL cholesterol (Goldman 1980)

- Magnesium (Nijenhuis 2005)

- Hypokalemia 5–8%

- Uricosuric, may increase gout

- Photosensitizing

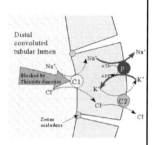

HCTZ VS CHLORTHALIDONE

- Since the Hypertension Detection and Follow-Up (HDFP) study in 1979, chlorthalidone alone has been used and not HCTZ in NIH trials (Saklayen 2016)

- Chlorthalidone continually found to reduce mortality in hypertensive patients, including ALLHAT, SHEP trials (Cooney 2015)

- HCTZ did not lower mortality compared to ACEi in 2nd Australian National Blood Pressure trial (Wing 2003)

- Dose switch: no weaning; use half as much chlorthalidone as HCTZ

ADJUNCTS & MONITORING

- Potassium magnesium citrate (Ruml 1998)

- Magnesium citrate

- Potassium chloride

- Serum electrolytes: baseline, after 2 and 4 wk, then annually

- RBC Mg^{2+}: baseline, after 2 wk, annually

- Glucose, LDL: baseline, annually

- Uric acid: in those at risk

ANTIHYPERTENSIVE DRUGS

- Rush to treat: what do the guidelines say? (Go 2014)

  - 140–159/90–99: lifestyle change first

  - >160/99: lifestyle change + drug

- What happens in practice?

  - "Pulling the trigger" on drug rx early, often

  - Evidence on advanced htn used ingenuously to promote drug use in patients with mild htn (Martin 2014)

ANTIHYPERTENSIVES IN THE ELDERLY

- Dementia in elderly patients due to drugs including antihypertensives in ~10% of cases (Larson 1987)

- Most major studies used atypical elderly populations: AFib, CKD, dementia/cognitive impairment usually excluded (Butt 2015)

- May increase risk of falling by exaggerating previously asymptomatic orthostatic hypotension (Butt 2015)

PROTON PUMP INHIBITORS

- Only approved by FDA for use for 1 yr maximum

- In reality, they are used more-or-else continuously once prescribed

- Rebound phenomenon and failure to very, very slowly wean people off leads to perception of drug failure/need to maintain

- Many adverse effects with chronic use

- Not treating the cause(s)

PROBLEMS W CHRONIC PPIs

- Impair β-carotene, vitamin B$_{12}$, iron, and magnesium absorption (Tang 1996; Marcuard 1994; Sarzynski 2011; Hess 2012)

- Induce esophageal, gastric, and small intestinal dysbiosis (Larner 1992; Yeomans 1995; Ssaltzman 1994)

- Increased risk of dysentery (Stockbruegger 1985), pneumonia (Mallow 2004), *Clostridium difficile* diarrhea (Dial 2005)

- Promote food allergies (Untersmayr 2005)

- Increase risk of osteoporotic fracture (de Vries 2011)

HYPERGASTRINEMIA/REBOUND

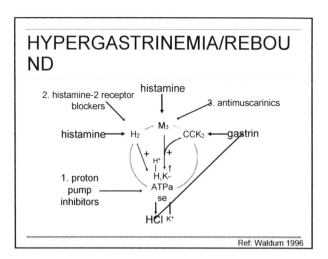

Ref: Waldum 1996

ANTIBIOTICS

- Many people (>40–50%) with colds/acute bronchitis, most of which are viral, still get antibx prescriptions (Gonzales 1997; Nyquist 1998)

- Recent study in Australia: 72% of sore throat pt given antibx, apprenticeship model of training leads to worse practice with time not improvement (Dallas 2016)

- ~25 million Rx for antibx for colds/yr in US (20% of all antibx Rx)

- Reasons: lack of alternatives, too rushed, parental/patient demands

- Outcome: drug resistance, worse/longer lasting dz, ↑mortality, ↑costs, ↑adv effects, ↑medicalization (Llor 2014)

OPIOIDS

The Perfect Storm:

- Massive push by Purdue Pharma to sell OxyContin 1996-2000 (sales from $48 million to $1.1 billion over that time; Van Zee 2009)

- Cannabis prohibition

- Ignoring non-pharmacologic approaches to pain

- The Opioid Pendulum (extremes in tx patterns vs. moderation)

- Toppling the Taliban = massive rise in heroin production in Afghanistan; drug war in Mexico in cities = massive growth in rural poppy production (Anonymous 2014)

HEROIN TO RX DRUGS

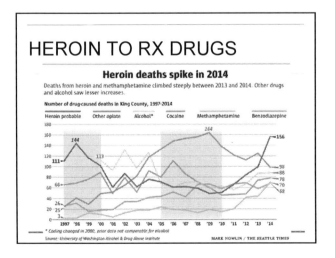

DEMOGRAPHICS OF OPIOIDS

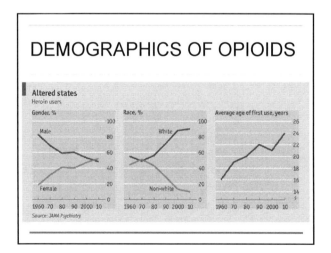

BENZODIAZEPINES

. Addictiveness of these drugs highly overlooked

. Degradation of sleep quality, though they reduce sleep latency, leads to degraded daytime function (Roehrs 2010)

. Efficacy is poor, they are now usually 2nd or 3rd line in recommendations for anxiety or insomnia but are far too often given 1st line

. Widespread misuse in the elderly, homeless populations, few guidelines, little monitoring (Murphy 2016)

CONSEQUENCES

. Inappropriate BZD use, esp. in the elderly and esp. long-acting BZD and long-term use, associated with (Airagnes 2016):

  . Falls

  . Delirium and other cognitive dysfunction, dementia (Larson 1987)

  . Acute respiratory failure

  . Car accidents

  . Dependence, withdrawal symptoms

ANTIPSYCHOTICS

. Overuse in elderly nursing home resident and children, esp. in foster care programs

. Used to control aggressiveness related to dementia, atypical depression

. Evidence base is weak for these indications

. CBT therapy can reduce need for meds in dementia

SSRI

. Second most prescribed category of drug, in ~10% of Americans

. Most prescribed by PCPs with limited mental health training

. Has led to a significant reduction in counseling use (from 33% to 20% from 1996 to 2005)

. Under prescribed (for mild depression that counseling, exercise, herbs would help) and overprescribed (people with severe depression often go long periods without treatment)

. Meta-analysis of trials submitted to FDA leading to drug approval: difference from placebo only reached clinical significant in those with the very worst depression (Kirsch 2008)

. Publication bias a huge problem (Turner 2008)

SSRI

. CBT + sertraline superior to either alone (Walkup 2008)

. *Hypericum* extract not superior to placebo in the Hypericum Depression Trial, but famously neither was sertraline!! (HDTSG 2002)

  . This probably means the study design was flawed, but also may just be because these agents don't work in mild depression

References

Airagnes G, Pelissolo A, Lavallée M, et al. (2016) "Benzodiazepine misuse in the elderly: Risk factors, consequences, and management" Curr Psychiatry Rep 18(10):89.

Anonymous (2014) "The great American relapse: An old sickness has returned to haunt a new generation" Economist Nov 20, http://www.economist.com/news/united-states/21633819-old-sickness-has-returned-haunt-new-generation-great-american-relapse [accessed 13 Mar 2017]

Avorn J, Everitt DE, Weiss S (1986) "Increased antidepressant use in patients prescribed beta-blockers" JAMA 255(3):357-60.

Butt DA, Harvey PJ (2015) "Benefits and risks of antihypertensive medications in the elderly" J Intern Med 278(6):599-626.

"Cooney D, Milfred-LaForest S, Rahman M (2015) "Diuretics for hypertension: Hydrochlorothiazide or chlorthalidone?" Cleve Clin J Med 82(8):527-33.

de Vries F, van Staa TP, Leufkens HG (2011) "Proton pump inhibitors, fracture risk and selection bias: Three studies, same database, two answers" Osteoporos Int 22(5):1641-2.

Dial S, Delaney JAC, Barkun AN, Suissa S (2005) "Use of gastric acid–suppressive agents and the risk of community-acquired Clostridium difficile–associated disease" JAMA 294(23):2989-95.

Everitt DE, Avorn J, Baker MW (1990) "Clinical decision-making in the evaluation and treatment of insomnia" *Am J Med* 89(3):357-62.

Go AS, Bauman MA, Coleman King SM, et al. (2014) "An effective approach to high blood pressure control: A science advisory from the American Heart Association, the American College of Cardiology, and the Centers for Disease Control and Prevention" *Hypertension* 63(4):878-85.

Goldman AI, Steele BW, Schnaper HW, et al. (1980) "Serum lipoprotein levels during chlorthalidone therapy. A Veterans Administration-National Heart, Lung, and Blood Institute cooperative study on antihypertensive therapy: mild hypertension" *JAMA* 244(15):1691-5.

Gonzales R, Steiner JF, Sande MA (1997) "Antibiotic prescribing for adults with colds, upper respiratory tract infections, and bronchitis by ambulatory care physicians" *JAMA* 278(11):901-4.

Goulding MR (2004) "Inappropriate medication prescribing for elderly ambulatory care patients" *Arch Intern Med* 164(3):305-12.

Hess MW, Hoenderop JGJ, Bindels RJM, Drenth JPH (2012) "Systematic review: Hypomagnesaemia induced by proton pump inhibition" *Aliment Pharmacol Ther* 36(5):405-13.

HDTSG = Hypericum Depression Trial Study Group (2002) "Effect of *Hypericum perforatum* (St John's wort) in major depressive disorder: A randomized controlled trial" *JAMA* 287(14):1807-14.

Kirsch I, Deacon BJ, Huedo-Medina TB, et al. (2008) "Initial severity and antidepressant benefits: A meta-analysis of data submitted to the Food and Drug Administration" *PLoS Med* 5(2):e45.

Larner AJ, Lendrum R (1992) "Oesophageal candidiasis after omeprazole therapy" *Gut* 33:860-1.

Larson EB, Kukull WA, Buchner D, Reifler BV (1987) " Adverse drug reactions associated with global cognitive impairment in elderly persons" *Ann Intern Med* 107(2):169-173.

Lazarou J, Pomeranz BH,Corey PN (1998) "Incidence of adverse drug reactions in hospitalized patients: A meta-analysis of prospective studies" *JAMA* 279(15):1200-5.

Liu GG,Christensen DB (2002) "The continuing challenge of inappropriate prescribing in the elderly: An update of the evidence" *J Amer Pharm Assoc* 42(6):847-57.

Llor C, Bjerrum L (2014) "Antimicrobial resistance: risk associated with antibiotic overuse and initiatives to reduce the problem" *Ther Adv Drug Saf* 5(6):229-41.

Mallow S, Rebuck JA, Osler T, et al. (2004) "Do proton pump inhibitors increase the incidence of nosocomial pneumonia and related infectious complications when compared with histamine-2 receptor antagonists in critically ill trauma patients?" *Curr Surg* 61(5):452-8.

Marcuard SP, Albernaz L, Khazanie PG (1994) "Omeprazole therapy causes malabsorption of cyanocobalamin (vitamin B12)" *Ann Intern Med* 120:211-5.

Martin SA, Boucher M, Wright JM, Saini V (2014) "Mild hypertension in people at low risk" *BMJ* 349:g5432.

Monane M, Avorn J, Beers MH, Everitt DE (1993) "Anticholinergic drug use and bowel function in nursing home patients" *Arch Intern Med* 153(5):633-8.

Murphy Y, Wilson E, Goldner EM, Fischer B (2016) "Benzodiazepine use, misuse, and harm at the population level in Canada: A comprehensive narrative review of data and developments since 1995" *Clin Drug Investing* 36(7):519-30.

Nijenhuis T, Vallon V, van der Kemp AW, et al. (2005) "Enhanced passive Ca(2+) reabsorption and reduced Mg(2+) channel abundance explains thiazide-induced hypocalciuria and hypomagnesemia" *J Clin Invest* 115(6):1651-8.

Nyquist AC, Gonzales R, Steiner JF, Sande MA (1998) "Antibiotic prescribing for children with colds, upper respiratory tract infections, and bronchitis" *JAMA* 279(11):875-7.

Rochon PA, Gurwitz JH (1995) "Drug therapy" *Lancet* 346(8966):32-6.

Rochon PA, Gurwitz JH (1997) "Optimising drug treatment for elderly people: The prescribing cascade" *BMJ* 315(7115):1096-9.

Roehrs T, Roth T (2010) "Drug-related sleep stage changes: Functional significance and clinical relevance" *Sleep Med Clin* 5(4):559–70.

Ruml LA, Wuermser LA, Poindexter J, Pak CY (1998) "The effect of varying molar ratios of potassium-magnesium citrate on thiazide-induced hypokalemia and magnesium loss" *J Clin Pharmacol* 38(11):1035-41.

Saklayen MG, Deshpande NV (2016) "Timeline of history of hypertension treatment" *Front Cardiovasc Med* 3:3.

Sarzynski E, Puttarajappa C, Xie Y, et al. (2011) "Association between proton pump inhibitor use and anemia: A retrospective cohort study" *Dig Dis Sci* 56(8):2349-53.

Shafi T, Appel LJ, Miller ER 3rd, et al. (2008) "Changes in serum potassium mediate thiazide-induced diabetes" *Hypertension* 52(6):1022-9.

Ssaltzman JR, Kowdley KV, Pedrosa MC, et al. (1994) "Bacterial overgrowth without clinical malabsorption in elderly hypochlorhydric subjects" *Gastroenterology* 106:615-23.

Stockbruegger RW (1985) "Bacterial overgrowth as a consequence of reduced gastric acidity" *Scand J Gastroent Suppl* 111:7-15.

Tang G, Serfaty-Lacrosniere C, Ermelinda Camilo M, Russell RM (1996) "Gastric acidity influences the blood response to a beta-carotene dose in humans" *Am J Clin Nutr* 64:622-6.

Turner EH, Matthews AM, Linardatos E, et al. (2008) "Selective publication of antidepressant trials and its influence on apparent efficacy" *N Engl J Med* 358(3):252-60.

Untersmayr E, Bakos N, Scholl I, et al. (2005) "Anti-ulcer drugs promote IgE formation toward dietary antigens in adult patients" *FASEB J* 19(6):656-8.

Van Zee A (2009) "The promotion and marketing of OxyContin: Commercial triumph, public health tragedy" *Am J Public Health* 99(2):221–7.

Waldum HL, Arnestad JS, Brenna E, et al. (1996) "Marked increase in gastric acid secretory capacity after omeprazole treatment" *Gut* 39:649-53.

Walkup JT, Albano AM, Piacentini J, et al. (2008) "Cognitive behavioral therapy, sertraline, or a combination in childhood anxiety" *N Engl J Med* 359(26):2753-66.

Wing LM, Reid CM, Ryan P, et al. (2003) "A comparison of outcomes with angiotensin-converting--enzyme inhibitors and diuretics for hypertension in the elderly" *N Engl J Med* 348(7):583-92.

Yeomans ND, Brimblecombe RW, Elder J, et al. (1995) "Effects of acid suppression on microbial flora of upper gut" *Dig Dis Sci* 40(suppl):81-95s.

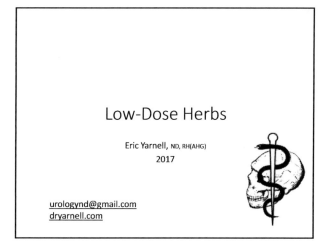

Low-Dose Herbs

Eric Yarnell, ND, RH(AHG)

2017

urologynd@gmail.com
dryarnell.com

Anticholinergics (Antimuscarinics)

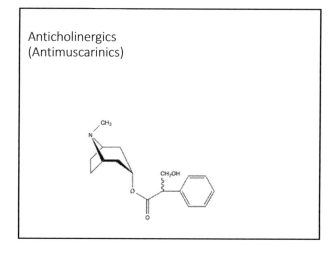

Mechanism

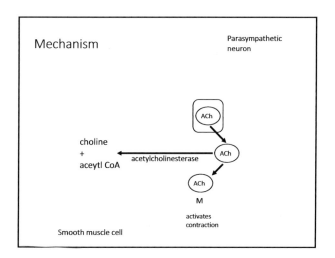

Parasympathetic neuron

choline
+
aceytl CoA

acetylcholinesterase

ACh
ACh
ACh

M

activates contraction

Smooth muscle cell

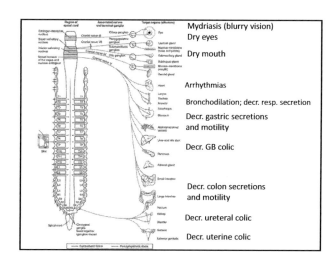

Mydriasis (blurry vision)
Dry eyes

Dry mouth

Arrhythmias

Bronchodilation; decr. resp. secretion

Decr. gastric secretions and motility

Decr. GB colic

Decr. colon secretions and motility

Decr. ureteral colic

Decr. uterine colic

Indications

- Smooth muscle spasms, severe
- Hypersecretion
- Parkinsonism (sx relief only)

Adverse Effects

- Xerostomia, xerophthalmia
- Flushing
- Mydriasis, blurry vision
- Confusion, memory loss
- Tachycardia
- Children, elderly more susceptible

Comparison

	Herb	Potency	Affinity	Usual starting dose*
Garryaceae	*Garrya spp (silk tassel)***	Mildest	GI	15–30 gtt
Solanaceae	*Atropa belladonna*	Moderate	GI, uterus	10 gtt
Solanaceae	*Datura stramonium*	Moderate-strong	Bronchioles	5 gtt
Solanaceae	*Hyoscyamus niger*	Strongest	GU, ureters	3 gtt

* 1:3 fresh plant tincture; adult dose   ** Bonus herb, not required to know for class

Comparators

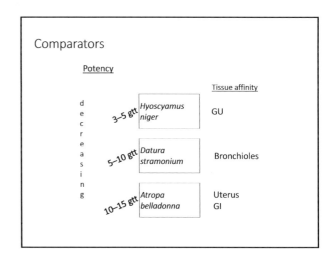

Potency

Tissue affinity

3–5 gtt	*Hyoscyamus niger*	GU
5–10 gtt	*Datura stramonium*	Bronchioles
10–15 gtt	*Atropa belladonna*	Uterus GI

decreasing

Solanaceae

Atropa belladonna
(belladonna) leaf,
root

(c) 2017 E. Yarnell

Tropane Alkaloids

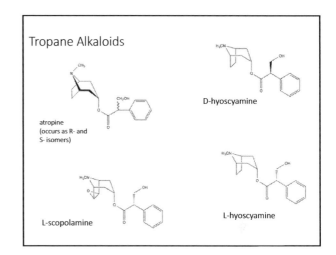

atropine
(occurs as R- and S- isomers)

D-hyoscyamine

L-scopolamine

L-hyoscyamine

Atropa and HCl

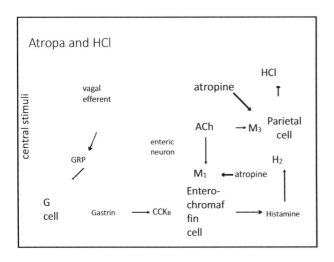

Datura

(c) 2017 E. Yarnell

Hyoscyamus niger

Garrya flavescens

▓Native to western US
▓Leaves are used
▓Milder than belladonna
▓Many interchangeable species

Ephedraceae

Ephedra sinica (má huáng 麻黄)

Protoalkaloids

(1*R*,2*S*)-(—)-ephedrine

(1*S*,2*S*)-(+)-pseudoephedrine

Ephedrine Actions

Alkaloids
α-1 adrenergic agonist
β-1 & 2 adren. agonist -> bronchodilating
Direct sympathomimetic

Tannins
Astringent
Antiviral
Diaphoretic

Indications

▓Asthma, acute
▓Allergies, acute
▓Otitis media, acute (tincture in the ear)
▓Enuresis
▓Urinary incontinence

Adverse effects

- Sympathetic excess symptoms:
  - Hypertension
  - Tachycardia
  - Restlessness, irritability
  - Insomnia
- CI: hypertension, BPH, insomnia, glaucoma, hyperthyroidism

Whole Herb vs. Ephedrine

Dose form	Ephedrine dose (mg)	K_a (1/h)	T_{lag} (h)	$t_{1/2}$ (h)	t_{max} (h)	C_{max} (ng/ml)
E. sinica caps	19.4	0.49	0.25	5.2	3.9	81
ephedrine tabs	20	1.73	0.38	5.74	1.69	73.9
ephedrine solution	22	2.35	0.18	6.75	1.81	79.4

K_a = absorption rate constant, T_{lag} = lag time, $t_{1/2}$ = elimination half-life, t_{max} = time to reach maximum concentration, C_{max} = maximum plasma concentration.

Refs: White 1997; Pickup 1976

Dosing

- Tincture (50% etoh, 1:3 w:v): 10–30 gtt up to qid in adults for acute treatment
- 5 drops tincture in the ear for otitis media, follow with cotton ball to prevent leakage (may want to warm it first to prevent nystagmus)
- Tea: 1—2 tsp/cup simmered for 15 min
- Do not use long-term
- Legal issues

Ephedra nevadensis

Ephedra References

Pickup ME, May CS, Senadagrie RS, Patterson JW (1976) "The pharmacokinetics of ephedrine after oral dosage in asthmatics receiving acute and chronic treatment" *Br J Clin Pharm* 3:123-34.
White LM, Gardner SF, Gurley BJ, et al. (1997) "Pharmacokinetics and cardiovascular effects of ma-huang (*Ephedra sinica*) in normotensive adults" *J Clin Pharmacol* 37:116-21.

(c) 2017 E. Yarnell

Rauwolfia serpentina

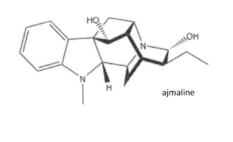

ajmaline

Apocynaceae

Rauwolfia serpentina
(Indian snakeroot)
root

(c) 2017 E. Yarnell

Actions

- Antihypertensive (central-acting vasodilator)
- Anti arrhythmic
- Calming
- Higher doses (>2 mg reserpine): antipsychotic

Reserpine

History of Rauwolfia

- Important historical medicine, but not clearly for htn
- First report of use to treat a human with htn (Vakil 1940)
- Soon became widely used for htn in India (Isharwal 2006)
- First published report about rauwolfia as an effective antihypertensive (Vakil 1949)

Rustom Jal Vakil, MD
(1911–1974)

Hypertension Breakthrough

- The first adequately powered clinical trial of antihypertensive therapy showing reduction in CV outcomes was VA Cooperative Study on Hypertension.

- n=143 American veterans with severe htn (diastolic BP 115–129 mmHg) x 1.5 yr on average

- Reserpine (0.25 mg dose: too high!!) + HCTZ + hydralazine vs. placebo

- 31 events (death, stroke, dissecting aneurysm, MI, CHF, fundal hemorrhage) in placebo vs. 2 in tx group (no deaths)

- Ref: Anonymous 1967

Dose

- Early studies used way too high of doses: 0.25–0.5 mg reserpine qd

- This led to frequent adverse effects: ED, lethargy, depression, Parkinsonism

- Lower dose 0.05 mg shown to be as effective with far fewer adverse effects in head-to-head randomized trial in VA system (Anonymous 1982)

- 0.1 mg reserpine + clomapide (old thiazide) as effective as enalapril with no difference in adverse effects in head-to-head randomized trial (Griebenow 1997)

- Loading dose: 0.1 mg reserpine qd-bid x 2 wk (in whole root extract)

- Maintenance dose: 0.05–0.1 mg qd (in whole root extract)

Rauwolfia references

Anonymous (1967) "Effects of treatment on morbidity in hypertension. Results in patients with diastolic blood pressures averaging 115 through 129 mm Hg" *JAMA* 202(11):1028-34.
Anonymous (1970) "Effects of treatment on morbidity in hypertension. II. Results in patients with diastolic blood pressure averaging 90 through 114 mm Hg" *JAMA* 213(7):1143-52.
Anonymous (1982) "Low doses v standard dose of reserpine. A randomized, double-blind, multiclinic trial in patients taking chlorthalidone" *JAMA* 248(19):2471-7.
Griebenow R, Pittrow DB, Weidinger G, et al. (1997) "Low-dose reserpine/thiazide combination in first-line treatment of hypertension: Efficacy and safety compared to an ACE inhibitor" *Blood Press* 6(5):299-306.
Isharwal S, Gupta S (2006) "Rustom Jal Vakil: His contributions to cardiology" *Tex Heart Inst J* 33(2):161-70.
Vakil RJ (1940) "Hypertension" *Med Bull* 8:495-503.
Vakil RJ (1949) "A clinical trial of *Rauwolfia serpentina* in essential hypertension" Br Heart J 11(4):350-5.

Papaveraceae

Sanguinaria canadensis (bloodroot)

Pharmacology

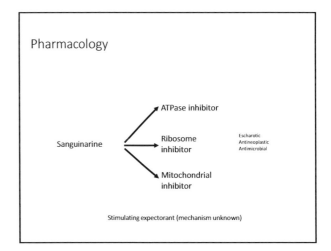

Stimulating expectorant (mechanism unknown)

Indications

- Gingivitis, periodontal disease (6 mon max)
- Cervical dysplasia (topical, 10 treatments over 3 wk)
- BCC (topical, low-grade easily-reached lesions only)
- Weak, wet cough (oral, short-term)

Adverse Effects

- Nausea and vomiting
- Topical use: painful destruction of healthy tissue

Dose

- Tincture or acetract (50% etoh, 1:5 w:v): 2–5 gtt tid
- Topical: with zinc chloride in ointment or paste, remove after 10 min and apply calendula or other healing agent

Sedatives and Strong Analgesics

Sedative Potency Ranking

Potency	Papaver somniferum
d e c r e a s i n g	Aconitum spp
	Cannabis sativa
	Pulsatilla/Anemone spp
	Gelsemium sempervirens
	Corydalis yanhusuo
	Piscidia piscipula

Aconitum napellus

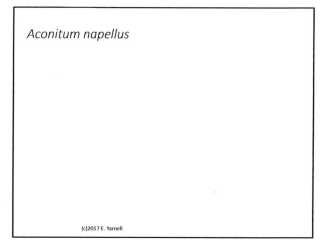

(c)2017 E. Yarnell

Aconitum carmichaeli

fù zǐ 附子

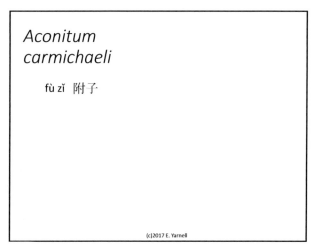

(c)2017 E. Yarnell

Aconite Alkaloids

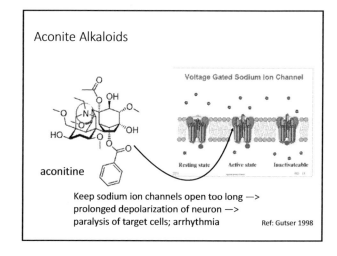

aconitine

Keep sodium ion channels open too long —>
prolonged depolarization of neuron —>
paralysis of target cells; arrhythmia

Ref: Gutser 1998

Alkaloids Compared

ALKALOIDS	ED50 (NOCICEPTIVE IN MICE)	Na+ CHANNEL AFFINITY (Ki)	ARRHYTHMO-GENICITY	LD50 (MICE)
aconitine, 3-acetylaconitine, hypaconitine	0.06 mg/kg	1.2 µM	high (30 nM)	0.15 mg/kg
lappaconitine	2.8 mg/kg	11.5 µM	bradycardia at 3 µM	5 mg/kg
delcorine, desoxydelcorine, karakoline, lappaconidine, lappaconine, lycoctonine	no effect	minimal (mM range)	none at 100 µM	>50 mg/kg

Ref: Gutser 1998

Aconitum columbianum

Gelsemium sempervirens

Gelsemine

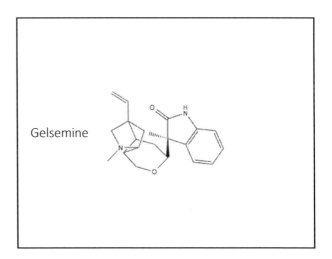

Anemone tuberosa

(c)2017 E. Yarnell

Pulsatilla vulgaris

Anemone occidentalis

(c)2017 E. Yarnell

Anemonin formation

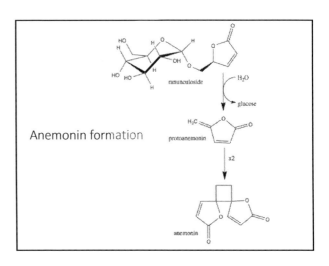

Sedatives/Analgesics References

Gutser UT, Friese J, Heubach JF, et al. (1998) "Mode of antinociceptive and toxic action of alkaloids of *Aconitum* spec" *Naunyn Schmiedebergs Arch Pharmacol* 357(1):39–48.

Pausinystalia yohimbe
yohimbe

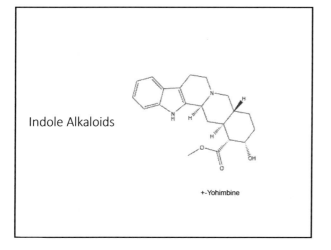

Indole Alkaloids

+-Yohimbine

Pharmacology

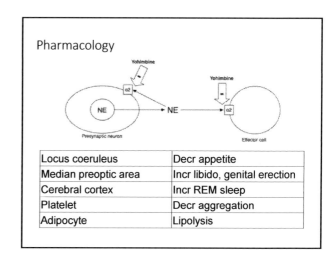

Locus coeruleus	Decr appetite
Median preoptic area	Incr libido, genital erection
Cerebral cortex	Incr REM sleep
Platelet	Decr aggregation
Adipocyte	Lipolysis

Clinical Aspects

- Increases libido and erectile function
- Requires consistent use

Dose

- Pure yohimbine HCl: 5.4 mg bid-tid
- Tincture, 1:5, 50% ethanol, 3–5 gtt bid-tid

Toxicology

- Therapeutic window is moderately narrow
- Can easily induce or aggravate anxiety or cause a panic attack
- Sympathetic overdrive symptoms including htn
- CI: panic disorder, major anxiety, PTSD, OCD, paranoia, hypertension (untreated)
- Drug-herb interactions: potentiates antidepressants (TCA, SSRI), avoid with MAOi and alcohol,

Taxus brevifolia
(Pacific yew)

Photo © 2013 E. Yarnell

Paclitaxel (Taxol)

Synthetic derivatives: docetaxel, cabazitaxel

Overprotective

Ref: Jordan 2004

Politics of Paclitaxel

- Basically US gov't (ie taxpayers) did most of the development and Bristol Meyers-Squibb got 5 years of exclusive marketing with mega-profits, which we didn't get much of
- Generic name really should be taxol, but again BMS was allowed to use that and shifted generic to unwieldy paclitaxel
- Very nice overview at
    - http://en.wikipedia.org/wiki/Paclitaxel

Whole Plant Use

- Needles over bark (for ecological reasons)
- Tincture of fresh needles 1:3, 3–5 gtt tid
- Paclitaxel better absorbed from whole *T. yunnanensis* than in isolation in rats (Jin 2013).
- "Inactive" taxanes enhance efficacy of paclitaxel in whole extracts (Ojima 1998).

Taxus References

Jin J, Cai D, Bi HC, et al. (2013) "Comparative pharmacokinetics of paclitaxel after oral administration of *Taxus yunnanensis* extract and pure paclitaxel to rats" *Fitoterapia* 90:1–9.
Jordan M, Wilson L (2004) "Microtubule as a target for anticancer drug" *Nature Rev Cancer* 4(1):253–265.
Ojima I, Bounaud PY, Takeuchi C, et al. (1998) "New taxanes as highly efficient reversal agents for multidrug resistance in cancer cells" *Bioorg Med Chem Lett* 8(2):189–194.

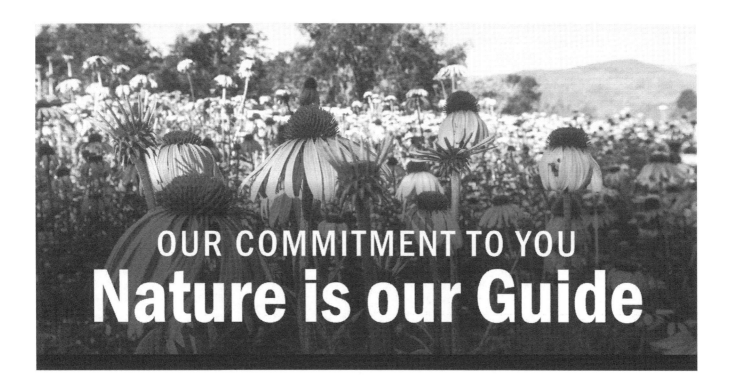
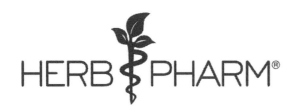
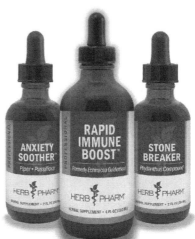

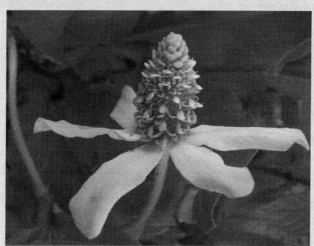

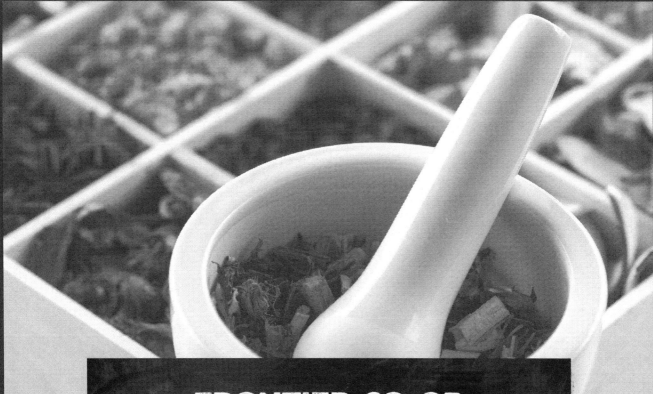
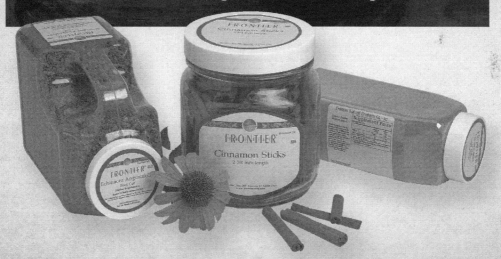

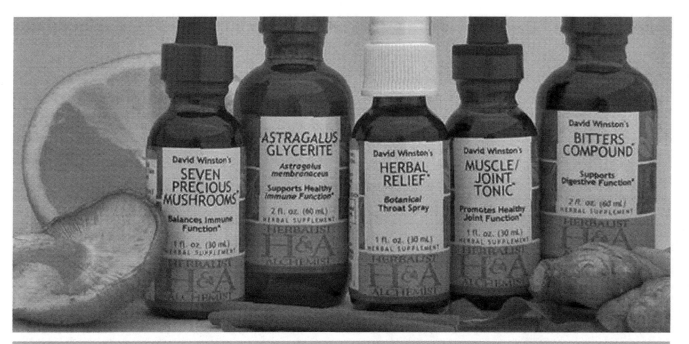
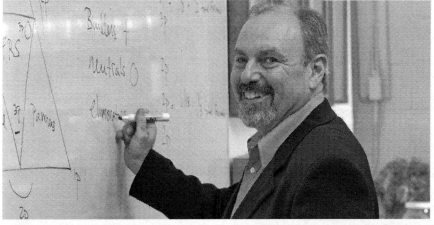
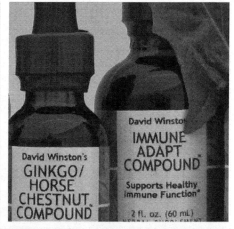
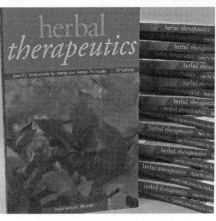

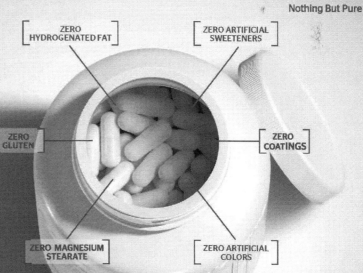

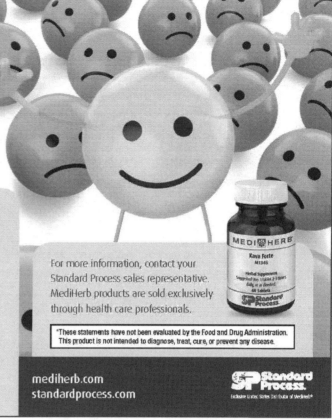
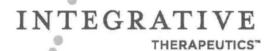
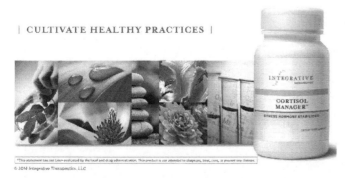

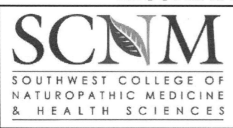

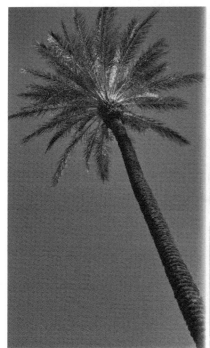
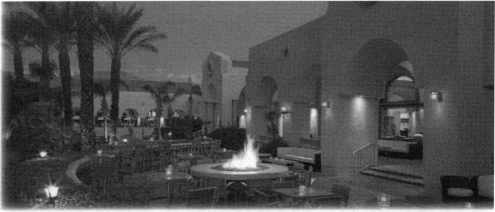
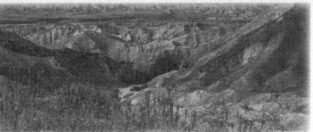
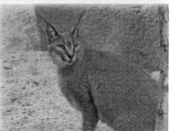

21ST CENTURY HOLISTIC NURSING:
RESHAPING Health & Wellness

American *Holistic Nurses* Association
37th Annual Conference • June 4 - 11th, 2017
Westin Mission Hills Resort & Spa
Rancho Mirage, CA

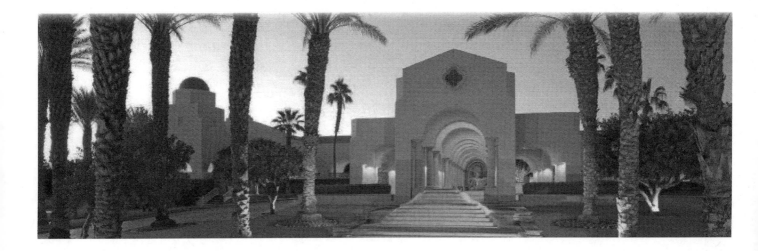

Thank you to our conference sponsors

Traditional Medicinals
www.traditionalmedicinals.com

Herb Pharm
www.herb-pharm.com

Frontier Co-op
www.frontiercoop.com

46993980R00155

Made in the USA
San Bernardino, CA
20 March 2017